Advances in Drug Research

Volume 8

Advances in
Drug Research

Series Editors

N. J. HARPER

Sterling Winthrop, Research and Development
Newcastle upon Tyne, England

and

ALMA B. SIMMONDS

Chelsea College
University of London, England

Volume 8
edited by Alma B. Simmonds

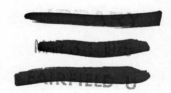

1974

ACADEMIC PRESS
LONDON   NEW YORK   SAN FRANCISCO
A Subsidiary of Harcourt Brace Jovanovich, Publishers

ACADEMIC PRESS INC. (LONDON) LTD
24–28 Oval Road
London NW1

US edition published by
ACADEMIC PRESS INC.
111 Fifth Avenue,
New York, New York 10003

Library of Congress Catalog Card Number: 64-24672
ISBN: 0-12-013308-3

PRINTED IN GREAT BRITAIN BY
WILLIAM CLOWES & SONS, LIMITED
LONDON, BECCLES AND COLCHESTER

Contributors to Volume 8

PAUL BASS, PhD
Professor in Pharmacology, Centre for Health Sciences, School of Pharmacy, University of Wisconsin, Pharmacy Building, 425 North Charter Street, Madison, USA

ALAN BENNETT, BPharm, PhD, MPS
Reader in Pharmacology, Department of Surgery, King's College Hospital Medical School, University of London, Denmark Hill, London, England

BARRY M. BLOOM, PhD
President, Pfizer Central Research, Groton, Connecticut, USA

DAVID PARKES, MD, MRCP
Senior Lecturer and Consultant Neurologist, King's College Hospital and the Maudsley Hospital, Denmark Hill, London, England

CATHERINE A. WILSON, BPharm, PhD
Lecturer in Pharmacology, Royal Veterinary College, University of London, Royal College Street, London, England

139947

Preface

In *Advances in Drug Research*, *Volume* 8, Dr Barry M. Bloom, a president of an international pharmaceutical company, analyses the reasons for the drop in the *Rate of Contemporary Drug Discovery* in the USA following changes in the regulatory processes for the introduction of new medicines. Although no one would deny the duty of government to protect its citizens, excessive concern for safety may delay the discovery of improved medicines for the many diseases that are, as yet, poorly treated. Dr Bloom's comments on the difficult balance between the need for safety and the need for better medicines merit serious consideration by all concerned with the discovery, development and approval of new medicines.

Dr David Parkes, a clinician closely associated with the treatment of patients with Parkinson's disease, reviews the pharmacology, toxicology, side effects and uses of *Amantadine*. Although not as dramatic as levodopa, it is generally more effective than the anticholinergics which have been in use since the 1880's. The unrelated antiviral properties which by chance led to its use in Parkinson's disease are also reviewed.

Drugs that antagonize the actions of prostaglandins are of great scientific and medical importance. The chapter on *Prostaglandin Antagonists* by Dr Alan Bennett, a pharmacologist well known in this field, is the most comprehensive and critical review available. It is written in a way which allows quick reference to all studies with prostaglandin antagonists in a particular tissue or species, and provides an assessment of their reliability and interpretation.

The complex interrelationships of *Hypothalamic Amines and the Release of Gonadotrophins and other Anterior Pituitary Hormones* is reviewed by a neuroendocrinologist, Dr Catherine A. Wilson. The extensive literature and often controversial findings regarding the exact roles of brain amine transmitters reflect the experimental difficulties in this field. Nevertheless, there may one day be counterparts to the many useful drugs affecting peripheral transmitters, which may selectively control the release of pituitary hormones. The review of the basic physiology of the neural control of gonadotrophins may inspire a new approach to fertility control.

New classes of nonanticholinergic *Gastric Antisecretory and Antiulcer Agents* have recently been discovered. Professor Paul Bass describes the interesting and potentially useful prostaglandin analogues and the gastric antisecretory antihistamines as well as the older drugs. He poses some searching and fundamental questions.

I should like to express my thanks to the authors for the excellence of their manuscripts and to Dorothy Sharp of Academic Press Inc. (London) Ltd for upholding the high standards of book production.

July 1974   ALMA B. SIMMONDS

Contents

The Rate of Contemporary Drug Discovery[1]

BARRY M. BLOOM, PhD.

Pfizer Central Research, Groton, Connecticut, USA

The growing distrust our society has manifested towards science and technology in recent years has caused additional constraints to be placed upon the process of innovation through new and more stringent government regulatory policies. Though subject to government regulation in the United States for many years, the pharmaceutical industry has felt the impact of regulation increasingly since the early 1960's, and certainly in ways that constrain research.

It is now a widely accepted fact that over the course of the past decade the rate at which important new therapeutic agents have emerged from industrial drug research laboratories and become available to medical practice in the USA has slowed considerably. The likely causes of this phenomenon have been discussed and debated at length. Not surprisingly, the main parties to the debate—the regulators and the regulated—often do not agree on the causes of the decline.

There are also differing views about a more profound question: Do we really need new drugs? Some feel that the use of therapeutic drugs in our society is already excessive and the number in use might better decrease. That, of course, makes the issue out to be whether we need *more* drugs, when in fact the proper cause for concern is that we need *better* drugs.

Three complementary views are at the core of the following discussion:

1. The slow down in the rate of emergence of new therapeutic agents has grave implications for the quality of future health care, especially as regards chronic-use drugs where our need for superior new therapeutic agents is greatest—for the treatment of such leading cripplers and killers as the cardiovascular and metabolic diseases.
2. The causes of the slow down in therapeutics progress are multiple and complex. The processes by which innovative drugs have been discovered are sometimes poorly understood—unfortunately, all too

[1] Presented at the Fifth Industrial Affiliates Symposium on the Effect of Regulatory Agencies on Scientific and Industrial Productivity, Stanford University, California, November 13-14, 1972. Updated for publication in "Advances in Drug Research", 1974.

often by those in the best position to influence the situation con-
structively.
3. Regulatory constraints are among the most prominent factors in the
recent decline of drug research productivity, although other
identifiable factors are certainly significant.

This analysis of the rate of introduction of new drugs into medical
practice in the USA is based on a list of the new single chemical
entities—the basic new therapeutic agents—approved and marketed
since 1941. The list *excludes* relatively minor products, such as new
salts of old drugs, specialty dosage forms, and combinations of previously
available drugs, so that it may focus upon the new therapeutic agents
most significant to medicine. For the years since 1940, broken down into
five-year periods, Fig. 1 shows that the rate of introduction of new

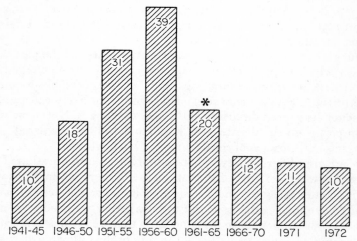

FIG. 1. Rate of introduction of new pharmaceuticals (1941–1972).
* Kefauver–Harris Amendment.

pharmaceuticals moved steadily upward, reaching a maximum during
the last half of the 1950's, when new entities were being introduced in
the USA at an average rate of almost forty per year. This same five-
year period (1956–1960) also is unsurpassed in terms of the *medical*
importance of the new compounds that emerged—the unprecedented
number of innovative and useful drugs that became available in that span
of time.

The sharp decline apparent in the graph coincides roughly with the
1962 passage of the Kefauver–Harris Amendments to the USA Food

and Drug Act, and more precisely with the preceding Kefauver hearings that profoundly influenced FDA regulatory practices. The net effect was a decline by half in the rate of new product emergence during the period 1961–1965, in comparison with the previous period. The rate further declined by almost half again in the most recent five-year period, reaching a low in 1969 when only seven compounds appeared on the list.

In seeking to analyse what happened during a period of dramatic progress in therapeutics to bring about such a sharp decline, the fact that major changes in the regulatory environment were taking place at that very time naturally suggests that perhaps the new regulations and the societal attitudes that brought them about were the cause.

Figure 2 details the rate of new product introductions, by drug category, for the five-year periods immediately preceding (1958–1962) and following (1963–1967) establishment of the new FDA regulations. It

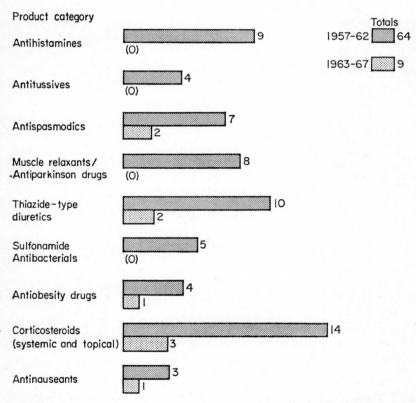

FIG. 2. New product introductions by drug category (1957–62; 1963–67).

is clear that in various well-established drug categories where a number of adequately useful agents already existed, the marketing of new products either ceased altogether or declined sharply following introduction of the new regulations.

Since the same phenomenon occurred in a number of other, minor classifications that we have *not* attempted to tabulate, one can calculate that *appreciably more than half of the decline in the rate of new product introductions that occurred after passage of the 1962 Amendments came about in this manner.*

There are a few therapeutic categories—among them some of the most important from the viewpoint of continuing medical need for superior new drugs—in which productivity has remained satisfactory, and Fig. 3 shows three such categories.

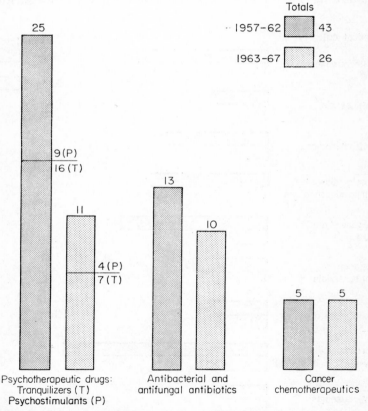

FIG. 3. Productivity of psychotherapeutics, antibiotics, and cancer chemotherapeutics (1957–62: 1963–67).

It is apparent in these specific cases that, during the five-year periods immediately pre- and post-1962, there was significantly less decline in the overall rate of appearance of new drugs, and important new medicines have continued to emerge.

But in the majority of therapeutic categories, including many of those where the need continues to be great, the rate of new product introduction in the USA declined substantially during the 1960's. An analysis of the list of basic New Drug Applications (NDA's) approved in the USA between 1966 and the end of 1972 certainly underscores this conclusion. Of the 80 basic new agents introduced during this most recent seven-year period, no less than 85 per cent were for central nervous system indications, infectious diseases, cancer chemotherapy or were corticosteroids—just four therapeutic categories.

TABLE 1

New ethical pharmaceutical product introductions 1950–1967

Year	Total new products	New single chemicals	Duplicate products	Compounded products	New dosage forms
1950	326	28	100	198	118
1951	321	35	74	212	120
1952	314	35	77	202	170
1953	353	48	79	226	97
1954	380	38	87	255	108
1955	403	31	90	282	96
1956	401	42	79	280	66
1957	400	51	88	261	96
1958	370	44	73	253	109
1959	315	63	49	203	104
1960	306	45	62	199	98
1961	260	39	32	189	106
1962	250	27	43	180	84
1963	199	16	34	149	52
1964	157	17	29	111	41
1965	112	23	18	71	22
1966	80	12	15	53	26
1967	82	25	25	32	14
TOTAL	5029	619	1054	3356	1527

Source "New Product Survey", Vol. 1 (1954) to Vol. 14 (1967), Paul DeHaen, Inc., New York, N.Y.

Obviously, during this same period, very few new drugs were introduced for the treatment of some of the most serious chronic diseases. For example: not one basic new drug for high blood pressure has obtained USA regulatory clearance (other than some diuretics) since 1963; not one new single-entity bronchodilator has come onto the USA market since 1961;[1] not one new nonsteroidal agent for the treatment of rheumatoid arthritis has been made available since 1965.

Even before the decline in the rate of emergence of basic new agents (in fact, as early as the mid-1950's), development efforts directed towards combination products began to receive significantly less emphasis in the pharmaceutical industry. And by the early 1960's, the same proved to be the case for new dosage forms of established drugs.

These facts—fewer incremental-improvement drugs in a number of well-exploited therapeutic categories, fewer combinations and secondary dosage forms—certainly indicate that the pharmaceutical industry has increasingly been directing its research towards discovering not merely new, but more *significant* new medicines. At the same time, expenditures for worldwide research and development towards ethical human pharmaceutical products by USA-headquartered firms more than trebled, going from 207·5 million dollars to 667·9 million dollars in the period between 1960 and 1972. So it hardly seems that industry's R and D (research and development) efforts are grossly misdirected or inadequate.

It is also a fact that, due in no small measure to the far-sighted government funding policies that have bolstered USA science education and academic basic research, industrial research organizations are presently staffed with better-trained, better-equipped and more experienced research scientists than ever before.

Where then are the causes of this serious decline in research productivity? The debate over this question has been intense in recent years, generating—as such debates often do—more heat than light.

Robert Dean, an authority on government regulatory matters at Smith, Kline and French, has characterized the nature of this past debate very well:

> *The reason for the decline isn't settled. The industry points at the Food and Drug Administration as the principal cause, and the FDA points right back, citing unimaginative research as the cause. One side says drug research is strangled by bureaucratic red tape; the other says, no, it's failing because it has strip-mined the old basic research and can't seem to find a new vein. As in all such things, the truth lies somewhere in between, mired in the metaphor.*

The notion that a lack of basic biological knowledge is contributing

[1] *Author's Note* During 1973 the FDA approved cromolyn sodium, an important new drug approved by the UK CSM four years earlier, and metaproterenol (orciprenaline), approved by the CSM in 1962.

Editor's Note See "Advances in Drug Research", Volume 5, 1970, for Disodium Cromoglycate.

to the difficulty we are experiencing in bringing forth important new drugs has its advocates—but may not be entirely valid. Superior new medicines were being discovered and developed at a faster rate ten years ago than they are today; yet in the intervening years, the National Institutes of Health have channelled vast funds into basic biomedical research, up to a present-day level that exceeds a billion dollars per year. Deficiencies in our basic knowledge of disease processes and drug action do operate against the development of new drugs, but it is not logical to argue that this factor alone brought about the present decline in research productivity.

A more persuasive view is that, inevitably, successful research efforts raise the prevailing standards in a given field of drug therapy. Thus, future research in that field must aim towards progressively more difficult goals. In other words, every good new drug makes the target area for subsequent discovery efforts just that much smaller and harder to hit. Drugs like the phenothiazine and benzodiazepine tranquilizers and the tricyclic antidepressants have upgraded the quality of treatment for the various mental illnesses to the point where significant new advances in that field are much more difficult to achieve. In some categories of therapeutics, this factor undoubtedly has contributed to the slowdown in progress. But the same reasoning does not explain the absence of new drugs to treat cardiovascular, pulmonary, and metabolic diseases, fields where much present-day therapy is clearly inadequate. The reasons for lack of success must lie elsewhere.

As the USA Food and Drug Administration has moved in recent years to discharge its prime responsibility to see to it that the medicines we have in this country are pure, efficacious and safe, it has, to some degree unwittingly, created a veritable labyrinth of regulations, requirements and guidelines. To successfully traverse the labyrinth requires a research capability that on occasion comes perilously close to the limits of our present corporate and even our national medical research resources.

The precise, unequivocal demonstration of drug efficacy over long time spans, using multiple control substances, in complex disease states like hypertension, angina pectoris and atherosclerosis, to name but a few, *sometimes* calls for clinical methodology which may be still undeveloped, untried or poorly understood. It *often* calls for clinical trial protocols that tax to the utmost the ability and willingness to cooperate of both patient and clinical investigator, and which take an inordinate period to complete. If this research consistently provided a greater understanding of the drug under study of practical benefit to patients, all the effort and time required and the sizeable drain upon limited clinical resources might be justified. There is basis for doubt, however, as to whether important additional insight is really being gained from the elaborate studies required today for the demonstration of efficacy.

Burdensome regulations can be tolerated when evaluating a new antibiotic agent, where the disease is commonly of short duration and drug efficacy is amenable to simple objective measurement. But these same regulations can prove to be the "straw that breaks the camel's back" in more complex and demanding clinical situations. This may be why useful new antibiotics are still appearing regularly, while new drugs for the treatment of hypertension are notable only by their absence.

Neither regulatory agency policy makers, industry drug research scientists, or academic medical experts appreciated the profound operational implications of this radical change in philosophy that we have undergone in recent years in regard to the assessment of efficacy of new human medicines. As Karl Beyer of Merck has put it, scientists find themselves: ". . . doing research on clinical research or on the fundamental aspects of something or other with the aid of new drugs we don't know much about. Understandably a lot of imponderables arise to confound the assessment of a drug under such conditions of investigation."

Other perceptive observers are also noticing that clinical investigation in the more complex fields is proving to be "the sticking point". Knowledgeable authorities from academic medicine, such as Louis Lasagna of the University of Rochester, have commented extensively on the nature of clinical evidence. In any given instance, they ask: What type should it be? How much is adequate? Is "more" necessarily "better"? How should it be evaluated? How much imperfection is tolerable in a clinical study?

The basic question is whether present-day requirements for "substantial evidence of efficacy" are excessive or not, when viewed in terms of what is feasible and cost-effective for present clinical methodology and resources. Increasingly, academic authorities are concluding that in some instances they are excessive. And to many observers, a basic difference in viewpoint as to what constitutes "substantial evidence" distinguished the highly regarded UK Committee on the Safety of Medicines from the FDA.

What can be done about problems such as these? To its great credit, the FDA Bureau of Drugs has come to recognize that while its prime responsibility is unquestionably to ensure to the American public that its marketed drugs are safe and efficacious, it also carries another important responsibility—to help drug research flourish in this country, thereby making useful new drugs available to medical practice as soon as possible. Commendable steps are currently being taken by the Agency, notably their current efforts in collaboration with outside consultants to identify practical means of simplifying and speeding up the process by which the enormous flow of incoming applications undergo technical and administrative review. Also noteworthy is their intent to accept more clinical data of foreign origin, providing that it is of appropriate quality.

Yet perhaps most important of all are the recent actions taken to identify and eliminate capricious judgements and judgement-makers within the Bureau, thereby squarely confronting a serious problem long overdue for attention. Many of the assessments made by technical reviewers involve judgements that really should not be left to a single individual to make.

An area where new initiatives on the part of FDA are needed involves the earliest stages of clinical investigation. Vital questions can often be answered by single-dose, or relatively short-term experiments in man, without incurring undue subject exposure. It ought to be possible to undertake such experiments without going through the entire sequence of preclinical investigations that must and do precede more prolonged or intensive clinical trials. Without such a change, the long information feedback loops between clinic and laboratory will continue to stultify the process of discovery.

This problem has an important counterpart in the academic setting, where clinical pharmacologists, working with compounds not intended as drugs, need to be relieved of some of the burdensome Investigational New Drug (IND) paperwork and delay introduced by the FDA review process even if they contemplate only the simplest kinds of experiments in man.

The pharmaceutical company research organizations sponsoring this work also must put forth the extra effort required to turn therapeutics progress back on again. Research scientists must become more proficient at determining whether a new experimental compound has the potential to justify its further development, and when it becomes apparent that the limitations of a compound outweigh its usefulness, it must be set aside without procrastination to conserve development resources.

Despite the inordinate difficulties that such research sometimes entails, our organizations must remain determined to deliver sorely needed new medicines. The cost-effectiveness of a "breakthrough" new drug for the prevention or treatment of heart attacks and stroke or rheumatoid arthritis would be enormous. Indeed, the advent of such a medicine could probably do more than any other single event to end the use of the word "drug" in a pejorative sense.

Finally, society itself must work to turn therapeutics progress back on again—political leaders, the media, consumer advocates, and the public at large. *Few* voices speak these days for the unfilled needs of patients with serious diseases where the potential of chemotherapy far exceeds that of other means of treatment. *Many* voices speak loudly of the risks inherent in drug research. The chorus is far out of balance, and the FDA can hardly find time from answering its many critics to exercise the sound, scientific judgement needed from it.

One can only hope that society will quickly come to realize that it is to its own great detriment to fail to place into proper perspective the problems of benefit and risk inevitably associated with the development and use of new drugs. To do otherwise would be to destroy one of the most important sources of man's well-being.

Amantadine

DAVID PARKES, MD, MRCP

*University Department of Neurology, King's College Hospital and the
Maudsley Hospital, London, England*

Abbreviations

DA, dopamine; NA, noradrenaline; 5-HT, 5-hydroxytryptamine; 5-HIAA, 5-hydroxyindoleacetic acid; 6-OH-DA, 6-hydroxydopamine; HVA, homovanillic acid; MAO, monoamine oxidase; DOPS, dihydroxyphenylserine.

1 Introduction

Amantadine (1-adamantanamine or 1-aminotricyclo-[3.3.1.1.^{3,7}]-decane) hydrochloride (1) is a stable, crystalline, water-soluble amine salt with a structure unrelated to that of any other antimicrobial or antiparkinsonian drug. The amine penetrates all cell membranes, including those of the nervous system. Its pronounced lipophilic nature is associated with the compact symmetrical hydrocarbon moiety. After oral administration, it is excreted unchanged in the urine, saliva, and milk. The blood to CSF ratio approaches 1:0·6. Amantadine has antiviral activity only against certain RNA viruses. It specifically blocks the penetration of sensitive strains into host cells (Hoffman *et al.*, 1965), and may also prevent viral uncoating after cellular entry (Kato and Eggers, 1969).

It is of proven value in viral diseases of man only in the prevention and treatment of influenza A$_2$ (Galbraith *et al.*, 1970). Its effect is incomplete but may be sufficient to reduce the serological response to infection due to diminution in virus numbers. There is no interference with antibody formation and, unlike many other antiviral drugs, amantadine is almost non-toxic. Amantadine may be of some value in certain slow virus

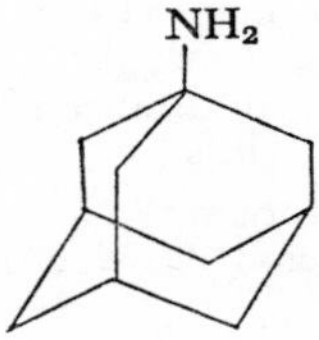

(1)

diseases, including Creutzfeldt–Jakob disease. This uncommon and fatal dementing illness may be arrested or even reversed. However, this is not finally established and there may be instead a non-specific alerting action of amantadine in elderly demented patients. The slight effect of amantadine in shortening the course of herpes zoster has not been explained, since the drug does not inhibit herpes virus hominis *in vitro* (Galbraith, 1973).

The activity of amantadine in Parkinson's disease is unrelated to the antiviral effect, and was found by chance by Schwab and his colleagues (1969), when the drug was given for influenza prophylaxis to a woman with Parkinson's disease. Although amantadine has a dramatic effect, equal to that of levodopa, in a few patients with Parkinson's disease (Barbeau *et al.*, 1971), in most patients the degree of improvement is slight. Amantadine may, however, be more effective than anticholinergic drugs. Optimum response to levodopa therapy is often limited by side effects, and amantadine in combination with maximally tolerated levodopa dosage has a slight but definite additional effect (Fehling, 1973).

Amantadine augments catecholamine metabolism and causes increased dopamine release from catecholamine neurones in response to the nerve impulse (Heikkila and Cohen, 1972). This is the likely explanation of its antiparkinsonian effect but it relieves only the signs and symptoms without changing the course of the disease.

2 Chemistry

The parent hydrocarbon, adamantane, occurs in small amounts in petroleum naphtha and can be obtained by a two-stage process from dicyclopentadiene. Hydrogenation of dicyclopentadiene under pressure using a nickel on kieselguhr catalyst yields a mixture of endo- and exo-trimethylene norbornane, which can be isomerized to adamantane by heating with aluminium chloride and hydrogen chloride (Schleyer, 1957; Dupont, 1964). Bromination (Landa *et al.*, 1955) followed by ammonolysis (Du Pont, 1964) yields amantadine. The preparation of adamantane derivatives has been extensively explored by Stetter (1954). Many adamantyl analogues of drugs have been prepared. Physical properties and pharmacological effects have been described (Stetter and Wulf, 1962; Stetter and Krause, 1967; Zinner and Dybowski, 1970; Stepanov and Isaev, 1970).

Of the many adamantyl derivatives, only amantadine hydrochloride has been widely assessed clinically for prophylaxis and treatment of influenza A_2 and as an antiparkinsonian drug. Aldrich *et al.* (1971) examined the *N*- and *C*-alkylated amantadines for antiviral activity against influenza A S-15 (swine) in mice. The *N*-methyl-, ethyl-, allyl-, dimethyl-, and diethyl-adamantanamines had activity comparable with that of amantadine. Substitution at the tertiary positions of the adamantane moiety affected activity adversely as did quaternization or *N*-oxidation of the *N*-dimethyladamantanamine. Replacement of the amine group of amantadine by H,OH,SH,CN,COOH,Cl or Br gave inactive compounds. Acyl derivatives of amantadine were usually less active than the parent compound, indicating the importance of a basic nitrogen for activity.

Separating the primary amino group from the bulky hydrocarbon by one methylene group gave an active compound and further substitution by methyl or ethyl at the α-position retained activity. The optical isomers of α-methyl-1-adamantanemethylamine, rimantadine (2) (found by Tsunoda *et al.*, 1965, to be more active than amantadine *in vitro* against influenza A Japanese 305 virus) were equipotent (Aldrich *et al.*, 1971).

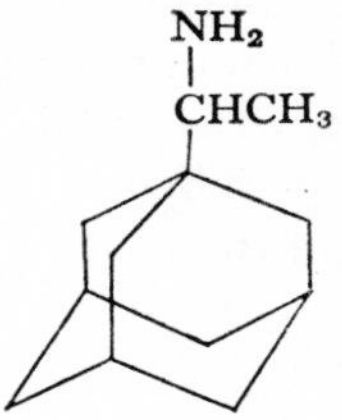

NH₂
|
CHCH₃

(2)

Lundahl and his colleagues (1972) studied adamantane-2-spiro-3'-pyrrolidine and several of its *N*-substituted derivatives. The *N*-alkyl substituted derivatives displayed antiviral action against influenza A, parainfluenza, Sendai, coxsackie, A_{21} and rhinovirus. This activity was comparable with that of spiropyrrolidines derived from other alicyclic compounds. The *N*-methyladamantane-2-spiro-3'-pyrrolidine (3) was superior to amantadine in level and spectrum of activity.

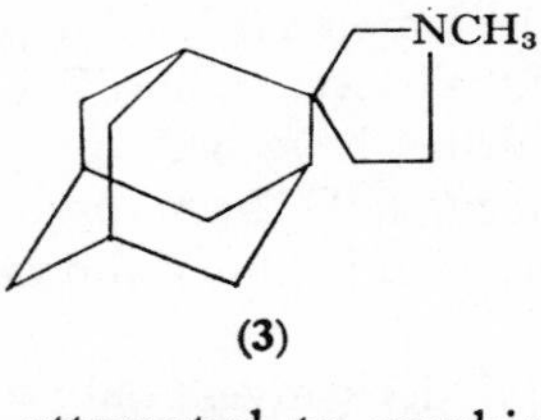

—NCH₃

(3)

Smejkal *et al.* (1972) attempted to combine the separate antiviral effects of thiosemicarbazones and aminoadamantane compounds in one molecule. Several such compounds had slightly greater anti-influenza virus activity than amantadine alone. Of various adamantyl residue substituted pyrimidines, 6-adamantyluracil had the greatest antiviral activity.

3 Pharmacokinetic studies

3.1 AMANTADINE DETERMINATION

A specific gas chromatographic method was developed for determining amantadine in body fluids and tissues by Bleidner *et al.* (1965). A more sensitive method of determination by radio chromatography with the use of ^{3}H-labelled amantadine was described by Uchiyama and Shibuya (1969), and Biandrate et al. (1972) described a simple, sensitive, and specific method for amantadine determination in human plasma. The compound is converted to its N-trichloracetyl derivative and determined by electron capture detector. The linearity of the method ranges from 25 to 1000 ng per ml of plasma. Plasma values in patients during chronic treatment with amantadine hydrochloride (200–300 mg daily) vary from 0·27 μg ml^{-1} to 0·77 μg ml^{-1} after one week of treatment, and 0·68 μg ml^{-1} to 1·01 μg ml^{-1} after three weeks. Clinical effect and drug levels have not been compared.

The drug is totally absorbed following oral dosage in all species studied (mice, rats, dogs, monkeys, and man), although the plasma clearance rate and tissue distribution show some differences. The urine is the major route of elimination in all species. Amantadine does not seem to be metabolized in man, slightly in the monkey and mouse, but more so in the dog and cat. Only the dog converts a portion of the administered drug in its N-methyl derivative.

3.2   METABOLISM IN MAN

Following oral administration of 2·5 mg kg^{-1} amantadine hydrochloride in man, maximal blood levels occur after 1 to 4 hours. The drug is totally absorbed from the gut, but it is not known whether absorption is delayed by the presence of food or whether there is any relationship between gastric emptying time and serum levels. It is excreted at a rate depending on the amount present in the body, so that levels rise until the rate of elimination approaches the rate of administration (Drill, 1958). The compound may be detected in the urine one week after a single dose (2 mg kg^{-1}). After a single dose, the cumulative amount recovered from the urine was 93 per cent, and the average observed excretion of amantadine in the urine was 92 per cent of the dose when 18 successive doses of 100 mg of the hydrochloride were given at 12-hour intervals (Bleidner et al., 1965). A saliva sample taken at 30 hours showed the compound to be present at a concentration approximating that in blood after a single dosage.

Rates of excretion in different individuals show considerable variations, with both fast and slow excretion rates. Some excrete as little as 27 per cent of the drug in 24 hours whilst fast excretors eliminate as much as 74 per cent in the same period.

The rate is influenced considerably by urinary pH (Geuens and Stephens, 1967). An initial dose of three times the daily maintenance dose will build up a stable body level in one day, and this body level will be about three times higher if the urine is kept alkaline by the administration of 4·2 g sodium bicarbonate three times daily. This is not suitable, however, for long-term treatment in view of the risk of renal deposits of calcium phosphate.

3.3 METABOLISM IN LABORATORY ANIMALS

In *mice*, the total percentage of unchanged amantadine recovered in the urine is high, and excretion is largely complete in about 12 hours. Only about 2 per cent of the dose is found in the faeces after an oral dose of 495 mg kg^{-1}. The incomplete recovery and the appearance of dose-related extraneous peaks in certain chromatograms indicate that some amantadine is metabolized. Amantadine is found in the heart, lung, kidney, and spleen and especially the liver of mice after oral dosage (Uchiyama and Shibuya, 1969). In *rats* a considerably lower percentage of the compound is recovered from the urine after a single oral dose than in mice. Recovery values of 16 and 18 per cent were obtained from 2 Sprague Dawley rats over a 70-hour collection period following single 10 mg kg^{-1} doses of the hydrochloride (Bleidner *et al.*, 1965).

In *dogs*, the average recovery of unchanged amantadine from urine following single oral doses of the hydrochloride is 19 per cent and less than 10 per cent of this amount is excreted as *N*-methylamantadine. This *N*-methyl compound occurs only in dog urine and blood (Bleidner *et al.*, 1965). Kidney, brain, lung, spleen, fat, heart, muscle, liver, and blood from a dog autopsied 24 hours following 30 successive daily doses of up to 50 mg kg^{-1} amantadine hydrochloride, contained less than one part per million of amantadine, indicating that the compound is completely metabolized or excreted within 24 hours in this species.

In African green *monkeys*, the average recovery of unchanged amantadine in the urine was 54 per cent following a single oral dose. There was no build-up of compound with successive doses. From the absence of total recovery following intravenous dosage and the presence of extraneous peaks in certain chromatograms, Bleidner *et al.* (1965) concluded that amantadine was metabolized to some degree in the monkey.

4 Toxicology studies

4.1 ACUTE AND CHRONIC TOXICITY IN ANIMALS

Vernier and his colleagues (1969) determined the acute and chronic toxicity of amantadine hydrochloride in the guinea-pig, mouse, rat, dog, rabbit, and monkey. Following oral, intraperitoneal and intravenous administration the oral LD 50 in the male *rat* was 1275 mg kg^{-1} and slightly lower in other rodents.

In *dogs* given 65 mg kg^{-1} by mouth, there were signs of central nervous stimulation at one hour, with tremors, myoclonic jerks, brief intermittent clonic convulsions, salivation, mydriasis, and a loss of pupillary response to light. This condition lasted 2–4 hours with recovery at 24 hours. With an oral dosage of 75 mg kg^{-1} in African green *monkeys* there were also signs of central nervous system stimulation, and clonic convulsions occurred. Other signs of CNS hyperexcitability occur in different animal species. In the *horse* amantadine causes tremors, hypersensitivity to stimuli, with brief intermittent clonic convulsions followed by prostration and death (Bryans *et al.*, 1966).

Chronic administration of amantadine hydrochloride to *rats* over a two-year treatment period moderately depressed gain in weight but other gross findings in these animals were unremarkable. Subsequent microscopy showed no amantadine-related histomorphologic alteration. Chronic studies in *monkeys* and *dogs* have not shown any evidence of organ toxicity.

Amantadine treatment had little effect on *rat* foetal development and post-natal growth apart from slight retardation of increase in body weight in high dosage (Kaito *et al.*, 1969; Kyo *et al.*, 1970). In the high dose group, the mortality rate of the foetus and the drop in body weight of surviving litter mates differed from controls by a very small amount. No deformities occurred in either group.

Studies of the effect of amantadine on reproduction in *rats* showed no difference in fertility, gestation, viability of foetus, and lactation index between treated and control animals except that in rats on high dosage (32 mg kg^{-1}) the fertility and lactation indices were a little depressed. Vernier and his colleagues (1969) concluded that amantadine hydrochloride was devoid of teratogenic and other adverse properties in the rat and rabbit under the conditions used. However, despite these findings, amantadine treatment cannot be recommended for pregnant women.

4.2   ACUTE AND CHRONIC TOXICITY IN MAN

Fahn and his colleagues (1971) described a 61-year-old man with postencephalitic parkinsonism who took a suicidal over-dosage of 2·8 g of amantadine hydrochloride. Some hours later he was found in an agitated state, waving his arms in the air, confused and incoherent. He was unable to stand and remained delirious all night. The next day he was unresponsive to questioning, combative, picking objects from the air, and rolling his eyes and head. Later he became orientated in person and place but was moderately dysarthric. He remained in an excited state with variable orientation for several days. Chlorpromazine (25 mg) was effective in quietening him. As well as this toxic psychosis, the patient also developed urinary retention with slight enlargement of the pupils. The pulse and blood pressure remained normal, and at no stage was the conscious level impaired. He eventually made a complete recovery.

The patient's parkinsonism with rigidity and tremor had been considerable prior to over-dosage, but at the height of amantadine intoxication the patient had no muscular rigidity and no tremor, although he was unable to stand without support. The signs of parkinsonism reappeared within 72 hours.

There was a mild metabolic disturbance perhaps due to ingestion of the hydrochloride, with minor changes in serum pCO_2 and pH suggesting a primary respiratory alkalosis and a mild metabolic acidosis. The patient was treated with intravenous fluids and also given diphenylhydantoin 100 mg i.m. for prophylaxis of possible convulsions which, however, did not occur.

Schwab et al. (1972) recorded somewhat similar findings, with the addition of coma, in a patient who took 100 capsules of 100 mg amantadine hydrochloride, and who survived after a period of confusion and ataxia.

Amantadine in high dosages (up to 600 mg daily) has little or no effect on blood pressure or heart rate in man, and does not cause cardiac arrhythmias. Pupillary responses have not been studied in detail. Temperature, sleep, appetite, hunger, and sexual functions are apparently not altered. Post-menopausal bleeding, a rare side effect of levodopa, has not been reported with amantadine, and also, in contrast to levodopa, amantadine in low or high dosage does not cause either emesis or involuntary movements. Signs of CNS excitation may occur in man but are less than with amphetamines. The interactions between amantadine and different antiparkinsonian drugs have been elucidated, but other possible interactions are not known. Central nervous system stimulants, including caffeine and amphetamine-type drugs should not be given in conjunction with amantadine.

5 Pharmacodynamic studies

In patients with Parkinson's disease DA levels in the striatum are reduced. DA acts as a neurotransmitter at certain strial synapses concerned with inhibition in the nigrostriatal pathway. The action of levodopa in Parkinson's disease is best attributed to the restoration of DA levels towards normal. NA depletion as well as DA depletion occurs in certain brain regions of patients with Parkinson's disease, but this may be a secondary phenomenon, and the NA precursor DOPS, unlike the DA precursor levodopa, is not of value in treatment.

5.1 GENERAL PHARMACOLOGY

5.1.1 *Anti-inflammatory effect*

The healing of herpetic lesions, and the shortening of fever in human influenza treated with amantadine, is probably not due to any antiviral effect. In rats, amantadine hydrochloride did not inhibit cotton pellet-induced granuloma formation nor reduce inflammation caused by polyvinyl alcohol–acacia solution lesions (Vernier *et al.*, 1969).

5.1.2 *Anti-pyretic effect*

In contrast to aminopyrine, which was consistently antipyretic and hypothermic under all experimental conditions used, amantadine hydrochloride caused inconstant effects on normal or elevated temperature of rats given pyrogens even at high dosage (Vernier *et al.*, 1969).

5.1.3 *Cardiovascular haemodynamic effects*

Amantadine hydrochloride up to 4.5 mg kg^{-1} i.v. over 2–3 seconds to anaesthetized dogs has no effect on arterial blood pressure. Higher doses of 13.5 mg kg^{-1} i.v. decreased mean arterial blood pressure by an average of 59 mm Hg (Vernier *et al.*, 1969). With this and higher dose levels, but not 6 mg kg^{-1} i.v., cardiac arrhythmias with ventricular extrasystoles always occurred, and similarly in the rabbit (Kaji *et al.*, 1966). These extrasystoles originated from a single focus, occurred in both awake and anaesthetized dogs, and the effect on cardiac rhythm was transient, completely reversible, and dose related. Single oral doses of amantadine hydrochloride (37 and 62 mg kg^{-1}) did not produce arrhythmias in dogs but 46 mg kg^{-1} orally in monkeys produced ventricular extrasystoles (Vernier *et al.*, 1969).

There is an increase in myocardial contraction force in anaesthetized and in spinal dogs given amantadine hydrochloride 1–3 mg kg^{-1} i.v. which appears to be adrenergically mediated, since it is prevented by prior reserpinization and restored by an intravenous infusion of NA. Amantadine hydrochloride at intravenous doses of from 0.5–4.5 mg kg^{-1} does not significantly affect the vasomotor responses to NA, phenethylamine, acetylcholine, carotid occlusion, or nicotine injection (Vernier *et al.*, 1969).

In DA-primed dogs, amantadine $(0.08 \text{ mg kg}^{-1}$ and above i.v.) caused dose-related pressor response (Grelak *et al.*, 1970). Without DA-priming, amantadine showed a small pressor response only at highest doses of amantadine. Grelak and his colleagues concluded that amantadine releases catecholamines from peripheral nerve storage sites, and probably has a similar action within the CNS. It seems unlikely that amantadine itself acts on adrenoceptors.

5.1.4 *Effect of amantadine on acetylcholine*

Amandadine has little, if any, anticholinergic effect and does not act like scopolamine, atropine, benztropine or other well-known centrally acting anticholinergic drugs (Grelak *et al.*, 1970; Simon *et al.*, 1970; Zetler, 1970; Vernier, 1971). Thus, amantadine has only $1:209\,000$ of the potency of atropine in causing antagonism of contractions of the guinea-pig ileum produced by acetycholine and has little effect on contractions to carbachol (Davies, 1971). It causes little or no antagonism of the acetylcholine-induced blood pressure response in dogs, and has no effect at a dosage of 40 mg kg^{-1} i.v. on oxotremorine-induced tremor in mice (Vernier, 1971), nor does it antagonize pilocarpine-induced saliva- tion in mice (Davies, 1971). Furthermore, amantadine has been found to increase acetylcholine levels in the CNS (Bak *et al.*, 1972).

Levodopa and amphetamine increased acetylcholine release from the exposed cortex (Beani *et al.*, 1968; Pepeu and Bartolini, 1968; Beani and Bianchi, 1970). Amantadine and amphetamine increased cortical acetyl- choline release in conscious, freely moving guinea-pigs, and both also stimulated locomotor behaviour (Beani and Bianchi, 1973). The effects of amantadine were still evident in guinea-pigs pretreated with reserpine or α-methyl-*p*-tyrosine, but were abolished by the combined inhibition of catecholamine synthesis and granular uptake by these two drugs. α-Methyl-*p*-tyrosine pretreatment alone prevented the effect of am- phetamine on both behaviour and acetylcholine release. A further difference between amantadine and amphetamine was that the former increased acetylcholine content in the caudate nucleus whilst ampheta- mines had no action. The authors concluded that the effects of amanta- dine in these animals were mediated via DA release, although a direct action of amantadine on the neurosecretory processes of cortical cho- linergic nerve endings could not be excluded.

Anticholinergic or antihistaminic drugs, such as benztropine, tri- hexyphenidyl and diphenhydramine are of some value in the treatment of parkinsonian rigidity, and this effect is usually attributed to the anticholinergic action of these compounds. However, these drugs also inhibit catecholamine re-uptake and an effect of these anticholinergic drugs on DA metabolism in human parkinsonism has not been excluded. The potency of anticholinergic drugs in inhibiting the re-uptake of ^{3}H-NA by hypothalamic homogenates is comparable to that of amantadine, and inhibition of ^{3}H-DA re-uptake in striatal homogenates is greater than that of amantadine (Coyle and Snyder, 1969; Snyder, 1970).

5.1.5 Effect of amantadine on 5-hydroxytryptamine

Smooth muscle contractions induced by 5-HT can be sensitized with different drugs (Sigg et al., 1963). In rat fundus strips 10^{-4} M of amantadine shifted the dose-response curve for 5-HT to the left by a factor of 10 (Weseman and Zilliken, 1967). Maximal sensitization was achieved by 10^{-3} M amantadine. With higher concentrations the fundus strip did not contract to 5-HT.

Using human blood platelets as a physiological and pharmacological model of the adrenergic neurone (Abrahams and Solomon, 1969; Born and Born, 1969), the effects of amantadine on 5-HT uptake and release were compared with those of amphetamine. Both drugs inhibited the uptake of ^{3}H-5-HT and both released recently acquired 5-HT from platelets. Amphetamine was 5–10 times more potent than amantadine (Lemmer, 1973). This is in contrast to brain tissue where the 5-HT concentration is unaffected or even increased by amantadine (Strömberg and Svensson, 1971; Baldessarini et al., 1972).

The relevance of 5-HT in pathogenesis, and changes in 5-HT metabolism to the treatment of parkinsonism, are uncertain. Chase and his colleagues (1972) showed that patient disability and CSF 5-HIAA concentration were increased by the 5-HT precursor L-5-hydroxytryptophan combined with an inhibitor of peripheral L-aromatic aminoacid decarboxylase. In particular, there was an increase in bradykinesia and rigidity.

5.2 EFFECT OF AMANTADINE ON CATECHOLAMINES

Amantadine affects the synthesis, accumulation, release, and re-uptake of catecholamines in the central and peripheral nervous system. These effects are slightly different in the heart and brain, where there are regional differences in the effects on DA and NA. Amantadine in most brain areas causes a slight increase in the rate of DA synthesis and also an increased release of both DA and NA (Scatton et al., 1970; Strömberg et al., 1970; Baldessarini, 1971; Min-Chu and Laverty, 1971; Voigtlander and Moore, 1971). Amantadine also inhibits the re-uptake of catecholamines (Vernier *et al.*, 1969; Fletcher and Redfern, 1970; Farnebo *et al.*, 1971; Thornburg and Moore, 1971; Baldessarini *et al.*, 1972; Herblin, 1972). All these actions result in an increased availability of transmitter but may occur only with higher concentrations of amantadine than are likely to be achieved in therapy. However, in low concentration, increased release of catecholamines, in response to nerve stimuli, is produced by amantadine.

5.2.1 *Dopamine synthesis*

Scatton *et al.* (1970) studied ^{3}H-DA synthesis by incubating slices of rat striatum with ^{3}H-L-tyrosine and measuring the ^{3}H-amine accumulation. Amantadine increased both ^{3}H-DA synthesis and release. Farnebo *et al.* (1971) too found that 10^{-5} M amantadine increased the ^{14}C-DA biosynthesis from ^{14}C-tyrosine in brain tissue. This increased synthesis was thought to be consequent to increased DA release produced by amantadine, which resulted in reduced end-product inhibition of tyrosine hydroxylase (Neff and Costa, 1966; Weiner and Rutledge, 1966) and thereby in an increased synthesis of DA.

5.2.2 *Dopamine and noradrenaline accumulation and release*

Amantadine hydrochloride 150 mg kg^{-1} had little effect on the levels of NA, DA, 5-HT and 5-HIAA in brain tissues of mice. The brain levels of these mono-amines and 5-HIAA showed little change although there was a significant reduction in the brain NA content at 105 minutes after amantadine was given (Strömberg and Svensson, 1971). At this time brain 5-HT was slightly increased and 5-HIAA slightly reduced. Amantadine decreased NA accumulation after levodopa administration in both cardiac and brain tissue. DA in the heart, but not the brain, was slightly increased after amantadine 50 or 150 mg kg^{-1}. Baldessarini and his colleagues (1972) also showed that amantadine had a different effect on heart and brain catecholamines in the rat. Large doses of amantadine slightly increased cardiac NA stores, but slightly decreased brain NA. The effect of amantadine on DA in both heart and brain was even less than on NA. No effect on 5-HT could be determined.

Amantadine 10^{-5} caused the release of small quantities of added DA in a synaptosome-rich fraction of the basal ganglia of rats (Heimans *et al.*, 1972), dextroamphetamine having a similar effect. This may not be relevant to the antiparkinsonian action of amantadine in man in view of the high concentration needed, but the possibility that this effect was secondary to blockade of re-uptake could not be excluded.

5.2.3 *Catecholamine re-uptake*[1]

One of the main mechanisms of inactivating released adrenergic neuro-transmitters is presynaptic neuronal membrane re-uptake. If this mechanism is inhibited, increased activation of post-synaptic DA and NA receptors may result. In order to test the ability of amantadine to inhibit this re-uptake mechanism, Strömberg and Svensson (1971) used 4-α-methylmetatyramine to deplete central and peripheral catecholamine stores. 4-α-Methylmetatyramine uses the membrane pump for entry into neurones and then causes intracellular catecholamine depletion (Carlsson *et al.*, 1969) and its action is prevented by substances which block the membrane pump. Amantadine prevents the catecholamine-depleting action of this compound by only 30 per cent in the heart and to no significant extent in the brain. This finding suggests that amantadine only inhibits this uptake mechanism at the level of the cell membrane to a very slight extent (Strömberg and Svensson, 1971).

Heimans *et al.* (1972) showed that amantadine caused dose-dependent blockade of DA re-uptake in a synaptosome-rich particulate fraction of rat basal ganglia homogenate; $3 \cdot 6 \times 10^{-6}$ M inhibited DA uptake by 50 per cent. Heikkila and Cohen (1972) found that amantadine was a very weak DA releasing agent in a number of brain areas. In contrast it caused a greater effect on the inhibition of ^{3}H-DA uptake. This was much greater in whole brain or cortex than in the neostriatum. Baldessarini and his colleagues (1972) showed that amantadine-induced inhibition of ^{3}H-NA re-uptake too was somewhat greater in the cerebral cortex than in the striatum. Re-uptake of ^{3}H-DA was inhibited less than ^{3}H-NA in both the cortex and the striatum and the doses required to affect re-uptake in these animal studies were higher than those used clinically.

5.2.4 *Ventricular and cisternal perfusion with amantadine*

Voigtlander and Moore (1971) studied the effect of amantadine-perfusion of the ventricular system on the efflux of ^{3}H-DA. Amantadine caused a selective and dose-related efflux of ^{3}H-DA from brain structures lining the cerebro-ventricular system. The caudate nuclei were probably the principal source. Amantadine also enhanced the efflux of DA resulting from electrical stimulus of the caudate nucleus. The magnitude of the amantadine-induced ^{3}H-DA efflux was dependent upon the concentration of amantadine perfused. Amantadine 10 μg ml^{-1} had no effect, but 30, 100, and 300 μg ml^{-1} caused a progressive increase in ^{3}H-DA

---

[1] See Iversen (1965), "The Uptake of Catecholamines" in "Advances in Drug Research", Vol. 2.

efflux. Following electrical stimulation of the caudate, the previously sub-threshold concentration of 10 μg ml^{-1} now caused a considerable increase in ^{3}H-DA efflux. This efflux of amine was substantially greater than that obtained by drug or electrical stimulation alone.

From these findings, Voigtlander and Moore considered that amantadine might increase ^{3}H-DA efflux from the brain in a number of different ways. The effect of active release or blockage of re-uptake could not be distinguished, but the efflux of ^{3}H-DA which accompanied high amantadine dosage was probably associated with the latter mechanism since similar concentrations block the transport of ^{3}H-DA into crude brain synaptosomes (Fletcher and Redfern, 1970; Thornburg and Moore, 1971). The same mechanism may also explain why amantadine potentiated the efflux of ^{3}H-DA induced by electrical stimulation.

Intracisternal (i. ci.) radio-labelled DA, levodopa, and NA were used by Symchowicz *et al.* (1973). When radio-labelled DA was given, amantadine pre-treatment resulted in higher radioactivity in all brain areas investigated. Increase in brain radioactivity was caused by a higher level of DA and its metabolites. Amantadine had no effect on the brain radioactivity concentration in experiments in which radio-labelled levodopa or NA were administered i.ci. Amantadine therefore seemed to affect brain DA in a different way and to a different degree than brain NA. These results are in contrast to those in striatal homogenates where intra-neuronal extragranular amines, in particular NA, are usually released by amantadine. The effect of amantadine at the nerve cell membrane is likely to be important, and the use of cultured neostriatal cells in maintenance media (Coyle *et al.*, 1973) will allow a study of DA metabolism using intact striatal neurones.

5.2.5 *Effects of amantadine on peripheral and central adrenergic systems*

Offermeier (1965) showed that amantadine potentiated the effect of NA on the isolated vas deferens of the rat (α-adrenergic response), as do inhibitors of catecholamine uptake like cocaine and imipramine. Amphetamine, unlike amantadine, did not cause this sensitization, but increased peristaltic activity of the vas deferens. Amantadine also potentiated the effect of NA on the guinea-pig tracheal chain (β-adrenergic response) (Offermeier, 1971).

The flexor hind limb reflex of acutely spinalized animals (Carlsson *et al.*, 1963; Andén *et al.*, 1966; 1967) is known to be highly dependent upon NA receptor activity, and this reflex is increased by dopa and other substances causing NA receptor stimulation either directly or indirectly. Farnebo and his colleagues (1971) found that amantadine 100 mg kg^{-1}

increased the strength of this reflex which was evoked by pinching the back paws. An increase was also found when these animals were given dopa, combined with the dopa decarboxylase inhibitor Ro4-4602 and this was potentiated by amantadine 25 mg kg^{-1} but not 5 mg kg^{-1}. However, amantadine 5 mg kg^{-1} potentiated the effects of dopa on this reflex in rats pretreated with reserpine and nialamide. The action of amantadine was blocked when the animal was pretreated with the tyrosine-hydroxylase inhibitor α-methyltyrosine methyl ester which depletes intraneuronal extra-granular catecholamine pools. Thus, it seems likely that amantadine has a releasing action on extra-granular stores in both the NA and DA nerve terminal systems. After combined reserpine-nialamide-dopa treatment extra-granular catecholamine stores are high and no stores of amines can occur in the granules.

5.2.6 *Effects of amantadine on monoamine oxidase*

Amantadine, and other indirectly acting sympathomimetic drugs like amphetamines, have common properties of causing both increased catecholamine release and inhibition of catecholamine re-uptake at nerve endings in the CNS (Lemmer, 1973). In addition, the effects of amphetamines and amantadine in behavioural studies in animals are, to some extent, similar, although amantadine has a lesser effect (Vernier *et al.*, 1969; Fibiger *et al.*, 1971; Strömberg and Svensson, 1971). Because of these facts an amphetamine-like action of amantadine has been proposed by many authors (Strömberg and Svensson, 1971; Farnebo *et al.*, 1971; Offermeier, 1971). However, in contrast to amphetamines amantadine has no inhibitory effect on monoamine oxidase either *in vitro* or *in vivo* (Blaschko *et al.*, 1937; da Prada *et al.*, 1965; Vernier *et al.*, 1969; Strömberg and Svensson, 1971; Baldessarini *et al.*, 1972).

Monoamine oxidase inhibitors are not effective treatment in parkinsonism: in experimental animals MAO inhibition will increase brain NA, but not DA, levels. Davies (1971) found that amantadine up to a final concentration of 10^{-4} M did not inhibit the MAO of beef brain mitochondria using kynuramine as a substrate. Pretreatment with the MAO inhibitor pheniprazine did not alter amantadine-stimulated motor activity in mice (Thornburg and Moore, 1972). In contrast, the stimulant action of dextro-amphetamine on motor activity in mice is enhanced by pretreatment with pheniprazine (Lew *et al.*, 1971). However, amantadine is not extensively metabolized in mice (Bleidner *et al.*, 1965) in contrast to amphetamine, and pheniprazine probably increases the effect of amphetamine in rodents by slowing its metabolism (Lew *et al.*, 1971). Vernier *et al.* (1969) and Baldessarini *et al.* (1972), also showed that amantadine had no effect on MAO; the latter workers demonstrated that amantadine had no effect on the deamination of ^{14}C-5-HT or ^{3}H-NA at high concentrations both *in vitro* and *in vivo*. Amantadine did not affect MAO activity in rat brain and liver in animals pretreated with iproniazid, which was given to facilitate the quantitative analysis of catecholamines and some of their metabolites, in selected brain regions (Symchowicz *et al.*, 1973).

The possibility that amantadine inhibits dopamine-β-hydroxylase is unlikely as amantadine has little effect on endogenous NA levels in the brain, and ^{3}H-NA formation from ^{3}H tyrosine is unaltered after amantadine administration (Strömberg and Svensson, 1971). The action of amantadine on dopa decarboxylase is not known. Decreased inactivation of DA could result from inhibition of the enzyme catechol-O-methyl transferase but amantadine has not been studied in this respect. McGeer *et al.* (1972) showed that amantadine had no significant effect on glutamic acid decarboyxlase using *in vitro* assays of homogenates of striata and other brain areas of rats.

5.3   EFFECT OF AMANTADINE ON ANIMAL BEHAVIOUR

5.3.1   *Effect on motor activity*

The relative importance of brain DA and NA in motor activity and, in particular, amphetamine-stimulated activity is, to some extent, controversial, but recent evidence favours a primary role for DA. Inhibition of dopamine hydroxylase with 1-phenyl-2-2'-thiazolyl-thiourea markedly depletes brain NA content but does not significantly alter the enhanced motor activity in mice following dextroamphetamine (Thornburg, 1972).

The effect of amantadine on spontaneous locomotor activity in animals has been investigated extensively (Vernier *et al.*, 1969; Svensson and Strömberg, 1970; Fliorio and Longo, 1971; Abuzzahab, 1971; Farnebo *et al.*, 1971; Strömberg and Svensson, 1971; Thornburg and Moore, 1972). Amantadine (25 mg kg^{-1}) significantly increases activity in rodents during the first part of a three-hour period, whilst a dosage of 50 mg kg^{-1} causes a significant effect for 3 hours, and 100 mg kg^{-1} is consistently more active during the last hour of the three-hour period (Fibiger *et al.*, 1971). Occasionally no increase in locomotor activity has been found, but the failure of Abuzzahab (1971) to demonstrate a significant increase in activity may have been due to toxic effects of high amantadine dosage. Strömberg and Svensson (1971) found an initial reduction in motor activity for 1 hour after 50, 100, and 150 mg kg^{-1} amantadine, followed by motor stimulation. Thornburg and Moore (1972) also found an initial suppression of motor activity at a dose of 160 mg kg^{-1}.

Maximal locomotor activity after amantadine is approximately one-tenth of that elicited by either dextro- or levo-amphetamine (Thornburg and Moore, 1972). Dextroamphetamine caused an immediate increase in locomotor activity in contrast to the 20–40 minutes period delay following amantadine injection by the same intraperitoneal route. High amphetamine dosage never elicited an initial depression of motor activity as occurred with amantadine.

Dextroamphetamine-stimulated motor activity in rodents is blocked by pretreatment with α-methyltyrosine, an inhibitor of catecholamine synthesis (Weissman et al., 1966; Dominic and Moore, 1969). Pretreatment with this compound did not affect amantadine-stimulated motor activity (Thornburg and Moore, 1972). In contrast, Strömberg et al. (1970) showed that the effect of amantadine on motor hyperactivity in rats was abolished by pretreatment with α-methyl-p-tyrosine methylester but not by pretreatment with reserpine which depletes intraneuronal granular catecholamine stores. Thornburg and Moore (1972) considered that amantadine-stimulated motor activity did not involve newly synthesized brain catecholamines, but according to Strömberg et al. (1970) catecholamines are required for the effect of amantadine in increasing motor activity. The initial hypokinesia and the time course in general of motor hyperactivity following amantadine is similar to that seen with combined dopa and extra-cerebral dopa decarboxylase inhibition (Strömberg, 1970).

5.3.2 Effect on stereotyped behaviour

There are many indications that stereotyped behaviour is the result of activation of the dopaminergic system in the corpus striatum. Amsler, in 1923, showed that apomorphine-induced compulsive gnawing in guinea-pigs and rats was prevented by destruction of the corpus striata. Ernst (1967) showed that dextroamphetamine also was able to bring about compulsive gnawing behaviour, although amphetamines probably acted by releasing endogenous DA in contrast to the direct DA receptor stimulant action of apomorphine. The dosages of apomorphine and levodopa required to elicit stereotyped behaviour are 10–100 times greater than those required to produce turning behaviour in rats (Ernst, 1967; Voigtlander and Moore, 1973). However, amphetamines may have an equal potency in causing both stereotyped and turning behaviour. Sniffing, gnawing, and rearing behaviour is dependent upon NA and well as DA receptor activity (Corrodi et al., 1970; Fuxe and Ungerstedt, 1970), although sniffing has been related mainly to DA receptor activity, and rearing to NA receptor stimulation.

Amantadine given alone does not produce stereotopies or only slightly affects the gross behaviour of animals. The ready production of such behaviour in rats and mice with amphetamines does not occur with amantadine. Davies (1971) detected no stereotyped activity following amantadine treatment, and Farnebo *et al.* (1971) found a very small amount of sniffing activity in rats given amantadine whilst gnawing was very uncommon. However, amantadine 5 mg kg^{-1} markedly potentiates the effects of dopa on rearing and sniffing in rats pretreated with reserpine and the dopa decarboxylase inhibitor Ro4-4602. After treatment with Ro4-4602 (**4**) alone the potentiating effects of amantadine are marked only with a dose of 25 mg kg^{-1}.

$$HO-\underset{\underset{HO\quad OH}{}}{\bigcirc}-CH_2NHNHCOCHCH_2OH$$
$$NH_2$$

(**4**)

Davies (1971) reported the unexpected finding that amantadine reduced rather than increased apomorphine-induced gnawing behaviour in both rats and mice, although this effect was only marked with comparatively high oral doses of 32 and 100 mg kg^{-1} amantadine. He also reported that amantadine antagonized and did not potentiate the dextroamphetamine-induced compulsive gnawing behaviour in mice, but to a lesser extent than apomorphine. Naylor and Costall (1971) found that amantadine did not potentiate amphetamine-induced stereotopies but Simon *et al.* (1970) found that amantadine at doses higher than 4 mg kg^{-1} i.p. in rats significantly increased the intensities of stereotopies such as licking and gnawing due to dextroamphetamine. This effect was dependent on the relative timing of injections and was not seen with a two-hour period between the injection of amantadine and amphetamine.

5.3.3   *Effect on animal rotation*

The turning of animals with unilateral striatal lesions is a useful method for investigating DA receptor activity (Andén *et al.*, 1966; Ungerstedt, 1968; 1971a; 1971b; 1971c). Lesions may be produced electrolytically or by a selective degeneration of the DA-producing neurone caused by 6-OH-DA injected locally in the nigrostriatal tract. Animals with unilateral lesions turn either to the operated or unoperated side in the presence of various drugs which alter DA receptor activity. The dose of levodopa necessary to produce a significant degree of turning is much lower than that required to increase locomotor activity in mice (Smith, 1963; Thut and Rech, 1970). Changes in NA receptor activity hardly influence animal rotation.

In rats with a 6-OH-DA induced unilateral degeneration of the nigro-neostriatal neurones (Ungerstedt, 1968; 1971a) supersensitivity of the DA receptors develops on the denervated side (Ungerstedt, 1971b). DA receptor stimulating agents, such as apomorphine (Andén et al., 1967) increase the DA receptor activity preferentially on the denervated side and the rat rotates to the intact side. In contrast, DA releasing agents such as amphetamine (Carlsson et al., 1966) increase DA receptor activity only on the intact side and the rat rotates to the denervated side. There is a progressive increase with time of the turning effect of apomorphine, and this may be due to the progressive development of unilateral receptor sensitivity (Voigtlander and Moore, 1973).

Amantadine 50 mg kg^{-1} i.p. in rats with unilateral 6-OH-DA lesions causes turning to the lesioned side, commencing after 15–20 minutes and lasting for 3–4 hours (Farnebo et al., 1971). Strömberg and Svensson (1971) also found that amantadine 50–150 mg kg^{-1} caused rotation to the side of the lesion in unilaterally striatomized rats. Rotatory behaviour was inhibited by previous DA receptor blockage, and when haloperidol 1 mg kg^{-1} was given 1 hour before amantadine, there was no alteration in the haloperidol-induced rotation to the unoperated side. Catechola-mine depletion caused by pretreatment with reserpine (100 mg kg^{-1}) also inhibited the effect of amantadine on turning behaviour. Strömberg and Svensson (1971) considered that amantadine facilitated dopaminergic transmission in the striatum in the same way as both levodopa and dextro-amphetamine since the turning effect of all these drugs was antagonized by haloperidol, which can be assumed to block striatal DA receptors (Andén et al., 1970). The turning effect of amantadine was inhibited after depletion of amines and inhibition of catecholamine synthesis, and so was likely to be indirect and not due to receptor stimulation, but mediated by the release of DA.

Voigtlander and Moore (1973) studied the comparative effects of apomorphine, levodopa, amantadine, amphetamines and other psycho-motor stimulants on turning behaviour of rodents. Dextro- and levo-amphetamine, and amantadine, increased turning to the lesioned side in contrast to apomorphine and levodopa, which caused contralateral turning. Amantadine 4–32 mg kg^{-1} caused fewer turns per minute than either amphetamine isomer 0·25–16 mg kg^{-1} (Fig. 1).

Farnebo et al. (1971) studied the effects of amantadine given together with levodopa in animals with unilateral electro-coagulation of the corpus striatum. Rotation caused by levodopa combined with the extracerebral dopa decarboxylase inhibitor Ro4-4602 was potentiated on the addition of amantadine. The turning behaviour of these animals is, in some respects, different from those with unilateral 6-OH-DA lesions. 6-OH-DA causes a selective destruction of DA-forming neurones whilst receptor areas as well as DA-forming neurones are destroyed non-selectively by electro-coagulation. In animals with unilateral electro-coagulation of the striatum, increased DA receptor activity caused by DA release (amphetamine) or receptor stimulation (apomorphine) in both cases results in rotation towards the operated side. The result of combined amantadine–dopa treatment on turning behaviour in 6-OH-DA lesioned animals may be different, since in these animals the turning effects of dopa due to extreme unilateral receptor supersensitivity may, to some degree, be reversed by amantadine.

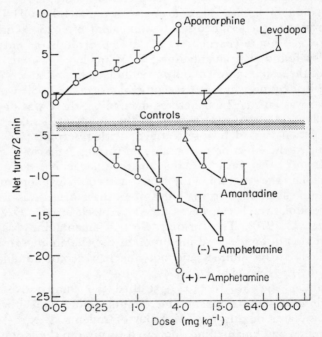

Fig. 1. Effects of various drugs upon the turning of mice with left striatal 6-hydroxydopamine lesions. Ten days or more after the lesions were made, mice were injected with the indicated doses of drugs and observed 30 minutes later. The horizontal line and crosshatching represent the mean and standard error of the pooled controls ($n = 88$). Each symbol represents the mean of the scores of at least 10 mice and the vertical lines denote 1 standard error. Solid symbols are significantly different from the controls ($p < 0.05$). Reprinted with permission from *Von Voigtlander and Moore*, 1973, Pergamon Press.

5.3.4 *Anticataleptic action of amantadine hydrochloride*

The anticataleptic action of amantadine hydrochloride 5–80 mg kg^{-1} s.c. in rodents was studied by Zetler (1970). Amantadine was active against trifluoperazine, haloperidol, bulbocapnine, paraoxon, pilocarpine, nicotine, and tetrabenazine-induced catalepsy. These cataleptogens are antagonized by anticholinergic drugs with the exception of tetrabenazine. Reversal of tetrabenazine-induced catalepsy showed that amantadine did not act in this respect as a central anticholinergic drug. The amantadine dose required to antagonize drug-induced catalepsy may be 5–10 times the human therapeutic dose, as with tetrabenazine-induced sedation in mice (Vernier *et al.*, 1969).

Pilocarpine and anticholinesterases such as paraoxon caused hypothermia as well as catalepsy. Amantadine increased hypothermia. In contrast, anticholinergic drugs abolished the hypothermia caused by central anticholinergic stimulation. The anticataleptic action of amantadine was similar to amphetamines, which, however, altered body temperature differently (Zetler, 1968).

TABLE 1

Anticataleptic action of amantadine and amphetamine

First injection	(s.c.) mg kg^{-1}	Second injection	(s.c.)^a mg kg^{-1}	Catalepsy^b
Amantadine	5	Trifluoperazine	2	12/15
(±)-Amphetamine	12	Trifluoperazine	2	7/15
Amantadine	40	Haloperidol	0·5	9/15
(±)-Amphetamine	10	Haloperidol	0·5	3/15
Amantadine	40	Bulbocapnine	30	10/15
(±)-Amphetamine	8	Bulbocapnine	30	5/15
Amantadine	40	Tetrabenazine	8	7/15
(±)-Amphetamine	4	Tetrabenazine	8	3/15

^{a} 10 min after the first injection.
^{b} Observations began 20 min after the first injection.
Doses refer to amantadine hydrochloride and dl-amphetamine sulphate.
Catalepsy results given as number of animals cataleptic: number injected.
Reprinted with permission from: Zetler (1970), Springer-Verlag, Berlin, Heidelberg, New York.

Simon *et al.* (1970) found that prochlorperazine-induced catalepsy in rats was antagonized by amantadine. Davies *et al.* (1973) found that conditioned avoidance behaviour in rats was inhibited by haloperidol 200 µg kg^{-1} s.c. which decreased the number of correct responses by approximately 55 per cent one hour after injection. Amantadine hydrochloride 12·5–50 mg kg i.p. reversed the inhibition due to haloperidol for 3 hours. Apomorphine 10 mg kg^{-1} i.p. reversed the effect of haloperidol for one hour. Levodopa 200 mg kg^{-1} i.p. had no immediate effect, but animals overcame the effects of haloperidol earlier. Benzhexol and atropine had no effect. Davies *et al.* (1973) considered that conditioned avoidance behaviour was a useful procedure for distinguishing between atropine-like and dopaminergic antiparkinsonian drugs. The action of amantadine was attributed to increased DA release, resulting in reversal of the competitive receptor block produced by haloperidol.

5.3.5   *Effect on experimentally induced rigidity*

Alpha and gamma motor activity was recorded in thin filaments from ventral roots supplying calf muscles in rats by Jurna *et al.* (1972). Alpha reflex activity was low and the gamma reflex activity was high in untreated animals. Amantadine increased alpha reflex discharges but did not cause rigidity. Reserpine 10 mg kg^{-1} increased alpha and reduced gamma activity in these animals; rigidity due to reserpine has been attributed to an increased and synchronized alpha motor activity and is abolished by levodopa (Roos and Steg, 1964; Jurna and Lanzer, 1969). Amantadine abolished the effect of reserpine on alpha and gamma reflex discharges.

Oxotremorine 48 μg kg^{-1} increased alpha reflex activity. In contrast to reserpine, it did not reduce but increased the gamma discharges. Amantadine abolished the effect of oxotremorine on the alpha motor system, but did not reduce gamma discharges. Oxotremorine raises the concentration of acetylcholine in the brain (Lundgren and Malmburg, 1968) and elicits rigidity based on alpha hyperactivity. The effect of amantadine on oxotremorine-induced rigidity was, however, attributed to a change in cerebral DA, and not acetycholine, metabolism (Jurna *et al.*, 1972).

5.3.6   *Mode of action of amantadine in parkinsonism*

Amantadine is relatively ineffective in increasing catecholamine synthesis, release, or re-uptake, as compared to amphetamines. Amantadine 3 mg kg^{-1} oral relieves parkinsonian akinesia and rigidity to as great or greater extent than either dextro (0·25 mg kg^{-1}) or levo (0·75 mg kg^{-1}) amphetamine (personal observation). Amantadine does not cause direct stimulation of DA or NA receptors (Farnebo *et al.*, 1971). The effect on brain DA is different from NA. Symchowicz *et al.* (1973) found that amantadine caused increases in brain radioactivity after radio-labelled

DA but not after radio-labelled NA i.ci. Farnebo *et al.* (1971) showed
that amantadine caused an increased release of ^{3}H-DA during electrical
field stimulation of slices of striatum. Heikkila and Cohen (1972)
considered that neither the direct release nor blockage of DA re-uptake
in the striatum accounted for the action of amantadine in patients with
Parkinson's disease and suggested that amantadine increased the amount
of DA liberated during the nerve impulse. Ventricular perfusion of
amantadine increases ^{3}H-DA efflux from the caudate nucleus during
electrical stimulation (Voigtlander and Moore, 1972) and this effect is
found with a concentration too low to cause DA release in the absence
of electrical stimulation. A model for increased release of neurotransmitter
during electrical stimulation is available in the cholinergic system where
it has been shown that guanidine (Otsuka and Endo, 1960) or tetraethyl-
ammonium ion (Benoit and Mambrini, 1970) increases the amount of
acetylcholine released during a single nerve impulse.

6 Amantadine in the treatment of Parkinson's disease

6.1 INTRODUCTION

James Parkinson in 1817 described the condition now honoured by his
name but it was not until the latter years of that century that any form of
effective treatment was known. Ogle in the Medical Times and Gazette
of 1865 suggested treatment with the Calabar bean, *physostigma venenosum*,
although the effect of this would be surely to increase rather than reduce
parkinsonian disability. Charcot is usually credited with the introduction
of anticholinergic drugs for the treatment of parkinsonism, first given
to reduce salivation. Erb (*Zeitschrift fur Therapie*, August 1887)
described hyoscine hydrobromide as "causing pronounced relief in
paralysis agitans attended with much aching pain". Anticholinergic
drugs remained the standard remedy for 80 years, until the importance
of dopamine deficiency in the striatum and the ability to reverse this was
realized. Levodopa alone or combined with a dopa decarboxylase
inhibitor is now established as the treatment of choice for most patients,
but some do not respond and other drugs which affect different aspects
of dopamine metabolism have been used. Of these only amantadine has
been widely assessed clinically; amphetamines have been barred largely on
account of possible misuse or addiction. The possibility that post-
synaptic as well as presynaptic events in the neostriatum can be altered
by drug therapy has as yet been almost totally neglected.

6.1.1 *Idiopathic Parkinson's disease*

In idiopathic Parkinson's disease there is degeneration of melanin pigmented neurones in the brain stem (Greenfield and Bosanquet, 1953). These cells manufacture DA, and DA depletion in the neostriatum is associated with symptoms of parkinsonism. In most untreated patients with Parkinson's disease, the DA metabolite HVA is in low concentration in the lumbar CSF. The therapeutic effect of levodopa is most likely due to reversal of striatal DA deficiency and levodopa causes an increase in CSF HVA concentration. A secondary role of cholinergic systems is demonstrated by the increase in parkinsonian disability caused by centrally acting anticholinesterases and the modest improvement brought about by anticholinergic drugs.

6.1.2 *Aetiology of Parkinson's disease*

The cause of Parkinson's disease is not known. Stephanis and Issidorides (1970) suggested there may be a disturbance in protein synthesis as well as changes in dopaminergic and cholinergic mechanisms. They postulated that an unknown agent stimulated the production of a new form of RNA; Issidorides submitted that this increase in RNA activity was inversely related to brain melanin content. Gomirato and Hyden (1963) described an increase in RNA in the glia of the globus pallidus early in the disease, with later an increase in RNA in the neurones in the same area. Neuronal degeneration linked to the vast group of abiotrophies, with as yet undetermined enzymic defects may be responsible (Lewis, 1971). Brown and Knox (1972) suggested that all cases of idiopathic Parkinson's disease were subsequent to encephalitis lethargica. Excess accumulation of heavy metals in the basal ganglia, abnormal MSH production, and a failure of the conversion of tyrosine to levodopa have also been suggested (Parkes *et al.*, 1972; Shuster *et al.*, 1973; Calne, 1970).

There is no direct evidence that any of these possibilities are associated with Parkinson's disease. However, if any are relevant there are several ways in which levodopa or amantadine might influence the cause as well as the symptoms of this disease. If RNA or protein synthesis is disturbed, the action of dopa on RNA synthesis may be important (Seale and Prasad, 1967) and dopa treatment may also affect MSH production. The chelating and antiviral effects of certain biogenic amines and amantadine (Fletcher *et al.*, 1965) may also be relevant in respect of metal containing co-enzymes concerned with catecholamine biosynthesis; or possible viral invasion of the nervous system.

6.1.3 *Treatment and disease progression*

There is no evidence that treatment of any kind affects either the cause or the progression of Parkinson's disease. The disability of patients taking anticholinergics is, on the whole, slowly progressive although some show little or no deterioration and others have an almost malignant course. Levodopa treatment does not affect disease progression (Hunter *et al.*, 1973) and there is no present indication that amantadine does.

6.1.4 *Parkinsonian syndromes*

Akinesia and rigidity occur in several diseases of the extrapyramidal system, but with the exception of Parkinson's disease there is not a selective degeneration of DA-forming cells. The results of treatment with amantadine are likely to be different from Parkinson's disease. Patients with cerebral arteriosclerosis and others with senile dementia are often akinetic and rigid and described as having arteriosclerotic parkinsonism but the exact pathological diagnosis may be difficult to establish in life and other clinical features are different to those in Parkinson's disease. Dementia in these conditions can make it difficult to assess changes in motor performance resulting from treatment.

6.1.5 *Drug-induced parkinsonism*

Phenothiazines and other neuroleptic drugs which reduce DA synthesis or block DA receptors can cause an akinetic and rigid state like Parkinson's disease, acute dystonic episodes, and akathisia, with restlessness and often discomfort of the limbs. These conditions improve on drug withdrawal but dyskinesias involving the face and mouth, which are often late in onset, occasionally are permanent.

6.1.6 *Score systems for disability assessment*

Hoehn and Yahr (1967), Godwin Austen *et al.* (1969), Webster (1968), Walker *et al.* (1972a), and many others, have introduced scoring systems for use in the determination of disability in patients with Parkinson's disease. These do not take into account the often considerable variation in symptoms and signs that may occur during one day, and there may be a seven-fold variation in the amplitude of tremor during a 24-hour period. Grading of the severity of disease (e.g. minor unilateral disability, bed- or chair-bound) is of value in showing disease progression. There is at present no biochemical test of use in the diagnosis of Parkinson's disease. The CSF HVA concentration is low in a number of disorders which may be confused with Parkinson's disease, including essential tremor (Curzon, 1973).

6.1.7 *Receptor supersensitivity*

After unilateral nigrostriatal lesions which destroy DA-forming cells but not DA receptors in animals, the development of unilateral receptor supersensitivity explains turning behaviour due to DA receptor stimulant drugs. Receptor supersensitivity is also likely to develop in human parkinsonism. A study of the possible use of DA-releasing drugs including amantadine, and DA receptor stimulating drugs such as apomorphine, to obtain some index of receptor supersensitivity in man has not yet been made.

6.2 AMANTADINE TREATMENT

Schwab *et al.* (1969) reported that 66 per cent of a group of 163 patients with Parkinson's disease improved after taking amantadine hydrochloride. Amantadine had been given to prevent influenza to a 58-year old woman with a moderately severe bilateral Parkinson's disease who then had a partial remission of her symptoms which returned on stopping the drug after 6 weeks. One hundred and seven parkinsonian patients were then given amantadine 200 mg daily and improved, 48 were unchanged and 3 were worse. In 5 patients the results were uncertain. A higher dosage than 200 mg had no additional benefit. Of those who improved, one-third showed a decline in response after 4–8 weeks, whilst in others benefit remained for 3–8 months. On amantadine withdrawal there was a prompt exacerbation of symptoms. Five patients who did not respond initially did so when amantadine was resumed 1–3 months later, whilst in other patients treatment was a failure from the onset. In 9 patients who stopped amantadine to begin levodopa, there was improvement on both drugs, 2 had no benefit from either and 1 patient was improved on levodopa but not on amantadine.

A quarter of patients described some side effects while taking amantadine (jitteryness, insomnia, abdominal uneasiness, loss of appetite, slight feeling of dizziness, and in one patient a feeling of depression). Side effects disappeared within 36 hours after amantadine was stopped. In some patients who may have been close to the limit of tolerance of anticholinergic drugs, the addition of amantadine potentiated the side effects of mental confusion and hallucination as the result of benzhexol and benztropine. Reducing the dosage of either anticholinergic drugs or amantadine abolished these particular side effects.

6.2.1   *Single drug treatment*

Thirteen patients with idiopathic Parkinson's disease were given amantadine 100 mg twice daily as a single treatment by Mann *et al.* (1971) and showed a moderate improvement in scores for bradykinesia, tremor and rigidity commencing on the second day. The improvement in bradykinesia and rigidity was greater than tremor. Eleven of the 13 patients improved by at least one stage of disease (Hoehn and Yahr, 1967), 3 by two stages, and 1 by four stages. The 2 patients who did not respond had a minor degree of disability due mainly to tremor, but otherwise there were no features distinguishing those patients who responded from those who did not.

6.2.2   *Intravenous amantadine treatment of Parkinson's disease*

Intravenous amantadine hydrochloride may cause venous thrombosis and use of this preparation in man has been limited. Fasano *et al.* (1970) described 16 patients with Parkinson's disease who each were given 100 mg amantadine intravenously. Two patients showed an excellent, 6 a good, and 2 a slight response. Five did not improve. In those who benefited there was improvement in rigidity and bradykinesia within 10 minutes of injection. A reduction in disability of 70 per cent occurred in some patients. This was a greater degree of benefit than that from oral amantadine, or from levodopa given intravenously and comparable degrees of improvement were only obtained after maintenance high dosage levodopa treatment by mouth. The effect of amantadine persisted for 24–48 hours and the only side effect was a transient sensation of heat in the face lasting 5–10 seconds. Cardiac arrhythmias did not occur with the dosage used.

6.2.3   *Amantadine combined with anticholinergic drugs*

In most placebo-controlled trials of amantadine, this has been given in combination with anticholinergic drugs (Dallos *et al.*, 1970; Fieshi *et al.*, 1970a; 1970b; 1970c; Parkes *et al.*, 1970a; Voller, 1970; Freedman *et al.*, 1971; MacFadyen *et al.*, 1972). Jorgensen *et al.* (1971) gave amantadine hydrochloride 200 mg daily to 149 parkinsonian patients for a three-week period. There was some evidence of improvement in over half—48 patients had a moderate to marked improvement, benefit was just detectable in 15, 27 showed no change and 24 deteriorated. As in other trials benefit occurred within 3 days of commencing amantadine. Patients had improvement in hand dexterity, walking, balance, and general mobility, as well as a sense of well-being and an ability to partake again in pastimes

TABLE 2

Amantadine therapy in the treatment of Parkinson's disease and post-encephalitic parkinsonism

Author	Population (out patients)	Number of patients	Amantadine hydrochloride daily dosage mg	Duration of observation	Overall improvement	Comments
1. Appleton *et al.* (1971)	Most patients idiopathic Parkinson's disease	19	200	6–11 months	Very good (3) All aspects of parkinsonism improved. Bradykinesia and rigidity most improvement	Failure of response not described
2. Campbell and Williams (1972)	24 patients with idiopathic Parkinson's disease	31	200	9–12 months	19 patients improvement wholly or partially sustained	8 patients lost initial benefit; 10 retained benefit; one patient died of heart failure
3. Castaigne *et al.* (1972)	4 post-encephalitic and 45 idiopathic Parkinson's disease	50	200–500	18 months	Very good 20%; good 36%; fairly good 26%; failure 18%. Maximum effect on akinesia, less effect on tremor	Diminution of activity seen in most patients
4. Labauge *et al.* (1972)	2 post-encephalitic	50		2–9 months	36 lasting improvement; 14 no improvement; good response 12; average response	Secondary response failure in 2 patients, not in others

		No.	Dosage (mg)	Duration	Response	
5. Nagaswami and Ranjini (1971)	Post-encephalitic, drug induced, and other forms of parkinsonism	38	200–300	24 weeks	Good initial improvement. No response 15%; poor response 9. Rigidity and akinesia responded well	Response mostly maintained
6. Parkes et al. (1971)	All patients idiopathic Parkinson's disease	26	200–600	1 year	29% mean reduction in total score after 1 year	Evidence not given of response failure
7. Rao and Pearce (1971)	15 idiopathic Parkinson's disease, 5 post-encephalitic	20	200–300	Up to 12 months	Nil 4; slight 6; good 6; excellent 4	8 patients showed partial response failure at 1–6 weeks. Decline not progressive
8. Schwab et al. (1972)	Disease aetiology not given	430	$(351)^a$–200 Some patients 300–500	Up to 900 days	64% improved. Marked improvement in a few cases	Response declines 30–60 days after commencement of amantadine
9. Sigwald et al. (1972)	Disease aetiology not given	58	100–500	1–20 months	Amantadine + levodopa: very good 10; nil 4. Amantadine alone: good 3; nil 3.	Response failure did not occur
10. Streifler and Kallay (1972)	32 "arteriosclerotic parkinsonism". 8 idiopathic Parkinson's disease, 9 post-encephalitic	28	200 in most cases	Over 1 year	No change 2; slight improvement 8; marked improvement 16; great improvement 2.	No response; failure

[a] 351 patients on a dosage of amantadine hydrochloride of 200 mg daily. Remaining patients on variable dosage up to 500 mg daily.

such as sewing and piano-playing. Tremor and rigidity, bradykinesia, posture, gait, arm-swing, facial aspect, speech, and self-care scores all improved as compared to placebo. Sudden withdrawal of amantadine caused a symptomatic worsening in several patients. Side effects were generally mild; 36 patients had specified side effects on amantadine and 46 patients had similar symptoms on placebo.

6.2.4   *Degree of improvement*

Improvement of 15–30 per cent in mean total disability scores has been found in most trials of amantadine (Dallos *et al.*, 1970; Appleton *et al.*, 1971). Many of the patients studied by Pearce (1971), and Pearce and Rao (1970), had an excellent response both in the short (3 months) and longer (1 year) term. Ten of these 20 patients showed substantial subjective and objective benefit and were able to carry out successfully several domestic chores and work which were previously impossible on anticholinergic drugs alone. However, 4 patients did not show any response. In contrast, Hunter *et al.* (1970a) found amantadine gave little or no therapeutic benefit and Greenburg (1971) reported that only 3 of 26 patients showed any improvement.

Barbeau *et al.* (1971) drew attention to the remarkable finding that in a small patient group the degree of improvement with amantadine hydrochloride was considerable, and similar in magnitude to that seen in these patients when on optimum levodopa treatment. Four of 64 patients had a 41–50 per cent and 4 a 50 per cent or greater degree of overall improvement with amantadine. Griffiths *et al.* (1971) described 4 patients, 3 of whom did extremely well on amantadine with no side effects, and 4 of 31 patients studied by Campbell and Williams (1972) made a dramatic response to amantadine. Morgan (1970) described two patients, aged 74 and 86, who made a very considerable and progressive improvement on amantadine. Eight days of treatment was necessary before any change was seen in one patient, but then progressive improvement occurred in the following eight weeks. Individual patients reported by Weiss *et al.* (1971) and Schwartz and Fahn (1970) were greatly improved by amantadine, and a woman was able to rise and walk alone for the first time for 5 years on the day of commencing amantadine therapy.

6.2.5   *Response to amantadine*

Twenty per cent of parkinsonian patients treated for a short period with amantadine show a good response, while a similar percentage show no response (Portera *et al.*, 1970). The factors which determine response to amantadine are not certain, and this is not related to age, sex, duration of disease or previous thalamolysis. However, Parkes *et al.* (1970a), and Jorgensen *et al.* (1971) found that the most severely disabled patients did best on amantadine treatment. The response to amantadine is not dependent on the presence of additional anticholinergic drugs, and patients with Parkinson's disease and post-encephalitic parkinsonism respond, at least initially, in a similar fashion. Improvement in akinetic-rigid syndromes in elderly demented patients with cerebral arterio-sclerosis or parenchymal brain disease is not established.

6.2.6 *Amantadine dosage*

Amantadine, 100, 300, and 500 mg daily, was given by Parkes *et al.* (1970b) to patients with Parkinson's disease, each dosage for a 2-week period. The patients described the preferred dose as 300 mg daily and this resulted in a 26 per cent reduction in the initial disability score. Nine of 43 patients did not respond to any amantadine dosage.

6.2.7 *Amantadine sulphate, citrate, and hydrochloride*

Amantadine hydrochloride is more rapidly absorbed than either the sulphate or the citrate (Voller, 1972) and produces a more rapid onset of effect with a comparatively high concentration of this form in the serum. There is probably no distinct clinical advantage in using one particular preparation, although Fünfgeld (1970) considered the clinical response to amantadine sulphate was superior to the hydrochloride. The excretory conditions for the sulphate and the hydrochloride are essentially similar.

6.3 LONG-TERM TREATMENT WITH AMANTADINE

In some patients there is a decline in initial response to amantadine after 4–12 weeks. In a group of 26 patients given amantadine 200–600 mg daily, alone, or combined with anticholinergic drugs over a period of one year, the mean reduction in total disability score was 17·3 per cent at three months. The improvement over one year (29·2 per cent) was not significantly greater statistically. Tremor, akinesia, rigidity and flexion of posture all improved in the long term. In this study there was no evidence of a decline in effect and on sudden withdrawal of amantadine after a year of treatment considerable deterioration occurred, indicating a persistent effect of this drug (Parkes *et al.*, 1971a). Campbell and Williams (1972) followed up 28 patients for 9–12 months of amantadine treatment.

TABLE 3

Effect of amantadine on disability scores

Feature	Initial	Scores Amantadine hydrochloride		
		100	300	500
General history	3·1	2·6	2·6	1·8
Walking history	3·8	3·3	2·6	2·4
Functional disability	6·7	7·1	5·9	5·5
Appearance	10·8	9·9	8·3	8·0
Tremor	5·6	4·1	3·4	3·3
Rigidity	7·6	6·0	5·4	5·4
Limb dexterity	10·0	8·0	6·9	7·1
Mood	1·9	2·1	1·4	1·7
TOTAL SCORE	49·8	43·5	36·9	35·5

Reduction in disability scores with amantadine hydrochloride 100, 300, and 500 mg per day in 43 patients with parkinsonism. Each dosage was given for 2 weeks and scores before treatment are shown. (Parkes *et al.*, 1970b—reprinted with permission.)

TABLE 4

Effect of amantadine on timed tests (in seconds)

Test	Controls aged		Initial	Amantadine HCl dose mg per day		
	21–26	50–69		100	300	500
Standing/sitting (5 times)	6	9	22	16	12	13
Walking 22 m	12	19	28	26	24	23
Eating 2 biscuits/10	6·6	12·8	20·1	18·1	18·3	18·1
Pegboard	9	14	29	26	25	29
Mittens	6	8	22	21	17	19
Writing set phrase	13	24	46	44	39	40
Finger movements:						
Right	11	15	26	21	18	20
Left	11	16	25	23	23	21
Pronation/supination						
Right	4	6	14	11	10	10
Left	4	6	15	13	12	10
TOTAL	83	130	247	219	198	203

Results of timed tests in 20 controls and in 43 parkinsonian patients on no treatment and a 100, 300, and 500 mg daily amantadine hydrochloride. (Parkes *et al.*, 1970b—reprinted with permission.)

The initial improvement was fully maintained in 10 of 19 patients who showed initial benefit. Two patients improved initially, but had some failure of response after a few weeks, and 6 patients showed a gradual deterioration in their score after 6–9 months of amantadine treatment. One patient died of heart failure 2 months after commencing amantadine.

Schwab *et al.* (1972) described 430 patients with Parkinson's disease who were treated with amantadine 200 mg daily, in a few cases for up to a 30-month period. Of 351 of these, 64 per cent showed a favourable response to amantadine but then in half of the patients there was some decline in therapeutic efficacy from between 30–60 days of starting treatment. In contrast, Nagaswami and Ranjini (1971) found no evidence of response failure to amantadine in patients with Parkinson's disease, although in patients with post-encephalitic parkinsonism amantadine improvement was short-lived. Streifler and Kallay (1972) found no marked difference between the degree of short-term and the degree of long-term benefit.

In patients studied by Appleton *et al.* (1971) the maximum rate of improvement in all aspects of parkinsonism occurred in the first 4 weeks of amantadine treatment. Thereafter, despite considerable individual fluctuations, considerable improvement persisted with no secondary failure of initial response for up to 11 months. These results are similar to those of Sigwald and Raymondeaud (1972) who found that amantadine caused a good degree of improvement in half of 58 patients and after several months of follow-up this initial effect did not lessen. However, levodopa was also given to these patients.

Castaigne *et al.* (1972) described the effects of amantadine in 50 patients seen at the Neurological Clinic of the Salpetrière. Not all these patients had idiopathic Parkinson's disease, but the results of amantadine treatment were considered to be good or very good in more than half. The initial effect was not always maintained for after an excellent initial response, this diminished in the first 4–12 days in 24 patients. A more delayed reduction of effect was found in 5 patients, after 2, 3, 4, 7, and 10 months of treatment respectively. In no case was this reduction of activity reversible by higher amantadine dosage. In contrast, there were 5 patients in whom the therapeutic action of amantadine was absent or weak initially, but then became apparent in one patient after 30 days, and in others after 3 months of treatment.

The secondary partial failure of response to amantadine after a few weeks' treatment was unexplained by Schwab *et al.* (1972). It was considered unlikely to be due to the natural progression of parkinsonism, which would not have been apparent over such a short period. Eventual partial depletion of transmitter in catecholamine neurones may occur in some patients, and if this is correct the effect of amantadine may be restored by levodopa. In patients with Parkinson's disease treated with levodopa there is also an apparent failure in response, although only after several years and not weeks of treatment (Hunter *et al.*, 1973). After 24 months of levodopa treatment a loss of benefit was detected, and after 36 months only 40 per cent of patients had maintained their initial improvement whilst the remainder had seriously deteriorated.

6.4 COMBINED AMANTADINE AND LEVODOPA THERAPY

The effect of the combination of amantadine with levodopa has been studied by many authors (Hunter *et al.*, 1970b; Sacks *et al.*, 1971; Critchley, 1972; Pollock and Jorgensen, 1972; Walker *et al.*, 1972b). The results of some of these trials are conflicting and the period for establishment of optimum levodopa therapy has been too short in many cases. Optimum levodopa dosage is dependent upon the side effects as well as the therapeutic effect of this drug.

In patients taking sub-optimal dosages of levodopa, there may be considerable additional clinical effects when amantadine is added as found by Völler (1970) in 90 patients treated for 6 weeks with amantadine hydrochloride in whom the therapeutic effect was increased when levodopa was added. Fieschi *et al.* (1970b) found that 11 of 20 patients preferred a combination of amantadine and levodopa to separate treatment; as in Völler's study, levodopa dosage was sub-optimal. Gomirato and Perfetti (1970) showed that the addition of amantadine to sub-optimal levodopa therapy resulted in some further clinical improvement in 7 patients, although there was no change in 3 others.

In patients on optimum levodopa therapy, the addition of amantadine may have very slight additional therapeutic effect, although Barbeau *et al.* (1971) were unable to demonstrate any useful synergistic effect of the two drugs, and Hunter *et al.* (1970b) and Godwin-Austen *et al.* (1970) found that when amantadine was given to patients taking optimum levodopa therapy there was no additional benefit. In patients studied by Scotti (1970a; 1970b) the optimal levodopa dosage was determined after several months of treatment by reducing the daily dosage by 1 g for one month. The latter addition of amantadine resulted in further clinical improvement in only 2 of these patients.

Walker *et al.* (1972b) studied patients who were taking a stable maximum tolerated dose of levodopa (mean dosage 3·58 g daily) and had been on this for at least 6 months before addition of amantadine 100 mg twice daily. A large battery of tests was used for evaluation and a combination of levodopa and amantadine was shown to be better than levodopa alone in respect of total functional disability scores, tremor of the arms and legs, gait, and a variety of activities of daily living. Fehling (1973) studied the effect of adding amantadine to optimum levodopa dosages in a controlled trial. Optimum levodopa dosage was determined by the side effects as well as the therapeutic effect in individual patients, and could not be expressed in terms of mg kg^{-1} body weight for all patients. Amantadine had a synergistic effect with levodopa under these conditions, at least during 4 weeks of observation. This synergistic effect was more pronounced in patients on low levodopa dosage than in patients on high dosage. The acute withdrawal of amantadine in patients on optimum levodopa therapy in some cases caused a temporary increase of the parkinsonian symptoms. The improvement when adding amantadine was only marginal in most patients, and there was no dramatic response, but several patients described subjective improvement. Side effects from adding amantadine to levodopa were minimal.

6.5 COMPARISON OF THE CLINICAL EFFECTS OF AMANTADINE, LEVODOPA, AND ANTICHOLINERGIC DRUGS

Anticholinergic drugs cause a slight improvement in rigidity in some patients with Parkinson's disease. There is little effect on bradykinesia (Duvoisin, 1967). Levodopa improves all the symptoms of parkinsonism with very substantial improvement in many patients. Amantadine improves the major symptoms of parkinsonism although to a much lesser extent than levodopa, although in most patients who respond to amantadine the degree of reduction in functional disability is greater than that with anticholinergic drugs. The reasons for individual patients' response to different antiparkinsonian drugs are not known.

Dallos *et al.* (1972) compared one month's treatment with levodopa 4 g daily, with one month of amantadine 400 mg daily, in two separate patient groups. In 34 patients with levodopa and 21 with amantadine, there was a 33 per cent improvement in tremor, rigidity, and akinesia on levodopa, as compared with 23 per cent on amantadine. Considerable further improvement with levodopa would be expected after one month of treatment, but no further improvement with amantadine. Of 30 patients treated with amantadine, 200 mg daily for two weeks and levodopa 3 g daily for a further 2 weeks, 19 patients responded to both drugs, 3 to amantadine alone, and 8 patients had no response to either (Parkes *et al.*, 1971c). Other patients would be expected to respond to levodopa in the long term. Barbeau *et al.* (1971) described patients who did not respond to amantadine but who did well on levodopa. Despite these exceptions, most patients respond to both amantadine and levodopa, or to neither; Pollock and Jorgensen (1972) found a highly significant correlation between the response to amantadine and the later response to levodopa.

Cox *et al.* (1973) studied the effect of drug order when amantadine

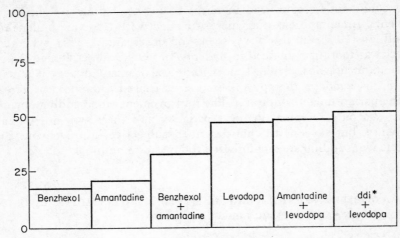

FIG. 2. Reduction of total disability by antiparkinsonian drugs. Diagrammatic representation showing percentage reduction in initial disability in different patient groups attending the Parkinson's disease clinic, King's College Hospital, from 1969–1973. Pretreatment disability mild to moderate in amantadine- and benzhexol-treated groups, and moderate to severe in others.
* ddi, Dopa decarboxylase inhibitor, "L-α-methyldopahydrazine," MK 486.

was given before, and after, levodopa treatment. Each was given for 6 weeks, and 6 weeks were allowed to elapse between the two treatment periods. Improvement occurred in patients given levodopa first, whereas no clinical effect was noted in patients treated first with amantadine. Levodopa was less effective in patients first given amantadine than in those given levodopa as the first drug. In contrast, amantadine was more effective in patients who had previously taken levodopa than in those who had not. The degree of disability in the two patient groups was comparable.

The separate effects of benzhexol 8 mg daily, amantadine 200 mg daily, and levodopa 750 mg to 3 g daily in the same patients were determined by Parkes et al. (1974). Patients were selected on account of the minor degree of their disability. Benzhexol and amantadine were given for 4 weeks, and levodopa for 6 months. Metaclopromide 30 mg daily was given to all patients taking levodopa to minimize nausea. The mean reduction in total disability score was 15 per cent from benzhexol and amantadine, and from levodopa 36 per cent. Benzhexol slightly lessened the rigidity and improved the flexion of posture of patients with Parkinson's disease, but had little effect on tremor or akinesia. Levodopa

TABLE 5

Comparative actions of antiparkinsonian drugs on total disability scores

	Amantadine 200 mg daily	Benzhexol 8 mg daily	Amantadine 200 mg and benzhexol 8 mg daily	Levodopa Mean 2·7 g daily
Initial score	31	31	31	31
Post-treatment score	27	27	19	20
Mean (%) improvement	15	15	40	36

Results of single drug treatment in 14 mildly disabled patients with parkinsonism. Treatment period: amantadine 4 weeks, benzhexol 4 weeks, and levodopa 6 months. (Data from Parkes *et al.*, 1974.)

and to a lesser extent amantadine caused improvement in all these symptoms. All but one of the patients who responded to amantadine responded to levodopa. There was no correlation between reduction in disability due to benzhexol and that due to amantadine.

6.6 EFFECTS OF AMANTADINE ON HOMOVANILLIC AND 5-HYDROXYINDOLE- ACETIC ACIDS

Roffler-Tarlov *et al.* (1971) found that amantadine had no effect on the HVA and 3,4-dihydroxyphenylacetic acid (dopac) concentrations in the mouse striatum. Pletscher *et al.* (1970) did, however, find a very minor increase in HVA levels following amantadine (25 mg kg^{-1}) in the brain of the rat and in the caudate nucleus of the rabbit, although Rinne *et al.* (1972) found that amantadine treatment for 9 days did not significantly alter the content of HVA in the rat brain.

In patients with Parkinson's disease treated with amantadine there is little or no change in the CSF concentration of HVA. The mean concentration of HVA in the CSF of 13 patients with Parkinson's disease was significantly less than that of 11 non-parkinsonian controls. The mean 5-HIAA concentration did not differ significantly between patients and controls (Parkes *et al.*, 1971a). (For non-parkinsonians: HVA 39 ± 13 ng ml^{-1}; 5-HIAA 23 ± 9 ng ml^{-1}. Parkinson's disease: HVA 12 ± 9 ng ml^{-1}; 5-HIAA 17 ± 12 ng ml^{-1}.) Amantadine 200 mg daily did not alter these values (post-amantadine HVA 12 ± 10 ng ml^{-1}; 5-HIAA 16 ± 12 ng ml^{-1}). Before amantadine treatment there was no significant relationship between the concentration of HVA and 5-HIAA, and total disability, akinesia, tremor, posture or rigidity scores. However, the patients who did well on amantadine with considerable reduction in total disability scores had a very low initial CSF HVA concentration and vice versa. Mawdsley *et al.* (1972) likewise found that the subnormal level of HVA in the CSF of 20 patients with Parkinson's disease (mean 21 ± 10 ng ml^{-1}) was not altered by amantadine treatment (post-amantadine 25 ± 11 ng ml^{-1}). The concentration of 5-HIAA within the CSF was normal both before and after amantadine treatment (16 ± 9 and 13 ± 7 ng ml^{-1} respectively). Rinne *et al.* (1972) also showed that amantadine treatment in 13 patients did not cause any significant change in the mean concentration of CSF HVA and in these patients there was no clear relationship between the concentration of HVA and clinical improvement. Amantadine did not cause any significant change in the concentrations of DA, HVA, or NA in the brain of a patient on amantadine therapy, given a last amantadine dose of 100 mg 7 hours prior to death. The DA concentration (μg g^{-1}) of the caudate nucleus of this amantadine-treated patient was 0·23 (control parkinsonian patient on no treatment 0·24) and of the substantia nigra 0·14 (controls 0·09).

Cox *et al.* (1973) found that amantadine hydrochloride had no effect on the CSF HVA concentration. When amantadine was given before a period of levodopa treatment, however, the expected rise in CSF HVA concentrations due to levodopa treatment did not occur. This was unexplained.

The CSF HVA concentration is, to some extent, an index of DA turnover in the brain, although at least following levodopa treatment, HVA also derives from metabolic activity in cerebral blood vessel walls (Goodwin *et al.*, 1970). The constant HVA concentration following amantadine indicates that this drug does not cause marked changes in cerebral DA turnover.

6.7   EFFECTS OF AMANTADINE IN DRUG-INDUCED DYSKINESIAS

Phenothiazines produce extrapyramidal symptoms in up to 40 per cent of patients who receive them. The frequency with which individual drugs cause movement disorders varies widely, and individual patient tolerance is very different (Ayd, 1961; Mindham *et al.*, 1972). Anticholinergic drugs are often given with long-term phenothiazine treatment, but the evidence that these or other antiparkinsonian drugs protect against phenothiazine-induced dyskinesia is conflicting. Mindham *et al.* (1972) found that orphenadrine was no more effective than placebo in treating fluphenazine-induced extrapyramidal disorders. In contrast, benzhexol may improve drug-induced dyskinesias (Dom *et al.*, 1971; Grove and Crammer, 1972). Levodopa has little or no effect on most drug-induced extrapyramidal reactions (Yaryura-Tobias *et al.*, 1970). The effect of amantadine is not established.

Kelly and Abazzahab (1971) found that rigidity, tremor, dystonia, and akathisia caused by haloperidol and phenothiazines was reduced in certain patients by amantadine 100–200 mg daily. Improvement in these symptoms was rapid, and the effect of akathisia was particularly marked. The degree of psychosis of these patients was not altered. Vale and Espejel (1971) found that patients with some features of tardive dyskinesia responded when given amantadine. Decker *et al.* (1971) reported that amantadine abolished involuntary movements of the face and lips in 6 chronic schizophrenics who had been given large amounts of antipsychotic drugs (not specified) for many years. These patients had intermittent rhythmic protrusion of the tongue, retrocolic dystonia, choreoathetoid movements of the toes, feet, fingers, and thumb, as well as antero-postero-rocking movements of the trunk. These movements ceased or were reduced within 4 days of commencing amantadine 300 mg daily and returned when this was stopped. However, further studies of these and other patients, including a controlled trial by Janowsky *et al.* (1972) led to the conclusion that amantadine did not improve any of the symptoms of tardive dyskinesia.

Nagaswami and Ranjini (1971) described 7 patients with a drug-induced extrapyramidal disorder who apparently responded to amantadine. Twenty psychotic patients with drug-induced parkinsonism as the result of butyrophenones or phenothiazines were given amantadine 400–600 mg daily by Rüther *et al.* (1973). Eleven patients showed a lessening of axial and limb rigidity and bradykinesia, and walking and speech were improved. The degree of symptomatic improvement was slight to moderate and amantadine had no effect on tremor.

Merrick and Schmitt (1973) studied 37 patients with phenothiazine-induced extrapyramidal syndrome who were given amantadine 100 mg twice daily for 3 weeks or benztropine mesylate 2 mg twice daily for 3 weeks followed by placebo and then the alternative active preparation. Most of these patients had schizophrenia and their psychotropic medication was continually unchanged. There was some improvement in rigidity, tremor, akathisia, dystonia, masking of facial expression, and rigidity of gait on amantadine and benztropine. Amantadine was a little more active in respect of facial expression and walking, although a lack of expression and parkinsonian gait occurred in only 50 per cent of these patients. Amantadine gave symptomatic relief of extrapyramidal symptoms within 4 hours of oral dosage. In addition to drug-induced parkinsonism, 6 patients had an oculogyric crisis. This improved within an hour of an oral dose of amantadine 100 mg; however, oculogyric crises may spontaneously resolve within this period with no treatment. Side effects of amantadine were few and a dry mouth occurred in only 1 patient, and a visual disturbance in 2, in contrast to the benztropine group in whom a dry mouth occurred in all and a visual disturbance in 15. Eleven patients in this study were given both amantadine and benztropine. There was no significant difference between the two medications in the same patient. Both drugs caused reversal of extrapyramidal symptoms, but amantadine was a little more active in speed of action and in the relief of rigidity.

In contrast to these findings, Mindham *et al.* (1972) found that amantadine was no more effective than placebo in the treatment of fluphenazine-induced dyskinesia and neither benzhexol 2–10 mg daily or amantadine 200 mg daily reversed the severe and persistent oral dyskinesias in 22 patients studied by Dynes (1970). These patients had long-standing parenchymal or vascular disease of the brain or schizophrenia, and the dyskinesia had been attributed to phenothiazine treatment which had been discontinued in 10 patients at least 6 months before study. No patient had more than a mild degree of tremor, rigidity or akinesia.

These results show a great disparity. Amantadine is probably of slight value in certain patients with drug-induced extrapyramidal disorders, but further studies are needed to identify which patients respond, and why.

6.8 OTHER EXTRAPYRAMIDAL DISORDERS

6.8.1 *Huntington's chorea, choreoathetosis and hemibalismus*

Scotti (1970c) described two patients with Huntington's chorea which was not improved by amantadine 200 mg daily. Five patients with Huntington's chorea, hemibalismus or athetosis treated by Parkes *et al.* (1971b) had no change in these involuntary movements when given amantadine 300 mg daily. In contrast, levodopa may have a slight effect in certain patients with chorea, and Barbeau (1969) showed that levodopa improved the akinesia and rigidity of juvenile patients with Huntington's chorea.

6.8.2 *Spasmodic torticollis*

Patients with spasmodic torticollis studied by Bigwood (1972), treated with amantadine for 7–10 days showed no change in the severity of neck movement. Gilbert (1971) found that a combination of haloperidol and amantadine in individual patients with spasmodic torticollis resulted in a cessation of involuntary movements. However, in contrast, a single patient with spasmodic torticollis showed an exacerbation of this when given amantadine 300 mg daily (Parkes *et al.*, 1971b).

6.8.3 *Progressive supranuclear palsy*

Scotti (1970c) treated a single patient with progressive supranuclear palsy with amantadine with no effect. Critchley (1972) also described a patient with this disorder, who had a slight improvement with levodopa but no additional benefit when amantadine was added. Two patients with progressive supranuclear palsy who were akinetic and rigid showed a very slight improvement in these features, together with some increase in the range of voluntary lateral, but not vertical, conjugate eye movements when given amantadine 300 mg daily (Parkes *et al.*, 1971b). There was no change in mental function. Treatment of patients with progressive supranuclear palsy with amantadine has little or no therapeutic value, and the effect of levodopa is almost certainly more marked (Mendell *et al.*, 1970).

6.8.4 *Oculogyric crises*

The effect of both amantadine and levodopa on oculogyric crises in patients with post-encephalitic parkinsonism is variable. Levodopa treatment provoked oculogyric crises in the first patient described by Cotzias *et al.* (1969), and also caused oculogyric crises for the first time in a patient with Wilson's disease (Barbeau and Friesen, 1970). Amantadine may increase the frequency of oculogyric crises in patients with post-encephalitic parkinsonism (Parkes *et al.*, 1971b), but in other patients with dystonia and oculogyric crises as a result of phenothiazines, amantadine may control oculogyric spasms (Merrick and Schmitt, 1973).

7 Side effects of amantadine treatment

The incidence of unwanted drug effect with amantadine is low (Rao and Pearce, 1971; Hacohen and Gurtner, 1972). CNS stimulant effects which are produced by high dosages in animals rarely occur with therapeutic dosages in man. Hallucinations and confusion occur in some patients, although these psychiatric disturbances are, in most cases, the result of combined treatment with anticholinergic drugs and amantadine. A patient reported by Schwab *et al.* (1969) had an epileptic seizure whilst taking 800 mg daily, and Critchley (1972) also described a patient with epilepsy during amantadine treatment. Dry mouth and urinary retention

TABLE 6

Side effects recorded during amantadine therapy in patients with parkinsonism

Author	Disease aetiology (Number of patients)	Mental disturbance Confusion	Hallucinations	Motor excitement	Livedo	Oedema	Miscellaneous
1. Appleton et al. (1971)	13 PD; 2 PEP (19)	—	3	—	—	1	Few and transient
2. Campbell and Williams (1972)	24 PD; 2 PEP (13)	—	1				Constipation Nausea (5)
3. Castaigne et al. (1972)	45 PD; 4 PEP (50)	Hypomanic behaviour 1	2	2		19	Insomnia (15) Restlessness (2)
4. Labauge et al. (1972)	2 PEP (50)	1	1	—	3	8	No orthostatic hypotension
5. Nagaswami and Ranjini (1971)	Various aetiology (38)	9	1	Many patients	Not described		Anorexia, Dizziness
6. Parkes et al. (1971)	26 PD (26)	Not recorded	Not recorded	—	23	15	Insignificant
7. Rao and Pearce (1971)	15 PD; 5 PEP (20)	Nil	Nil				Myalgia (1) Shivering (1) Giddiness (1) Rash (1)
8. Schwab et al. (1972)	(430)	19	—	Increased tremor	8	3	54 patients had one side effect and 31 two or more
9. Sigwald et al. (1972)	(58)	Not reported					Orthostatic hypotension frequent (L-dopa additionally)
10. Streifler and Kallay (1972)	32 ASP 8 PD 9 PEP (49)	Paranoid symptoms 1		Restlessness Excitement	2	Not described	Insomnia (2) Vertigo (1) Stomach ache (1)

PD, idiopathic Parkinson's disease; PEP, post-encephalitic parkinsonism; ASP, arteriosclerotic parkinsonism.

TABLE 7

Side effects accompanying amantadine dosages

Side effect	Amantadine dosage (mg d^{-1})		
	100	300	500
Nausea	5	3	3
Vomiting	2	1	0
Diarrhoea	2	0	0
Stomach ache	4	1	1
Giddiness	7	6	6
Headache	6	1	4
Confusion	7	5	11
Nightmares	5	7	9
Difficulty falling asleep	5	4	9
Early waking	5	7	7
Dry mouth	6	10	11
Palpitations	9	1	3
Focusing difficulty	0	3	7
Jitteryness	4	4	4
Hallucinations	0	3	6
No side effects	26	23	21

Side effects in 43 patients with Parkinson's disease on amantadine 100, 300, and 500 mg daily. (Parkes *et al.*, 1970b—reprinted with permission.)

which are sometimes caused by anticholinergic drugs are not produced by amantadine. Nausea, vomiting, and involuntary movements which may result from levodopa are not caused by amantadine. Addiction and tolerance to amantadine has not been reported. Amantadine does, however, cause the unique side effect of livedo reticularis of the skin, with leg oedema in some patients.

7.1 HALLUCINATIONS AND CONFUSION

All drugs which are used to treat parkinsonism occasionally cause hallucinations and mental confusion (Yahr and Duvoisin, 1968; Schwarz and Fahn, 1970). In the case of amantadine, disordered awareness and hallucinations are very uncommon when the drug is given by itself, although more frequent in patients on combined treatment with anticholinergic drugs. Amantadine-induced mental confusion is more common in patients with akinetic rigid syndromes accompanying senile dementia or cerebral arteriosclerosis than in patients with idiopathic Parkinson's disease, and some of the former patients may be hallucinated before any drug treatment.

Schwab *et al.* (1969) reported hallucinations in a few of 163 patients given amantadine, who previously may have been close to the limits of tolerance of anticholinergics. Parkes *et al.* (1970a) reported confusion and nightmares in 2 of 35 patients given amantadine 200 mg daily, whereas 7 of these patients had similar effects whilst on placebo. Mental confusion becomes increasingly common with higher amantadine dosage. With 100 mg daily, none of 26 patients were hallucinated, but 3 patients given 300 mg daily and 6 given 500 mg daily were (Parkes *et al.*, 1970b). In a group of patients studied by Dallos *et al.* (1970) the summation of amantadine 200 mg daily with benzhexol or orphenadrine caused visual hallucinations in a few patients. Of 30 patients with Parkinson's disease described by Voller (1970), treated also with anticholinergic drugs, only one developed hallucinations with amantadine. Two patients described by Martin (1970) developed visual hallucinations on a combination of anticholinergic drugs with amantadine. These ceased on amantadine withdrawal. Sigwald *et al.* (1970) found nocturnal confusion in 6 of 57 patients treated with amantadine.

In elderly patients treated with amantadine for prophylaxis against influenza A_2, the drug rarely causes hallucinations when given for a short period in 200 mg daily dosage (Leeming, 1969). In contrast, when amantadine is given to elderly patients with akinetic rigid syndromes accompanying diffuse vascular and parenchymal brain disease, hallucinations are more common. Such a patient described by Herson (1970) developed considerable mental deterioration when given amantadine 200 mg daily.

Coloured Lilliputian hallucinations in parkinsonian patients on amantadine therapy were described by Harper and Knothe (1973). The first patient was a woman of 66 with an apallidal syndrome as the result of coal-gas poisoning. Four days after commencing amantadine 200 mg daily she developed startling visual hallucinations including an apparition of a clothes-line with babies' clothes pegged thereon. She was not disorientated in time or space, and her symptoms subsided within 48 hours of amantadine withdrawal. The second patient had cerebrovascular disease and also developed Lilliputian hallucinations seeing tiny red people walking up a hand held in front of her. The third patient, with Parkinson's disease, saw little green men. All these patients were also taking anticholinergic drugs.

7.2   CNS STIMULATION

7.2.1   *Parkinson's disease*

Restlessness, nervousness, and irritability occurred together with other side effects in 22 per cent of patients given amantadine by Schwab *et al.*

(1969). These stimulant properties may account for the increase rather than decrease in tremor reported in some patients. Sigwald *et al.* (1970) found that amantadine caused nervous tension with increased tremor in 4 of 57 patients, and also insomnia in 4 patients. Several drugs with CNS stimulant properties including amphetamines, ephedrine, and methylphenidate, like amantadine, will increase the efflux of catecholamines into CSF perfusates (Carr and Moore, 1970), and the weak central stimulant effect of amantadine, with insomnia in a few patients, may be due to the effect of this drug on catecholamine metabolism.

7.2.2 Antidepressant action of amantadine

Because of one theory of biogenic amine disturbance in the affective disorders (Schildkraut and Ketty, 1967), Vale and his colleagues (1971) studied the antidepressant activity of amantadine in 40 depressed patients. Amantadine 100–200 mg daily was given for 4 weeks and resulted in a modest improvement in depression as compared to placebo. Comparing the mean scores for improvement with other antidepressants, amantadine was less effective than amitriptyline.

7.2.3 Alerting effects of amantadine

In elderly subjects with cerebral atherosclerosis or parkinsonism amantadine has an alerting effect (Vitetta, 1971). Domenichini *et al.* (1972) studied the awakening effect of amantadine after ketamine anaesthesia. This phencyclidine-related drug, used as an intravenous anaesthetic, leads to disagreeable dreams, and wakening may be prolonged. Amantadine 300 mg i.v. at the end of operation has a considerable alerting effect, as shown by the patient's ability to read and write. This action of amantadine has not yet been further evaluated. Ersmarck and Lidvall (1973) gave amantadine 200 mg daily to patients suffering from narcolepsy. All these had earlier received amphetamines with symptomatic relief but amantadine was no more effective than placebo and did not reduce the frequency of narcoleptic attacks. The alerting effect of levodopa in hepatic coma (Parkes *et al.*, 1970c) with a transient increase in conscious level and an increase in dominant EEG frequency, has not been reported with amantadine.

7.3 INVOLUNTARY MOVEMENTS

The patient described by Fahn *et al.* (1971) had chorea resulting from levodopa, but after amantadine 2·8 g, involuntary movements did not occur although his previous rigidity and tremor were abolished. Amantadine, unlike levodopa, does not cause involuntary movements and patients given combined treatment with anticholinergic drugs do not develop athetosis, chorea, or abnormal postures. The addition of amantadine does not affect the severity of involuntary movements resulting from levodopa treatment (Godwin-Austen *et al.*, 1970). However, Weiss *et al.* (1971) reported an unusual patient with dyskinesia induced by levodopa that persisted after withdrawal, and was then exacerbated by amantadine 200 mg per day. There is one case report of involuntary movements, similar to those produced by levodopa, resulting from amantadine treatment; Pearce (1971) described a woman of 68 who developed gross linguo-facial dyskinesia with amantadine 200 mg daily, which produced a considerable improvement in the signs of parkinsonism. Abnormal tic-like movements of the hand, shoulder, and arm occurred in a patient on amantadine described by Martín (1970), but this patient may also have been taking phenothiazines and the involuntary movements persisted despite amantadine withdrawal.

7.4   LIVEDO RETICULARIS

Shealy *et al.* (1970) first described livedo reticularis in parkinsonian patients treated with amantadine. This skin disorder results in a marbled fishnet-like appearance, and though first described in 1895, it had not been previously attributed to drug usage. Williams and Goodman (1925) classified livedo into three groups.

1. *Cutis marmorata*, a transient mottled appearance due to cold, appearing in many normal people and disappearing with warming, due to a physiological response of vasomotor constriction of the small arterioles.
2. *Idiopathic livedo reticularis* is a more permanent skin discolouration.
3. *Livedo reticularis symptomatica* characterized by persistent mottling with evidence of other diseases involving the peripheral vascular system.

Diseases associated with this last variety of livedo were described by Champion (1965) and include collagen disorders, arterial embolization, thrombocytopoenia, and cryoglobulinaemia.

Ten of 34 patients described by Silver and Sahs (1972) developed livedo during amantadine treatment. The first appearance of livedo was 1–14 months after the start of therapy. Both sexes were affected. Nine had skin changes in the legs, and all patients had livedo in the arms. Livedo was mainly distal and more severe when the limbs were exposed to cold; it disappeared with the limb elevated. Four patients developed ankle oedema either 1–2 months before, or simultaneously with the development of livedo. Once established, there was no apparent increase in the severity of livedo with continued treatment.

Urinary analysis, haemoglobin, haematocrit, and erythrocyte count, leucocyte count, and differential ESR, platelet count, liver function tests, rheumatoid factor, protein electrophoresis, antinuclear antibodies, cryoglobulins, and cryofibrinogens and skin biopsies were all normal apart from increased levels of serum cryofibrinogens in 3 patients.

Vollum *et al.* (1971) found that livedo was present in 60 per cent of the normal population over the age of 50, although only to a minor extent. After 6–8 weeks' amantadine treatment 90 per cent of patients with Parkinson's disease showed either an exaggeration of livedo or an increase in its extent, or developed it for the first time. There were no signs of hepato-splenomegaly or lymphadenopathy to suggest a generalized disorder and blood pressure was within the normal range. Skin biopsies done in 6 patients were normal in 5 although one had a small venule partially occluded by organizing thrombus with an associated inflammatory cell infiltrate, mainly lymphocytic, with no other evidence of vasculitis. Extensive investigations to exclude an underlying systemic disorder or a lupus erythematous-like syndrome were all negative. Adrenaline or NA injection into the skin in 6 amantadine-treated patients caused vasoconstriction with a loss of the livedo pattern and pallor. Intradermal injection of isoprenaline caused an accentuation of the vascular pattern. The normal adrenergic responses indicated that amantadine did not cause alpha-receptor blockade of the dermal vessels, although dose-response curves in many patients would be necessary to confirm this.

Livedo reticularis does not persist after amantadine withdrawal, and in view of the normal haematological and other findings, it is probable that livedo is a physiological and not pathological response to amantadine. Local catecholamine release due to amantadine might cause vasoconstriction of certain arterioles of the skin in such a manner that livedo reticularis is produced (Silver and Sahs, 1972). However, Labauge *et al.* (1972) reporting livedo in 3, and oedema in 8, of 50 parkinsonian patients treated with amantadine, considered that livedo was an allergic phenomena in view of urticaria in one patient.

7.5 OEDEMA

Sigwald *et al.* (1970) described leg oedema first appearing after 6 weeks of amantadine treatment. Oedema persisted throughout the day with little or no morning regression, and slight oedema might also occur in the hands. Oedema is frequently accompanied by livedo and both persist during amantadine treatment if dosage is unchanged, although both regress over 4–8 weeks when amantadine is withdrawn. The severity of oedema is not related to the presence or severity of livedo (Vollum *et al.*, 1971). Up to 10 per cent of patients treated with amantadine (200–500 mg daily) develop oedema. There are no signs of cardiac, liver, or kidney disease in patients with oedema. In other forms of physiological or pathological livedo, oedema does not occur.

Parkes *et al.* (1971a) investigated total body water exchangeable sodium and potassium content in patients with Parkinson's disease before and during amantadine treatment. Total body water, extracellular fluid, and total exchangeable sodium content were similar in 19 patients with parkinsonism who had not been given amantadine, and in 11 immobile age and sex matched controls who did not have Parkinson's disease. Amantadine 300 mg daily did not alter these values. The 24-hour exchangeable potassium was slightly lower in the 19 non-amantadine treated patients than controls. After 3 weeks' amantadine there was a slight rise in total body potassium, so that potassium content was similar in patients and controls. The development of oedema in 6 patients on amantadine was not accompanied by a rise in total body water or change in electrolytes. Oedema may result from a peripheral fluid shift due to increase in vascular permeability in skin but not muscle blood vessels.

7.6 MISCELLANEOUS EFFECTS

7.6.1 *Plasma growth hormone*

The effect of levodopa on the dopaminergic tubero-hypophysial system has been held responsible for the vaginal bleeding in some post-menopausal women on this drug, because functionally these neurones are concerned with the regulation of gonadotrophin secretion (Fuxe *et al.*, 1969). In the growth hormone releasing system dopaminergic neurones are probably involved and a single oral levodopa dose can cause a considerable rise in plasma levels of growth hormone (Boden *et al.*, 1972). Kytömäki *et al.* (1973) studied how amantadine and levodopa stimulated growth hormone secretion. A considerable rise in plasma growth hormone concentration (four-fold to ten-fold) was found after levodopa i.v. in patients with Parkinson's disease and other neurological disorders. The concentration of plasma growth hormone was highest 45 minutes after the injection. The oral dose of 1 g of levodopa also caused a significant increase in plasma growth hormone, although this was less than that following injection of levodopa 1·5 mg kg^{-1} i.v. In contrast, however, oral dosage of 0·5 g of levodopa or 100 mg of amantadine has no effect. Plasma insulin levels were nearly unchanged after amantadine and levodopa, and blood sugar levels were also unchanged. The effect of higher amantadine dosage on plasma growth hormone has not been established. The functional integrity of the dopaminergic tubero-hypophysial system in patients with Parkinson's disease is an important observation which indicates that this disease does not involve non-specifically DA-forming, but specifically melanin-forming neurones.

7.6.2 *Effect of amantadine on dopa metabolism*

Peaston *et al.* (1973) reported a metabolic study of the effects of amantadine hydrochloride on the fate of orally administered L-2-^{14}C-dopa in three subjects with Parkinson's disease. This was given before and after a 4-week period of amantadine 100 mg daily and serum and urinary distribution of radioactivity determined in catecholamine, dopa, methoxydopa, and phenol–carboxylic acid fractions. Variations in L-2-^{14}C-dopa metabolism in normal and non-amantadine treated parkinsonian subjects were not reported. In the patients studied, amantadine moderately decreased serum and urine radioactivity and markedly decreased the urinary, but not serum catecholamine fraction. There was a two-fold rise in urinary phenol carboxylic acids fraction. These findings suggested that amantadine may decrease extracerebral metabolism of levodopa and reduce the extent of its metabolism to its catecholamine metabolites.

7.6.3 *Effect of amantadine on the blink reflex*

An abnormally brisk reflex was described in extrapyramidal syndromes by Guillain *et al.* (1924) and a light tap to the glabella causes reflex closure of the eyelids in patients with parkinsonism. With repeated tapping, blinking persists rather than disappears in almost 100 per cent of patients with Parkinson's disease (Pearce *et al.*, 1968). Changes in blink reflex with levodopa and amantadine were found by Penders and Delwaide (1971) and Messina *et al.* (1972) in patients with parkinsonism. Both drugs produced some recovery of the normal habituation of the blink reflex with repeated stimuli, levodopa being more effective than amantadine. Classical anticholinergic drugs produced no change in this reflex.

8 Antiviral action of amantadine hydrochloride

8.1 INTRODUCTION

A large number of chemical compounds are active against viruses (Bauer, 1972) but very few are of value in medicine because of unacceptable toxicity, or the drug does not work in man. Most of these drugs, which are effective against a few DNA viruses only, interfere with viral DNA synthesis. In contrast, amantadine interferes with cell entry of certain strains of RNA-containing viruses. It is of proven value in prevention and treatment of only one viral disease in man, influenza A_2 (Galbraith et al., 1970).

Influenza viruses comprise three groups A, B, and C, not related antigenically, with different epidemiological characteristics. Specific immunity to influenza develops following infection but may decline within a year or two. Influenza is one of the few infectious diseases in man to cause short-term explosive mass outbreaks. There are epidemics of influenza A regularly at intervals of 2–3 years, and these may affect up to 50 per cent of the population of all age groups. During the winter of 1968–1969, 17·5 million adults were suffering from influenza in the German Federal Republic (Schwarz, 1969). Symptoms include headache, with chills, sweats, malaise and fatigue, as well as muscle aches and pains, photophobia, nasal stuffiness or discharge, and laryngeal and tracheal infection. Most patients recover in 1–2 weeks but in aged or chronically disabled subjects there is an appreciable morbidity and mortality.

8.1.1 Mechanisms of antiviral action

Hoffman et al. (1965) found that amantadine did not cause either inhibition of absorption of virus to cells or inhibition of virus release, and did not alter multiplication of intracellular virus tissue. Amantadine specifically blocked the penetration of sensitive strains of virus into the host cell in tissue culture. Once absorbed onto the cell surface the virus remained attached in an infectious form. The mode of action of amantadine is unique amongst antiviral agents. These results in tissue culture resemble those observed with specific virus antibody. However, whilst antibody reacts directly with virus, the antiviral activity of amantadine is not due to a direct action on the virus, but to an action on the host cell, although the specificity of action is virus and not host-system related.

The prevention of cellular entry to RNA viruses produced by amantadine (Jackson, et al., 1963; Davies et al., 1964; Grunert et al., 1965) may be the result of blockage of receptor areas of cell membranes where viruses normally enter (Dales and Choppin, 1962). Alternatively, amantadine may bind sensitive strains of virus to areas of the cell surface (if these exist) not susceptible to penetration (Hoffmann et al., 1965). Electron microscope studies have shown that amantadine does not interfere with attachment of virus to the cell, but prevents viral penetration (Fletcher *et al.*, 1965; Fletcher and Yusa, 1967). Electron microscope studies suggest that intact influenza particles are taken into cells by phagocytosis (Dales and Choppin, 1962). This engulfment process is prevented by ammonium chloride and various amines as well as by amantadine. The effect can be nullified by simply washing the cells and amines may interfere with the penetration process by causing ionic changes at the cell surface.

Kato and Eggers (1969) found in a fowl plague virus–chick embryo cell system, that amantadine had no direct inactivating effect on virus infectivity, and virus adsorption to cells was not inhibited. Uncoating of virus after cell entry was, however, markedly inhibited by amantadine. The virus was labelled by neutral red. This dye is incorporated into certain virions and renders them photosensitive. Loss of photosensitivity occurs shortly after the virus infects cells and can be used as an indicator of uncoating: 90 per cent of infective centres become photoresistant after 1 hour in control culture as compared to 30 per cent resistant in amantadine-treated cultures.

8.1.2 *Viral inhibition by amines*

The multiplication of various influenza virus strains, rubella virus, adenovirus, and polio virus, is inhibited by adrenaline and noradrenaline, ammonium salts, and halogenophenethylamines (Oxford and Schild, 1967). These amines all act at an early stage in the virus growth cycle. Only the halogenophenethylamines have detectable viricidal effects, especially marked for rubella virus. Ammonium acetate and amantadine are active *in vivo*, and reduce the incidence of lung lesions in mice following intranasal infection by an influenza strain; neither compound inhibits growth of a rubella strain in the rabbit lung. Adrenaline and NA have less antiviral activity for influenza viruses than other amines, with the exception of the action of NA on influenza B virus.

8.1.3 *Interferon and amantadine*

Lavrov *et al.* (1968) found that amantadine produced an inhibitory effect on reproduction of the viruses in chick embryo cells when combined with an inhibitor of nucleic acid synthesis (5-fluorouracil) useful against influenza A/WSN virus, or with an inhibitor of protein synthesis (DL-ethionine) useful against fowl plague virus. Multiplication of WSN virus in chick embryo cells was inhibited both by interferon and amantadine, and in the presence of both inhibitors, infectious virus was not detected. Interferon and amantadine influence different stages in viral development, and their synergistic effect was only observed with a low multiplicity of infection. Amantadine by slowing down or completely blocking penetration of the cells by virus particles reduces the number of infected cells in the culture, whilst interferon reduces the number of newly formed virus particles (Hallum and Younger, 1966).

8.2 SPECTRUM OF ANTIVIRAL ACTIVITY

Amantadine hydrochloride inhibits virus multiplication of influenza A, the Sendai strain of para-influenza, pseudo-rabies virus and rubella (Davies *et al.*, 1964; Neumayer *et al.*, 1965; Hoffmann *et al.*, 1965). Resistant viruses include influenza B, Newcastle disease virus, mumps, para-influenza strains 1, 2, and 3, herpes simplex virus and many others. Antiviral action is found in tissue culture and in ovo, in experimental infections of animals and in man, although the degree of antiviral activity is different in different systems. The most consistent antiviral activity is obtained whan amantadine is added before infection, although in plaque inhibition systems in tissue culture, and against certain strains of influenza in mouse infections, continuous treatment with amantadine starting some time after infection provides a significant antiviral effect.

8.2.1 *Sensitivity of different strains*

The Japan/305/57 strain of influenza shows a marked inhibition of multiplication with amantadine 1.6 μg ml^{-1} and complete absence of haemagglutinin production at 25 μg ml^{-1}, whereas the AA/2/60 strain is only slightly affected (Neumayer *et al.*, 1965). Influenza A$_2$/Hong Kong/ 50/68 virus production is completely blocked by amantadine 10 μg ml^{-1} and even at 0.4 μg ml^{-1} there is a one-log reduction in haemagglutinin titre (McGahen *et al.*, 1968). If amantadine is given before infection with WSN influenza, complete suppression of plaque formation is obtained by 0.8–1.6 μg ml^{-1} of the drug but higher dosage is necessary to reduce plaque formation when added immediately after the virus.

Schild and Sutton (1965) found that amantadine hydrochloride in tissue culture and in experimental infections in mice was ineffective against influenza A/PR8, had a minimal effect on NWS influenza A and FM$_1$, a slight effect on two Singapore influenza strains, a greater effect of A$_2$/Tokyo/1/62 and most effect on A$_2$/Scot/49/57. Tyrrell *et al.* (1965), using organ cultures of human tracheal and nasal tissues, found that destruction of cilia and viral multiplication were slightly delayed but not prevented by amantadine: the inhibition of influenza A$_2$(Pak/1/67) was much greater than that of A$_2$ Copenhagen.

The antiviral effect of amantadine is dependent upon the size of the inoculum. In one-step multiplication cycle experiments using the A_2 strain Japan/305/57, when many infectious virus particles are added for each cell present in tissue culture, the maximum effect of amantadine is a one-log drop in virus production (Davies *et al.*, 1964). Many cells become infected and produce virus despite the presence of an adequate amount of the drug.

8.2.2 *Resistance to amantadine*

Cochran *et al.* (1965) showed that influenza virus A_2/Japan/305/57 became resistant to amantadine after one passage in calf kidney cell culture in the presence of the drug. However, Grunert *et al.* (1965) using influenza A/Swine/S15 failed to demonstrate resistance to amantadine with eight serial passages through mice treated with the drug, and Hoffman *et al.* (1965) found that after 8 serial passages of influenza A/NWS in mono-layers in the presence of 25 μg ml^{-1} of amantadine resistance to amantadine did not occur. Sabin (1967) considered that a high percentage of the virus particles in the original culture may have been drug-resistant.

8.2.3 *Antiviral action against Rubella*

In animal and tissue culture studies amantadine has an effect on rubella virus comparable to that observed against some strains of influenza A_2 (Maassab and Cochran, 1964; Cusamano *et al.*, 1965). However, amantadine does not protect against naturally occurring rubella. Twenty-two of 149 amantadine-treated children and 5 of 161 placebo-treated children under 15 developed rubella during an epidemic and in older children the incidence of rubella in drug and placebo groups was similar (Tyler and Kessler, 1964).

8.3 HUMAN INFLUENZA

8.3.1 *Assessment of antiviral action*

Volunteers selected to assess the prophylactic value of amantadine must be susceptible to challenge, and since the main purpose of an anti-influenza drug is to prevent disease without necessarily preventing infection, only tests with a disease-producing strain can yield information on this point (Sabin, 1967). Patients in placebo and drug groups should be matched for antibody status prior to infection. The haemagglutination inhibiting antibody system is concerned with natural immunity although complement fixation antibody titres, directed against viral core antigens, rise during infection.

8.3.2 Experimentally induced influenza

Hornick et al. (1966) studied prison volunteers with little or no pre-existing immunity to a moderately virulent influenza strain, shown by the absence of neutralizing antibodies, given amantadine 200 mg daily. Five of the 29 drug-treated volunteers developed a febrile illness of moderate severity when challenged with Rockville 1/65 strain, as compared to severe illness in 6 and moderately severe illness in 7 of 29 placebo-treated volunteers. Using a less virulent A_2 influenza strain (Scot-59/57) which in tissue culture tests by Schild and Sutton (1965) was found to be the most highly susceptible strain to amantadine, Tyrrell et al. (1965) found no effect of amantadine in adult volunteers. When an attenuated strain of A_2 influenza virus was given to student volunteers, Jackson et al. (1963) found it difficult to evaluate the infrequent and mild respiratory manifestations. The chief effect of amantadine was a slight reduction in the number in whom antibody developed. The results of these studies are unimpressive, although with a moderately virulent strain of A_2 influenza virus there was some reduction in illness severity if not in infection rate produced by amantadine.

8.3.3 Influenza epidemics

A large study of amantadine in the prophylaxis of influenza was conducted in Leningrad during the outbreak of A_2 Hong Kong influenza in 1969, involving a double-blind placebo controlled trial among several thousand young men. The incidence of clinical disease among amantadine-treated students was half that among control students living in the same schools (Smorodintsev et al., 1970).

In a study in Michigan in 1968–1969, the mass immunization of schoolchildren against influenza was followed by a reduced incidence of this disease, not only among schoolchildren, but in the entire population, perhaps due to the fact that immunization of the children weakened the chain of transmission within the community (Monto et al., 1970). The results of the trial of amantadine in Leningrad in 1969 suggested that the large-scale use of this drug may have a similar effect as this mass immunization. Thus the incidence rate of clinical influenza among control students was 7·8 per cent as compared with 4 per cent among amantadine-treated students living in the same buildings. This rate was considerably lower than the rates among other control students studying at the same schools but living at home (21·4 per cent).

Galbraith and his colleagues (1969c) found that amantadine definitely protected the household contacts of patients with influenza, although in the following year, during the A_2/Hong Kong outbreak, no protective effect was found in a similar study; both strains were equally sensitive in laboratory tests (Galbraith et al., 1969a). In Helsinki during the Hong Kong epidemic of 1969, subjects with initially low antihaemagglutinin titres received no protection from amantadine (Oker-Blom et al., 1970) and high protection may be only afforded to subjects who already have some basic immunity.

The use of amantadine hydrochloride as a prophylactic against naturally occurring influenza may result in a reduction of duration of fever, more rapid recovery, and less frequent complications in patients who eventually develop influenza (Maté et al., 1971; Kitamoto, 1971; Galbraith et al., 1973).

8.3.4 Influenza prophylaxis in hospital in-patients

The prophylactic effect of amantadine hydrochloride in preventing hospital-acquired influenza infection was evaluated during an outbreak of influenza $A(H_3N_2)$ infection by O'Donoghue et al. (1973). All patients admitted to a hospital medical and neurology service over a 30-day period were investigated, and 50 given amantadine and 61 untreated. Fourteen patients acquired either clinical or subclinical influenza. Seven clinical and 5 subclinical infections occurred in untreated patients, while only 2 subclinical infections occurred in patients on amantadine. Amantadine prophylaxis resulted in an 80 per cent protective effect.

8.3.5 Treatment of influenza

Galbraith et al. (1971) studied the therapeutic activity of amantadine 200 mg daily during an epidemic of influenza caused by A_2/Hong Kong/68. A hundred and fifty-three patients with serologically proven influenza A_2 were studied in the family environment. Of these 72 received amantadine and 91 placebo. The mean duration of fever was significantly reduced in treated individuals compared with those receiving placebo but there was no effect on other influenzal symptoms.

8.3.6 Rimantadine and amantadine-spiro compounds

Beare et al. (1972) studied the effect of N-methyladamantane-2-spiro-3'-

pyrrolidine maleate in the protection of volunteers against challenge with A_2/Hong Kong influenza strain. The effect of this compound may have been greater than that of amantadine, although a direct comparison was not done. Another analogue of amantadine, rimantadine, has also been shown to be potentially useful in the treatment of established influenza A infections (Wingfield *et al.*, 1969; Togo *et al.*, 1970).

8.3.7 *Antibody response during amantadine treatment*

Hornick *et al.* (1966) found that amantadine given to 58 prison volunteers who had little or no pre-existing antibody to an influenza strain did not protect against infection, as shown by the development of haemagglutination-inhibition antibody, but the post-infection antibody levels with amantadine were significantly lower than those developed by subjects given placebo. In a trial by Smorodintsev *et al.* (1970), a four-fold antibody rise occurred in 25 per cent of amantadine-treated and 51 per cent of placebo-treated volunteers who all had a low antibody titre prior to inoculation with a live influenza strain. In amantadine-treated subjects with initially high serum antibody, influenza virus killed by heating still produces antibody in 14 per cent of subjects (Stanley *et al.*, 1965). Lower post-challenge antibody levels after amantadine probably result from inhibition of virus multiplication and diminution in antigenic stimulation.

In therapeutic studies on the whole, there has been no evidence of reduction of the levels of circulatory influenza antibodies in infected individuals who receive amantadine (Galbraith *et al.*, 1969a; 1969b; 1971) although in one study a reduction of the antibody response was observed in treated volunteers who were artificially infected with influenza A_2/Rockville/1/65 (Bloomfield *et al.*, 1970).

Antibody responses during amantadine treatment in animals were studied by Muldoon and Jackson (1967). Amantadine given by different routes and at several dosages had no effect on the rate or titre of antibody synthesis to 2 antigens, bovine serum albumin and an influenza A_2 strain. In contrast, 6-mercaptopurine did affect antibovine serum albumin synthesis.

Amantadine hydrochloride was evaluated by Killen *et al.* (1969) as a possible immunosuppressive drug for prolonging the survival of kidney grafts in the dog. The severity of rejection shown by histological examination of control animals and amantadine-treated ones after bilateral nephrectomy and then renal homotransplantation was not affected by amantadine, and mean survival times were unaltered.

8.4 CREUTZFELDT–JAKOB DISEASE

In this uncommon fatal illness there are signs of higher cortical dysfunction with dementia, and also a movement disorder with pyramidal and extrapyramidal features, together with myoclonus. There are also other consequences of diffuse cerebral and cerebellar pathology such as seizures, ataxia and mutism. One clinico-pathological type, sub-acute spongiform encephalopathy (SSE; Nevin *et al.*, 1960), is transmittable to primates (Gibbs *et al.*, 1968). Braham (1971) described one patient with fairly typical clinical characteristics of Creutzfeldt–Jakob disease, who showed some improvement in 9 months of amantadine treatment but eventually died. No autopsy was done. Sanders and Dunn (1973) described two patients with Creutzfeldt–Jakob disease. One made an initial improvement, lasting two months, with amantadine therapy, but eventually died. In this patient pathological changes were typical of SSE. The second patient had deteriorated for 30 months prior to amantadine therapy (an unusually long time course for the clinical diagnosis to be substantiated). However, he made an apparent recovery when given amantadine. Hamoen (1973) described a single patient who may have been suffering from Creutzfeldt–Jakob disease; he was demented and eventually became comatose, but regained full consciousness when given amantadine 200 mg daily. Dementia was not affected by this treatment. Withdrawal, and later replacement of amantadine, was accompanied by deterioration of conscious level and a further period of recovery. The final outcome in this case was not reported.

There seems little doubt that amantadine has some action in Creutzfeldt–Jakob disease, although the specificity of this has not been established. The use of amantadine is justified in an otherwise universally fatal condition, although it seems essential to start amantadine treatment as soon as a clinical diagnosis can be made before permanent brain damage has occurred (Sanders and Dunn, 1973). However, a patient with typical neurological and EEG changes of SSE treated with amantadine 200 mg daily by Herishanu (1973) showed no improvement and the EEG was not altered.

In Creutzfeldt–Jakob disease there is often considerable wasting of muscles, and this fact led Norris (1972) to use amantadine to treat 18 patients with muscle wasting due to amyotrophic lateral sclerosis. In none of these was there any detectable alteration in the clinical course apart from distinct worsening of 2 patients.

Cochran (1971) studied the action of amantadine in scrapie in mice. Scrapie is a "slow virus" disease, characterized pathologically by a spongiform encephalopathy. Mice were inoculated intracerebrally with

Chandler strain mouse-adapted scrapie. This was fatal to all inoculated mice, and mean survival times were not altered when treatment with 0·05 per cent amantadine diet was started either before inoculation or 90 days after.

8.5   SUBACUTE SCLEROSING PANENCEPHALITIS

Dawson (1933) first described what is now called subacute sclerosing panencephalitis (SSPE). Intranuclear inclusion bodies are often found in the brains of affected patients and are composed of myxovirus-like particles (Shaw *et al.*, 1967). Rubeola virus antigen has been found in brain tissue (Freman *et al.*, 1967) and rubeola virus antibodies have been demonstrated in very high titres in serum and CSF (Connolly *et al.*, 1967; Sever and Zeman, 1968). An encephalitogenic agent has been transferred to ferrets from brain biopsy material (Katz *et al.*, 1968) and measles virus has been isolated from a brain biopsy (Barbosa *et al.*, 1969). Recently the disease has been transferred to dogs (Notermans *et al.*, 1973). Other possible aetiological factors were suggested by Baguley and Glasgow (1973). It is not certain why a rare disease such as SSPE is associated with such a ubiquitous infection as measles. There may be differences between the measles-like virus associated with SSPE and the wild virus (Payne and Baublis, 1971), or the immunological reaction to the measles virus may be abnormal (Dayan and Stokes, 1972).

Haslam *et al.* (1969) used amantadine to treat SSPE in 5 patients. These children, aged 5–11, had a progressive disturbance of higher mental function and a movement disorder, in most cases with myoclonus. They were given amantadine 10 mg kg^{-1} daily. Progressive deterioration occurred in all. However, the clinical course was apparently prolonged and amongst living patients at the time of the report the average length of survival was 22 months from the onset of therapy. This was in contrast to the life expectancy in most published series of one year, or less, following diagnosis. However, a chronic and relapsing course has occurred in some patients. Haslam and his colleagues considered that amantadine hydrochloride may prolong life and stabilize the disease progress, perhaps by preventing the spread of virus. However, there have been no reports of recovery of proven cases of SSPE with amantadine treatment. Further evaluation of treated patients and early institution of amantadine therapy is needed. Amantadine is not effective in human measles (Dickinson *et al.*, 1967) although it has some inhibitory *in vitro* activity against rubeola virus.

8.6 CONGENITAL RUBELLA SYNDROME

The congenital rubella syndrome is a multi-organ disturbance with evidence of chronic viral infection. There are a variety of abnormalities in the immunoglobulins of these infants, most commonly a moderate elevation of serum IgM. Infants with this syndrome have high titres of antibodies which neutralize rubella virus, and persistent viraemia as well as virus excretion from the throat may occur (Hancock *et al.*, 1968; Plotkin *et al.*, 1966).

Amantadine is inhibitory to rubella virus *in vitro* (Maassab and Cochran, 1964) but the drug may fail to protect against naturally occurring rubella and in children with the congenital rubella syndrome attempts to eradicate the virus have, on the whole, been unsuccessful (Schubert *et al.*, 1966; Plotkin *et al.*, 1966). A patient described by Hancock *et al.* (1968), however, showed clinical improvement with decrease in lymphadenopathy and hepatosplenomegaly, and improvement in liver function tests after 3 weeks of amantadine hydrochloride 4 mg kg^{-1}. When amantadine was stopped the patient became clinically worse with recurrence of respiratory and other symptoms. In contrast, amantadine treatment was unsuccessful in a Negro infant with hypogammaglobulinaemia and a congenital rubella syndrome described by Plotkin *et al.* (1966). Virus excretion was not abolished and the clinical course of the illness was not altered. However, amantadine was given for the comparatively short period of 10 days; amantadine appears to affect only the early stages of rubella virus infection of the cell (Plotkin, 1965; Oxford and Schild, 1965).

8.7 HERPES ZOSTER

Herpes zoster (shingles) virus infection of the nervous system causes an acutely painful skin lesion in dermatome distribution with accompanying skin eruption along the course of sensory nerves. Pain may precede the skin lesion by some days, and elderly patients may develop the distressing condition of post-herpetic neuralgia with persistent pain. The skin lesions are often accompanied by fever and malaise. Uncomplicated segmental shingles responds to continuously applied topical 35–40 per cent idoxuridine in dimethylsulphoxide and another thymidine analogue, trifluorothymidine is useful in the treatment of zoster involving the eye (Juel-Jensen, 1973). Amantadine may be of some slight value in herpes. Galbraith (1973) found in a double-blind placebo-controlled trial of 100 patients there was no difference in duration of pain between amantadine and placebo-treated groups, when pain disappeared during a 28-day observation period. However, pain lasted more than 28 days in a greater number of patients on placebo than on amantadine (15 as compared to 7). The mode of action of amantadine was not explained, but may not have been due to any antiviral action, since amantadine has no effect on herpes virus hominis, a similar virus to the varicella-zoster virus.

9 Effect of amantadine on the EEG

Parkinson's disease

The EEG of patients with Parkinson's disease shows no gross abnormality (England *et al.*, 1959). The EEG of demented akinetic and rigid patients with cerebral arteriosclerosis may, in contrast, show a considerable excess of slow frequencies (Nevin, 1967). In a few patients, almost

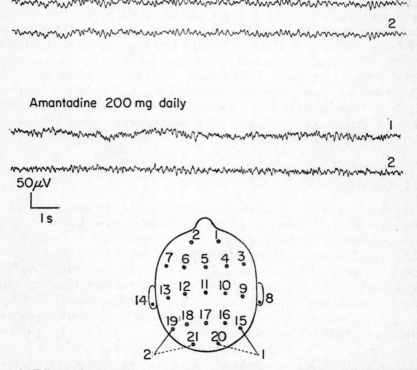

FIG. 3. Effects of amantadine on the EEG. Parieto-occipital tracing from a patient with idiopathic Parkinson's disease before and after amantadine hydrochloride (200 mg daily) treatment for 14 days.

certainly in the latter diagnostic category, amantadine has a considerable effect upon the EEG.

In patients with idiopathic Parkinson's disease treated with single drug therapy with amantadine, Mann *et al.* (1971) found this had no gross effect on the EEG, and Porterra *et al.* (1970) found no change in the visual analysis of EEG tracings in patients with parkinsonism before and after amantadine therapy. Fünfgeld (1970), however, found an abnormal

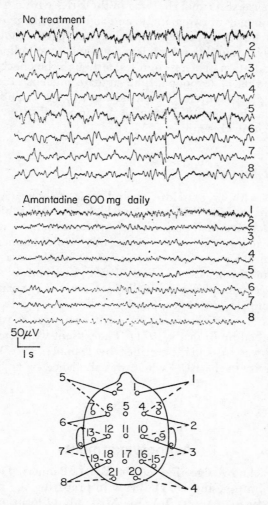

FIG. 4. Effect of amantadine on the EEG. EEG recording from a patient with Creutzfeldt–Jakob disease before and after amantadine hydrochloride (600 mg daily) for 72 hours.

EEG with excessive slow activity in 16 of 25 untreated patients with parkinsonism. Many of these patients may have had arteriosclerotic parkinsonism rather than idiopathic Parkinson's disease. After amantadine treatment the EEG returned to normal in 5 patients. One patient developed focal epileptiform potentials on a low dosage of amantadine citrate, but the patient did not have epilepsy and this EEG abnormality disappeared when amantadine dosage was reduced. Van Manen (1972) found an increase of normal rhythms in the EEG with overall increase in dominant frequency in two akinetic and rigid patients given amantadine, but there was, however, no detectable EEG change in another 8 patients. Puca *et al.* (1973) found that both levodopa and amantadine increased the number and duration of sleep spindles, although the effect of amantadine was less than that of levodopa. The caudate nucleus is involved in the mediation of sleep spindles (Buchwald *et al.*, 1961) and the action of amantadine on sleep spindles may be due to an effect on catecholamine metabolism within this area.

Creutzfeldt–Jakob disease

Most patients with Creutzfeldt–Jakob disease at some stage of the illness develop a characteristic EEG pattern which consists of diffuse slowing of background activity with periodic bisynchronous sharp wave complexes which occur at intervals of 0·5–2 seconds (Goldhammer *et al.*, 1972). There is a consistent pattern of evolution of EEG abnormality with the progression of the illness (Abbott, 1959; Lee and Blair, 1973). The interval between complexes gradually increases while normal background rhythms disappear, to be replaced by diffuse irregular slow activity. Amantadine may partially reverse the EEG changes as was the case in a patient described by Braham (1971). The patient with Creutzfeldt–Jakob disease, who was in coma, described by Hamoen (1973) had repetitive triphasic activity in the EEG which was abolished by amantadine.

Acknowledgments

I gratefully acknowledge the help of Dr A. Bennett, Dr A. Galbraith, Dr R. N. P. Sutton, and Dr D. Tarsy in preparing the manuscript, and Mrs P. Asselman, Mrs I. Jebson, Miss M. O'Rourke, and Mrs M. Spencer for secretarial assistance. Miss B. Conlin of the Medical Information Department of Geigy (UK) Limited also gave invaluable help.

References

Abbot, J. (1959). *Electroencephalogr. Clin. Neurophysiol.* **11**, 184.

Abrahams, W. C. and Solomon, H. M. (1969). *Clin. Pharmacol. Ther.* **10**, 702.

Abuzzahab, F. X. (1971). *Fed. Proc.* **30**, 381.

Aldrich, P. E., Hermann, E. C., Meier, W. E., Paulshock, M., Prichard, W. W. W., Snyder, J. A. and Watts, J. C. (1971). *J. Mednl. Pharm. Chem.* **14**, 535.

Amsler, C. (1923). *Naunyn-Schmiedeberg's Arch. Exp. Pathol. Pharmakol.* **97**, 1.

Andén, N. E., Dahlström. A., Fuxe, K. and Larsson, K. (1966). *Acta Pharmacol. Toxicol.* **24**, 263.

Andén, N. E., Corrodi, H., Fuxe, K. and Hökfelt, T. (1967). *Eur. J. Pharmacol.* **2**, 59.

Andén, N. E., Butcher, S. G., Corrodi, H., Fuxe, K. and Ungerstedt, U. (1970). *Eur. J. Pharmacol.* **11**, 303.

Appleton, D. B., Eadie, M. J. and Sutherland, J. M. (1971). *Med. J. Aust.* **58**, 707.

Ayd, F. J. Jr. (1961). *J. Amer. Med. Ass.* **175**, 1054.

Baguley, Diane and Glasgow, G. L. (1973). *Lancet*, **ii**, 763.

Bak, I. J., Hassler, R., Kim, J. S. and Kataoka, K. (1972). *J. Neurol. Transmiss.* **33**, 45.

Baldessarini, R. J. (1971). *Biochem. Pharmacol.* **20**, 1769.

Baldessarini, R. J., Lipinski, J. F. and Chace, K. V. (1972). *Biochem. Pharmacol.* **21**, 77.

Barbeau, A. (1969). *Lancet*, **ii**, 1066.

Barbeau, A. and Friesen, H. (1970). *Lancet*, **i**, 1180.

Barbeau, A., Mars, H., Botez, M. I. and Joubert, Marie (1971). *Can. Med. Ass. J.* **105**, 42.

Barbosa, L. H., Fuccillo, D. A., Sever, J. L. and Zeman, W. (1969). *Nature (Lond.)*, **221**, 974.

Bauer, D. J. (ed.) (1972). "Chemotherapy of Virus Diseases", vol. 1. Pergamon, Oxford.

Beani, L. and Bianchi, C. (1970). In "Drugs and Cholinergic Mechanisms in the CNS" (Eds E. Heilbronn A. Winter), pp. 369–386. Research Institute of National Defence, Stockholm.

Beani, L. and Bianchi, C. (1973). *Neuropharmacology*, **12**, 283.

Beani, L., Bianchi, C., Santinoceto, L. and Marchetti, P. (1968). *Int. J. Neuropharmacol.* **7**, 469.

Beare, A. S., Hall, T. S. and Tyrrell, D. A. J. (1972). *Lancet*, **i**, 1039.

Benoit, P. S. and Mambrini, J. (1970). *J. Physiol. (London)*, **210**, 681.

Biandrate, P., Tognoni, G., Belvedere, G., Frigerio, A., Rizzo, M. and Morselli, P. L. (1972). *J. Chromatogr.* **74**, 31.

Bigwood, G. F. (1972). *New Engl. J. Med.* **286**, 1161.

Blaschko, H., Richter, D. and Schlossman, H. (1937). *Biochem. J.* **31**, 2187.

Bleidner, W. E., Harmon, J. B., Hewes, W. E., Lynes, T. E. and Hermann, E. C. (1965). *J. Pharmacol. Exp. Ther.* **150**, 484.

Bloomfield, S. S., Gaffney, T. E. and Schiff, G. M. (1970). *Amer. J. Epidemiop.* **91**, 568.

Boden, G., Lundy, L. and Owen, O. (1972). *Neuroendocrinology*, **10**, 309.

Born, G. and Born, R. (1969). Blood platelets as pharmacological systems. Abstr. 4th Intern. Congr. Pharmacol. Basel, 14–18 July.

Braham, J. (1971). *Brit. Med. J.* **iv**, 212.

Brown, E. L. and Knox, E. G. (1972). *Lancet*, **i**, 974.

Bryans, J. T., Zent, W. W., Grunert, R. R. and Boughton, D. C. (1966). *Nature (London)*, **212**, 1542.

Buchwald, N. A., Wyers, E. J., Lauprecht, C. W. and Heuser, G. (1961). *Electroencephalogr. Clin. Neurophysiol.* **13**, 531.

Calne, D. (1970). *In* "Parkinsonism: Physiology, Pharmacology, and Treatment". Arnold, London.

Campbell, A. M. G. and Williams, M. J. (1972). *Brit. J. Clin. Pract.* **26**, 19.

Carlsson, A., Magnusson, T. and Rosengren, E. (1963). *Experientia*, **19**, 359.

Carlsson, A., Fuxe, K., Hamberger, B. and Lindqvist, M. (1966). *Acta Physiol. Scand.* **67**, 481.

Carlsson, A., Corrodi, H., Fuxe, K. and Hökfelt, T. (1969). *Eur. J. Pharmacol.* **5**, 367.

Carr, I. A. and Moore, K. E. (1970). *Biochem. Pharmacol.* **19**, 2671.

Castaigne, P., Laplane, D. and Dordain, G. (1972). *Nouv. Presse Med.* **1**, 533.

Champion, R. H. (1965). *Brit. J. Dermatol.* **77**, 167.

Chase, T. N., Ng., L. K. Y. and Watanabe, A. M. (1972). *Neurology*, **22**, 479.

Cochran, K. W. (1971). *Fed. Proc.* **30**, 679.

Cochran, K. W., Maasab, H. R., Tsunoda, A. and Berlin, B. S. (1965). *Ann. N.Y. Acad. Sci.* **130**, 432.

Connolly, J. H., Allen, I. V., Hurvitz, L. J. and Millar, J. H. D. (1967). *Lancet*, **i**, 542.

Corrodi, H., Fuxe, K., Ljungdahl, Å. and Ögren, S.-O. (1970). *Brain Res.* **24**, 451.

Cox, B., Danta, G., Schnieden, H. and Yuill, G. M. (1973). *J. Neurol. Neurosurg. Psychiat.* **36**, 354.

Coyle, J. T. and Snyder, S. H. (1969). *Science*, **166**, 899.

Coyle, J. T., Jacobowitz, D., Klein, D. and Axelrod, J. (1973). *J. Neurobiol.* **4**, 461.

Critchley, E. (1972). *Practitioner*, **208**, 499.

Curzon, G. (1973). *Proc. Roy. Soc. Med.* **66**, 873.

Cusamano, C. L., Sever, J. L., Schiff, G. M. and Huebner, R. J. (1965). *Clin. Res.* **13**, 41.

Dales, S. and Choppin, P. W. (1962). *Virology*, **18**, 489.

Dallos, V., Heathfield, K. and Stone, P. (1970). *Brit. Med. J.* **iv**, 24.

Dallos, V., Heathfield, K., Stone, P. and Allen, F. (1972). *Postgrad. Med. J.* **48**, 354.

Da Prada, M., Bartolini, G. and Pletscher, A. (1965). *J. Pharmacol. Exp. Ther.* **158**, 394.

Davies, J. (1971). Proceedings of the VIROFRAL (amantadine) symposium, Lidingö, pp. 19–28.

Davies, W. L., Grunert, R. R., Haff, R. F., McGahen, J. W., Neumayer, E. M., Paulshock, M., Watts, J. C., Wood, T. R., Hermann, E. C. and Hoffmann, C. E. (1964). *Science*, **144**, 862.

Davies, J. A., Jackson, B. and Redfern, P. H. (1973). *Neuropharmacology*, **12**, 735.

Dawson, J. R. (1933), *Amer. J. Pathol.* **9**, 7.

Dayan, A. D. and Stokes, M. I. (1972). *Brit. Med. J.* **ii**, 374.

Decker, B. L., Davis, J. M., Janowsky, D. S., Yousef, M. K. and Sekerke, H. J. (1971). *New Engl. J. Med.* **285**, 860.

Dickinson, P. C. T., Chang, T. W. and Weinstein, L. (1967). *In* "Antimicrobial Agents and Chemotherapy" (Ed. Gladys L. Hobby), pp. 521–526. American Society for Microbiology, Ann Arbor, Michigan.

Dom, R., Van Lommel, R. and Baro, F. (1971). *Acta Psychiat. Scand.* **47**, 399.

Domenichini, E., Carbonera, D., Pagnin, A. and Scherini, A. (1972). *Curr. Ther. Res.* **14**, 707.

Dominic, J. A. and Moore, K. E. (1969). *Arch. Int. Pharmacodyn.* **178**, 166.

Drill, V. A. (1958). *In* "Pharmacology in Medicine". McGraw-Hill, New York.

Dupont de Nemours and Co. (1964). U.S. Patent 373,825, June 9th.

Duvoisin, R. C. (1967). *Arch. Neurol. (Chicago)*, **17**, 124.

Dynes, J. B. (1970). *Dis. Nerv. Syst.* **31**, 854.

England, A. C., Schwab, R. S. and Petterson, E. (1959). *Electroencephalogr. Clin. Neurophysiol.* **11**, 723.

Ernst, A. M. (1967). *Psychopharmacologia*, **10**, 316.

Ersmark, B. and Lidvall, H. (1973). *Psychopharmacologia*, **28**, 308.

Fahn, S., Craddock, G. and Kumin, G. (1971). *Arch. Neurol. (Chicago)*, **25**, 45.

Farnebo, L. O., Fuxe, K., Goldstein, M., Hamberger, B. and Ungerstedt, U. (1971). *Eur. J. Pharmacol.* **16**, 27.

Fasano, V. A., Urciuoli, R. and Broggi, G. (1970). *Minerva Med.* **61**, 2895.

Fehling, C. (1973). *Acta Neurol. Scand.* **49**, 245.

Fibiger, H. C., Fox, M., McGeer, E. G. and McGeer, P. L. (1971). *J. Pharm. Pharmacol.* **9**, 724.

Fieschi, C., Nardini, M., Casacchia. M., Reitano, M., Tedone, M. E., Ferrari, P. and Robotti, E. (1970a). *Sist. Nerv.* **22**, 126.

Fieschi, C., Nardini, M., Casacchia, M., Tedone, M. E. and Robotti, E. (1970b). *Lancet*, **i**, 945.

Fieschi, C., Nardini, M., Casacchia, M., Tedone, M. E. and Reitano, M. (1970c). *Lancet*, **ii**, 154.

Fletcher, R. D. and Yusa, A. (1967). *Virology*, **31**, 382.

Fletcher, R. D., Hirschfield, J. E. and Forbes, M. (1965). *Nature (London)*, **207**, 664.

Fletcher, Elisa A. and Redfern, P. H. (1970). *J. Pharm. Pharmacol.* **22**, 957.

Florio, V. and Longo, V. G. (1971). *Physiol. Behav.* **6**, 465.

Freedman, B. E., Getz, E., MacGregor, J. MacW. and Ames, F. R. (1971). *S. Afr. Med. J.* **45**, 435.

Freman, J. M., Magoffin, R. L., Lennette, E. H. and Herndon, R. M. (1967). *Lancet*, **ii**, 129.

Fünfgeld, E. W. (1970). *Deut. Med. Wochenschr.* **95**, 1834.

Fuxe, K. and Ungerstedt, U. (1970). *In* "Symposium on Amphetamine and Related Compounds" (Eds Costa and Garattini), pp. 83–86. Tamburini, Milan.

Fuxe, K., Hökfelt, T. and Nilsson, C. (1969). *Neuroendocrinology*, **5**, 107.

Galbraith, A. W. (1973). *Brit. Med. J.* **iv**, 693.

Galbraith, A. W., Oxford, J. S., Schild, G. C. and Watson, G. I. (1969a). *Bull. W. H. O.* **41**, 671.

Galbraith, A. W., Oxford, J. S., Schild, G. C. and Watson, G. I. (1969b). Paper presented at the Second Conference on Antiviral Substances of the New York Academy of Sciences.

Galbraith, A. W., Oxford, J. S., Schild, G. C. and Watson, G. I. (1969c). *Lancet*, **ii**, 1026.

Galbraith, A. W., Oxford, J. S., Schild, G. C. and Watson, G. I. (1970). *Ann. N. Y. Acad. Sci.* **173**, 29.

Galbraith, A. W., Oxford, J. S., Schild, G. C., Potter, C. W. and Watson, G. I. (1971). *Lancet*, **ii**, 113.

Galbraith, A. W., Schild, G. C., Potter, C. W. and Watson, G. I. (1973). *J. Roy. Coll. Gen. Pract.* **23**, 34.

Geuens, H. and Stephens, R. L. (1967). Fifth International Congress of Chemotherapy, Vienna, Austria, vol. II/2, pp. 703–713. Verlag d. Wiener Med. Akademie, Wien, 1967.

Gibbs, C. J. Jr., Gajdusek, D. C., Asher, D. M., Alpers, M. P., Beck, E., Daniel, P. M. and Matthews, W. B. (1968). *Science*, **161**, 388.

Gilbert, G. J. (1971). *New England J. Med.* **284**, 896.

Godwin-Austen, R. B., Tomlinson, E. B., Frears, C. C. and Kok, H. W. L. (1969). *Lancet*, **ii**, 165.

Godwin-Austen, R. B., Frears, C. C., Bergmann, S., Parkes, J. D. and Knill-Jones, R. P. (1970), *Lancet*, **ii**, 383.

Goldhammer, Y., Bubis, J. J., Sarova-Pinhas, I. and Braham, J. (1972). *J. Neurol. Neurosurg. Psychiat.* **35**, 1.

Gomirato, G. and Hyden, H. (1963). *Brain*, **86**, 773.

Gomirato, G. and Perfetti, C. (1970). *Rev. Biol.* **16**, 247.

Goodwin, F. K., Brodie, H. K. H., Murphy, D. L. and Bunney, W. E. (1970). *Lancet*, **i**, 908.

Greenburg, J. (1971). *P. Med. J.* **74**, 54.

Greenfield, J. S. and Bosanquet, F. D. (1953). *J. Neurol. Neurosurg. Psychiat.* **16**, 213.

Grelak, R. P., Clark, R., Stump, J. M. and Vernier, V. G. (1970). *Science*, **169**, 203.

Griffiths, A. V., Parker, W. N. B. and Palmer, R. M. (1971). *Practitioner*, **207**, 679.

Grove, L. and Crammer, J. L. (1972). *Brit. Med. J.* **i**, 276.

Grunert, R. R., McGahen, J. W. and Davies, W. L. (1965). *Virology*, **26**, 262.

Guillain, G., Alajouanine, Th. and Marquézy, R. (1924). *C.R. Soc. Biol. (Paris)*, **91**, 364.

Hacohen, H. and Gurtner, B. (1972). *Schweiz. Med. Wochenschr.* **102**, 583.

Hallum, J. and Younger, J. (1966). *J. Bacteriol.* **92**, 1047.

Hamoen, A. M. (1973). *Brit. Med. J.*, **iii**, 272.

Hancock, M. P., Huntley, C. C. and Sever, J. L. (1968). *J. Pediat.* **72**, 636.

Harper, R. W. and Knothe, Barbara (1973). *Med. J. Aust.* **i**, 444.

Haslam, R. H., McQuillen, M. P. and Clark, D. B. (1969). *Neurology*, **19**, 1080.

Heikkila, R. E. and Cohen, G. (1972). *Eur. J. Pharmacol.* **20**, 156.

Heimans, R. L. H., Rand, M. J. and Fennessy, M. R. (1972). *J. Pharm. Pharmacol.* **24**, 875.

Herblin, W. F. (1972). *Biochem. Pharmacol.* **21**, 1993.

Herishanu, Y. (1973). *J. Amer. Geriat. Soc.* **21**, 229.

Herson, R. N. (1970). *Lancet*, **ii**, 721.

Hoehn, M. M. and Yahr, M. D. (1967). *Neurology*, **17**, 427.

Hoffmann, C. E., Neumayer, E. M., Haff, R. F. and Goldsby, R. A. (1965). *J. Bacteriol.* **90**, 623.

Hornick, R. B., Togo, Y. and Dawkins, A. T. (1966). Abstracted: *Bacteriol. Proc.* 131.

Hunter, K. R., Stern, G. M., Laurence, D. R. and Armitage, P. (1970a). *Lancet*, **i**, 1127.

Hunter, K. R., Stern, G. M., Laurence, D. R. and Armitage, P. (1970b). *Lancet*, **ii**, 566.

Hunter, K. R., Laurence, D. R., Shaw, K. M. and Stern, G. M. (1973). *Lancet*, **ii**, 929.

Issidorides, M. (1970). *Nature (London)*, **225**, 962.

Jackson, G. G., Muldoon, R. L. and Akers, L. W. (1963). *Antimicrob. Ag. Chemother.* **3**, 703.

Janowsky, D. S., El-Yousef, M. K., Davis, J. M., Sekerke, H. J., Morris, D. R. and Decker, B. (1972). *New England J. Med.* **286**, 785.

Jorgensen, P. B., Bergin, J. D., Haas, L., Cuningham, J. A. K., Norah, D. D., Pollock, M., Robinson, R. G. and Spears, G. F. S. (1971). *N.Z. Med. J.* **73**, 263.

Juel-Jensen, B. E. (1973). *Brit. J. Hosp. Med.* **10**, 402.

Jurna, I. and Lanzer, G. (1969). *Naunyn-Schmiedeberg's Arch. Exp. Pathol. Pharmakol.* **262**, 309.

Jurna, I., Grossmann, W. and Nell, T. (1972). *Neuropharmacology*, **11**, 559.

Kaito, H. E., Okamoto, I. and Kyo, I. (1969). *Gendai no Rinsho.* **3**, 782.

Kaji, M., Yanaga, T., Ito, M., Arita, M., Saeki, K., Tanour, M. and Mashiba, H. (1966). *Fukuoka Acta Med.* **57**, 251.

Kato, N. and Eggers, Hans J. (1969). *Virology*, **37**, 632.

Katz, M., Rorke, L. B., Masland, W. S., Koprowski, H. and Tucker, S. H. (1968). *New England J. Med.* **279**, 793.

Kelly, J. T. and Abuzzahab, F. S. (1971). *J. Clin. Pharmacol.* **11**, 211.

Killen, D. A., Hattori, H. and Zukoski, C. F. (1969). *Surgery*, **66**, 550.

Kitamoto, O. (1971). *Jap. J. Tuberc. Chest. Dis.* **17**, 1.

Kyo, I., Okamoto, E. and Kaito, H. (1970). *Gendai no Rinsho*, **4**, 44.

Kytömäki, O., Nousiainen, R., Pekkarinen, A., Rinne, U. K. and Viljanen, M. (1973). *J. Neurol. Transmission*, **34**, 145.

Labauge, R., Peguret, C., Blotman, F., Temple, D. and Attia, J. D. (1972). *J. Med. Montpellier*, **7**, 142.

Landa, S., Kriebel, S. and Knobloch, E. (1955). *Chem. Abstr.* **49**, 1598.

Lavrov, S. V., Eremkina, E. I., Orlova, T. G., Galegov, G. A., Soloviev, V. D. and Zhdanov, V. M. (1968). *Nature (London)*, **217**, 856.

Lee, R. G. and Blair, R. D. G. (1973). *Electroencephalogr. Clin. Neurophysiol.* **35**, 133.

Leeming, J. T. (1969). *Brit. Med. J.* **1**, 313.

Lemmer, B. (1973). *Eur. J. Pharmacol.* **21**, 183.

Lew, C., Iversen, S. D. and Iversen, L. L. (1971). *Eur. J. Pharmacol.* **14**, 351.

Lewis, P. D. (1971). *Brit. Med. J.* **iii**, 690.

Lundahl, K., Schut, J., Schlatmann, J. L., Paerels, G. B. and Peters, A. (1972). *J. Med. Chem.* **15**, 129.

Lundgren, G. and Malmburg, M. (1968). *Biochem. Pharmacol.* **17**, 1051.

MacFadyen, D. J., Picton, T. W., Zeldowicz, L. and McGreer, P. L. (1972). *J. Clin. Pharmacol.* **12**, 274.

McGahen, J. W., Neumayer, E. M., Grunert, R. P., Davies, W. L. and Hoffmann, C. E. (1968). Paper presented at a Seminar on Symmetrel, December 12, 1968, Delaware, U.S.A.

McGeer, E. G., Fibiger, H. C. and McGeer, P. L. (1972). *Biochem. Med.* **6**, 189.

Maassab, H. F. and Cochran, K. W. (1964). *Science*, **145**, 1443.

Mann, D. C., Pearce, L. A. and Waterbury, L. D. (1971). *Neurology*, **21**, 958.

Martín, F. (1970). *Rev. Clin. Espan.* **118**, 371.

Maté, J., Simon, M. and Juvancz, I. (1971). *Ther. Hung.* **19**, 117.

Mawdsley, C., Williams, I. R., Pullar, I. A., Davidson, D. L. and Kinloch, N. E. (1972). *Clin. Pharmacol. Ther.* **13**, 575.

Mendell, J. R., Chase, T. N. and Engel, W. K. (1970). *Lancet*, **i**, 593.

Merrick, E. M. and Schmitt, P. P. (1973). *Curr. Ther. Res., Clin. Exp.* **15**, 552.
Messina, C., Di Rosa, A. E. and Tomasello, F. (1972). *J. Neurol. Sci.* **17**, 141.
Min-Chu, L. and Laverty, R. (1971). *Proc. Univ. Otago Med. Sch.* **49**, 14.
Mindham, R. H. S., Gaind, R., Anstree, B. H. and Rimmer, L. (1972). *Psychol. Med.* **2**, 406.
Monto, A. S., Cavallaro, J. J. and Keller, J. B. (1970). *Arch. Environ. Health*, **21**, 408.
Morgan, L. (1970). *Med. J. Aust.* **14**, 652.
Muldoon, R. L. and Jackson, G. G. (1967). *Proc. Soc. Exp. Biol. Med.* **126**, 26.
Nagaswami, S. and Ranjini, R. (1971). *J. Kans. Med. Soc.* **72**, 465.
Naylor, R. J. and Costall, B. (1971). *Life Sci.* **10**, 909.
Neff, N. H. and Costa, E. (1966). *Life Sci.* **5**, 951.
Neumayer, E. M., Haff, R. F. and Hoffman, C. E. (1965). *Proc. Soc. Exp. Biol. Med.* **119**, 393.
Nevin, S. (1967). *Proc. Roy. Soc. Med.* **60**, 517.
Nevin, S., McMenemey, W. H., Behrman, S. and Jones, D. P. (1960). *Brain*, **83**, 519.
Norris, F. H. (1972). *Brit. Med. J.* **ii**, 349.
Notermans, S. L. H., Tijl, W. F. J., Willems, F. T. C. and Sloof, J. L. (1973). *Neurology*, **23**, 543.
O'Donoghue, J. M., Ray, G. C., Terry, D. W. Jr. and Beaty, H. N. (1973). *Amer. J. Epidemiol.* **97**, 276.
Offermeier, J. (1965). *In* "Serotonin and its Derivatives", p. 89. Toben Offset, Nÿmegen.
Offermeier, J. (1971). *In* "Parkinson's Disease. A New Approach to Treatment" (Eds. G. F. B. Birdwood, S. S. B. Gilder and C. A. S. Wink), p. 85. Academic Press, London and New York.
Oker-Blom, N., Hovi, T., Leinikki, P., Palosuo, T., Pettersson, R. and Suni, J. (1970). *Brit. Med. J.* **iii**, 676.
Otsuka, M. and Endo, M. (1960). *J. Pharmacol. Exp. Ther.* **128**, 273.
Oxford, J. S. and Schild, G. C. (1967). *Brit. J. Exp. Pathol.* **48**, 235.
Parkes, J. D., Zilkha, K. J., Calver, D. M. and Knill-Jones, R. P. (1970a). *Lancet*, **i**, 259.
Parkes, J. D., Zilkha, K. J., Marsden, P., Baxter, R. C. H. and Knill-Jones, R. P. (1970b). *Lancet*, **i**, 1130.
Parkes, J. D., Sharpstone, P. and Williams, R. (1970c). *Lancet*, **ii**, 1341.
Parkes, J. D., Baxter, R. C. H., Curzon, G., Knill-Jones, R. P., Knott, P. J., Marsden, C. D., Tatersall, R. and Vollum, Dorothy (1971a). *Lancet*, **i**, 1083.
Parkes, J. D., Knill-Jones, R. P. and Clements, P. J. (1971b). *Postgrad. Med. J.* **47**, 116.
Parkes, J. D., Zilkha, K. J., Knill-Jones, R. P., Clements, P. J. and Baxter, R. (1971c). *Int. Z. Klin. Pharmakol. Ther. Toxikol.* **4**, 356.
Parkes, J. D., Branfoot, A. C., Marsden, C. D. and Vollum, D. (1972). *Lancet*, **ii**, 1373.
Parkes, J. D., Baxter, R. C., Marsden, C. D. and Rees, J. E. R. (1974). *J. Neurol. Neurosurg. Psychiat.* (In press.)
Payne, F. E. and Baublis, J. V. (1971). *Perspect. Med. Virol.* **7**, 179.
Pearce, J. (1971). *Brit. Med. J.* **iii**, 529.
Pearce, J. and Rao, N. S. (1970). *Lancet*, **ii**, 1091.
Pearce, J., Aziz, H. and Gallagher, J. C. (1968). *J. Neurol. Neurosurg. Psychiat.* **31**, 501.

Peaston, M. J. T., Bianchine, J. R. and Messiha, F. S. (1973). *Life Sci.* **13**, 237.
Penders, C. A. and Delwaide, P. J. (1971). *J. Neurol. Neurosurg. Psychiat.* **34**, 674.
Pepeu, G. and Bartolini, A. (1968). *Eur. J. Pharmacol.* **4**, 254.
Pletscher, A., Bartholini, G. and Prada, M. Da. (1970). *Méd. et Hyg. (Genève)*, **933**, 1500.
Plotkin, S. A. (1965). *Arch. Gesamte. Virusforsch.* **16**, 438.
Plotkin, S. A., Klaus, R. M. and Whitely, J. P. (1966). *J. Pediat.* **68**, 1085.
Pollock, M. and Jorgensen, P. (1972). *Aust. N.Z. J. Med.* **3**, 252.
Portera, A., Varela de Seijas, E., Mara, P., Ramírez Echevarría, T. J. and Amaya Pombo, C. (1970). *Rev. Clin. Espan.* **117**, 579.
Puca, F. M., Bricolo, A. and Turella, G. (1973). *Electroencephalogr. Clin. Neurophysiol.* **35**, 327.
Rao, N. S. and Pearce, J. (1971). *Practitioner*, **206**, 241.
Rinne, U. K., Sonninen, V. and Hyyppä, M. (1972). *Experientia*, **28**, 57.
Roffler-Tarlov, S., Sharman, D. F. and Tegerdine, P. (1971). *Brit. J. Pharmacol. Chemother.* **42**, 343.
Roos, B. E. and Steg, G. (1964). *Life Sci.* **3**, 351.
Rüther, E., Fusmann-Hegenwald, M. and Eben, E. (1973). *Activ. Nerv. Super.* **15**, 2.
Sabin, A. B. (1967). *J. Amer. Med. Ass.* **200**, 943.
Sacks, O., Schwartz, W. F. and Messeloff, C. R. (1971). *Clin. Pharmacol. Ther.* **12**, 301.
Sanders, W. L. and Dunn, T. L. (1973). *J. Neurol. Neurosurg. Psychiat.* **36**, 581.
Scatton, B., Ceramy, A., Besson, M. J. and Glowinski, J. (1970). *Eur. J. Pharmacol.* **13**, 131.
Schild, G. C. and Sutton, R. N. P. (1965). *Brit. J. Exp. Pathol.* **46**, 263.
Schildkraut, J. J. and Ketty, S. S. (1967). *Science*, **156**, 21.
Schleyer, P. von R. (1957). *J. Amer. Chem. Soc.* **79**, 3292.
Schubert, G. S., Schiff, G. and West, C. (1966). Society for Pediatric Research, p. 159.
Schwab, R. S., England, A. C., Poskanzer, D. C. and Young, R. R. (1969). *J. Amer. Med. Ass.* **208**, 1168.
Schwab, R. S., Poskanzer, D. C., England, A. C. and Young, R. R. (1972). *J. Amer. Med. Ass.* **222**, 792.
Schwarz, G. A. and Fahn, S. (1970). *Med. Clin. N. Amer.* **54**, 773.
Schwarz, H. G. (1969). *Arbeitsmed. Sozialmed. Arbeitshyg.* **4**, 231.
Scotti, G. (1970). *Lancet*, **i**, 1394.
Scotti, G. (1970b). *Sist. Nerv.* **22**, 144.
Scotti, G. (1970c). *Sist. Nerv.* **22**, 232.
Seale, R. V. and Prasad, K. N. (1967). *Anat. Rec.* **168**, 259.
Sever, J. L. and Zeman, W. (1968). *In* Conference on measles virus and subacute sclerosing panencephalitis. Neurology, vol. 18, no. 1, part 2.
Shaw, C. M., Buchan, G. C. and Carlson, C. B. (1967). *New England J. Med.* **277**, 511.
Shealy, C. N., Weeth, J. B. and Mercier, D. (1970). *J. Amer. Med. Ass.* **212**, 1522.
Shuster, S., Thody, A. J., Goolamali, S. K., Burton, J. L., Plummer, N. and Bates, D. (1973). *Lancet*, **i**, 463.
Sigg, E. B., Soffer, L. and Gyermek, L. (1963). *J. Pharmacol. Exp. Ther.* **142**. 13.
Sigwald, J. and Raymondeaud, C. (1972). *Nouv. Press. Med.* **1**, 1237.
Sigwald, J., Raymondeaud, C. and Piot, C. (1970). *Rev. Neurol.* **122**, 145.

Silver, D. E. and Sahs, A. L. (1972). *Neurology*, **22**, 665.
Simon, P., Malatray, J. and Boissier, J. R. (1970). *J. Pharm. Pharmacol.* **22**, 546.
Smejkal, F., Budesinsky, Z., Sluka, J. and Kuchar, M. (1972). *In* "Advances in Antimicrobial and Antineoplastic Chemotherapy" (Eds. M. Hejzlar, M. Semonsky, and S. Masak), p. 879. Urban and Schwarzenberg, Munchen.
Smith, C. B. (1963). *J. Pharmacol. Exp. Ther.* **142**, 343.
Smorodintsev, A. A., Karpuhin, G. I., Zlydnikov, D. M., Malyseva, A. M., Svecova, E. G., Burov, S. A., Hramcova, L. M., Romanov, J. U. A., Taros, L. J., Ivannikov, J. G. and Novoselov, S. D. (1970). *Bull. W. H. O.* **42**, 865.
Snyder, (1970). *Biol. Psychiat.* **2**, 367.
Stanley, E. D., Muldoon, L. W., Akers, L. W. and Jackson, G. G. (1965). *Ann. N.Y. Acad. Sci.* **130**, 44.
Stepanov, F. M. and Isaev, S. D. (1970). *Zh. Organ. Khimii.* **6**, 1195.
Stephanis, C. N. and Issidorides, M. (1970). *Nature (London)*, **225**, 962.
Stetter, H. (1954). *Angew Chem.* **66**, 217.
Stetter, H. and Krause, M. (1967). *Tetrahedron Lett.* **19**, 1841.
Stetter, H. and Wulff, C. (1962). *Chem. Ber.* **95**, 2302.
Streifler, M. and Kallay, U. (1972). *Harefuah*, **82**, 1.
Strömberg, U. (1970). *Psychopharmacologia*, **18**, 58.
Strömberg, U., Svensson, T. H. and Waldeck, B. (1970). *J. Pharm. Pharmacol.* **22**, 959.
Strömberg, U. and Svensson, T. H. (1971). *Acta Pharmacol. Toxicol.* **30**, 161.
Svensson, T. H. and Strömberg, U. (1970). *J. Pharm. Pharmacol.* **22**, 639.
Symchowicz, S., Korduba, C. A. and Veals, J. (1973). *Eur. J. Pharmacol.* **21**, 155.
Thornburg, J. E. (1972). *Fed. Proc.* **31**, 530 Abs.
Thornburg, J. E. and Moore, K. E. (1971). *Pharmacologist*, **13**, 202.
Thornburg, J. E. and Moore, K. E. (1972). *Neuropharmacology*, **66**, 675.
Thut, P. D. and Rech, R. H. (1970). *Pharmacologist*, **12**, 227.
Togo, Y., Hornick, R. B., Felitti, V. J., Kaufman, M. L., Dawkins, A. T. Jr., Kilpe, V. E. and Claghorn, J. L. (1970). *J. Amer. Med. Ass.* **211**, 1149.
Tsatsas, G., Costakis, E., Casadio, S., Lumachi, B. and Marazzi-Uberti, E. (1969). *Ann. Pharm. Fr.* **27**, 363.
Tsunoda, A., Maassab, H. F., Cochran, K. W. and Eveland, W. E. (1965). *Antimicrob. Ag. Chemother.*, 553.
Tyler, E. T. and Kessler, W. B. (1964). Paper read at the Symposium on Aspects of Antiviral Therapy, Wilmington, Delaware, Oct. 22–23.
Tyrrell, D. A. J., Bynoe, M. L. and Hoorn, B. (1965). *Brit. J. Exp. Pathol.* **46**, 370.
Uchiyama, M. and Shibuya, M. (1969). *Chem. Pharm. Bull.* **17**, 841.
Ungerstedt, U. (1968). *Eur. J. Pharmacol.* **5**, 107.
Ungerstedt, U. (1971a). *In* "6-Hydroxydopamine and Catecholamine Neurones" (Eds T. Malmfors and H. Thoenen), p. 101. North-Holland, Amsterdam.
Ungerstedt, U. (1971b). *Acta Physiol. Scand. Suppl.* **367**, 69.
Ungerstedt, U. (1971c). *Acta Physiol. Scand. Suppl.* **367**, 49.
Vale, S. and Espejel, M. A. (1971). *New England J. Med.* **284**, 673.
Vale, S., Espejel, M. A. and Dominguez, J. C. (1971). *Lancet*, **ii**, 437.
Van Manen, J. (1972). *Psychiat. Neurol. Neurochem.* **75**, 49.
Vernier, V. G. (1971). Paper presented at the Wilmington Symposium on amantadine, Delaware.
Vernier, V. G., Harmon, J. B., Stump, J. M., Lynes, T. E., Marvel, J. P. and Smith, D. H. (1969). *Toxicol. Appl. Pharmacol.* **15**, 642.

Vitetta, M. (1971). *Minerva Med.* **62**, 3984.

Voigtlander, P. F. Von and Moore, K. E. (1971). *Science*, **174**, 408.

Voigtlander, P. F. Von and Moore, K. E. (1973). *Neuropharmacology*, **12**, 451.

Voller, Gert. (1970). *Deut. Med. Wochenschr.* **95**, 934.

Voller, Gert. (1972). *Muench. Med. Wochenschr.* **114**, 1066.

Vollum, Dorothy, Parkes, J. D. and Doyle, D. (1971). *Brit. Med. J.* **ii**, 627.

Walker, J. E., Albers, J. W., Tourtellotte, W. W., Henderson, W. G., Potvin, A. R. and Smith, A. (1972a). *J. Chronic Dis.* **25**, 149.

Walker, J. E., Potvin, A., Tourtellotte, W., Albers, J., Repa, B., Henderson, W. and Snyder, D. (1972b). *Clin. Pharmacol. Ther.* **13**, 28.

Webster, D. D. (1968). *Modern Treatment*, **5**, 257.

Weiner, N. and Rutledge, C. (1966). *In* "Mechanisms of Release of Biogenic Amines" (Eds. Von Euler, Rossell and Uvnäs), p. 307. Pergamon, London.

Weiss, J. L., Ng, L. K. Y. and Chase, T. N. (1971). *Lancet*, **i**, 1016.

Weissman, A., Koe, B. K. and Tenen, S. S. (1966). *J. Pharmacol. Exp. Ther.* **151**, 339.

Wesemann, W. and Zilliken, F. (1967). *J. Pharm. Pharmacol.* **19**, 203.

Williams, C. M. and Goodman, H. (1925). *J. Amer. Med. Ass.* **85**, 955.

Wingfield, W. L., Pollock, D. and Grunert, R. R. (1969). *New England J. Med.* **281**, 579.

Yahr, M. D. and Duvoisin, R. C. (1968). *Med. Treatment*, **5**, 283.

Yaryura-Tobias, J. A., Wolpert, A., Dana, L. and Merlis, S. (1970). *Dis. Nerv. Syst.* **31**, 60.

Zetler, G. (1968). *Int. J. Neuropharmacol.* **7**, 325.

Zetler, G. (1970). *Naunyn-Schmiedeberg's Arch. Pharmakol.* **266**, 276.

Zinner, G. and Dybowski, U. (1970). *Arch. Pharm.* **303**, 488.

Prostaglandin Antagonists

ALAN BENNETT, BPharm, PhD, MPS

Department of Surgery, King's College Hospital Medical School, London, England

1 Introduction

Prostaglandin antagonists have become available over the last few years and their value as pharmacological tools and as potential therapeutic agents is now recognized. Since the review by Eakins and Sanner in 1972, no dramatic advances have been made, but more is now known about their actions, selectivity and possible therapeutic uses (Sanner, 1974). The potency of the prostaglandin antagonists now available is low compared, for example, with blockade of acetylcholine by atropine, but they are sufficiently active to be useful. The term "prostaglandin antagonist" is used here to mean a compound which selectively antagonizes the actions of prostaglandins at their site of action and not compounds such as aspirin which depress the formation of prostaglandins by inhibiting prostaglandin synthetase. The antagonists of prostaglandin to be discussed here mainly belong to three chemically unrelated classes, 7-oxaprostaglandins, dibenzoxazepine hydrazides, and polyphloretin phosphate.

The most common natural prostaglandins (**1**) are named as derivatives of prostanoic acid, a C-20 straight chain acid having C-8 and C-12 linked so as to form a cyclopentane ring. These PGs have a double bond at C-13 and a 15α-hydroxyl group. Each is known by a letter signifying a particular substitution pattern of the ring and a subscript numeral denoting the number of bouble bonds in the side chains. These may occur at C-5 and C-17 in addition to the one at C-13. The subscript in PGF_α refers to the 9α-hydroxyl group.

Fried *et al.* (1969; 1971), having observed that the synthetic 7-oxa-prostaglandins possessed smooth muscle stimulating activity, prepared 7-oxaprostaglandins which were without oxygen functions at positions 9 and 11 and at positions 9, 11, and 15. They also prepared various homologues including those with four-membered or six-membered cycloalkane rings. These were tested as agonists and also as antagonists of PGE_1 on guinea-pig ileum, rabbit duodenum and gerbil colon. They found that the degree of hydroxylation determined whether the compound was an agonist or antagonist. Compounds with an oxygen function (hydroxyl or carbonyl) at C-9 and C-11 were agonists, whether or not there was also a C-15 hydroxyl group. Compounds without oxygen functions at C-9 and C-11 and with a C-15 hydroxyl might be agonist or antagonist, and compounds devoid of oxygen functions at C-9, 11, and

15 were said to be "pure antagonists", although other work shows that this is not always so (see sections 2 to 5). The most selective antagonist found by Fried and his colleagues was 7-oxa-13-prostynoic acid (2). It has been separated into its optical isomers (Fried *et al.*, 1971) but their actions have not so far been studied.

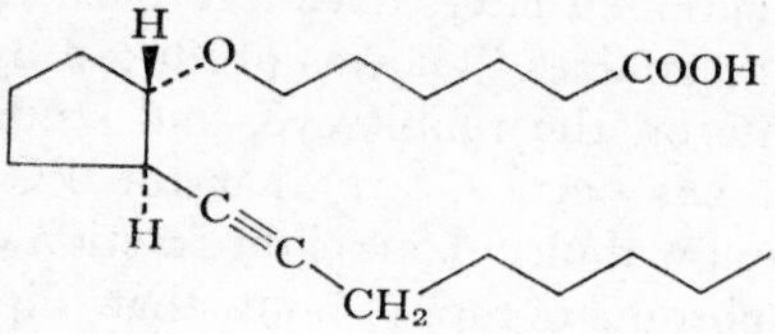

(2)

Coyne and Cusic (1968) synthesized a series of 1-acyl-2-(10,11-dihydrodibenz[b,f][1,4]oxazepine-10-carbonyl)hydrazines (3) which they found to possess anticonvulsant and analgesic properties. Sanner (1969) provided the first evidence that one of these substances (SC-19220) antagonizes PGs. Other related substances are also PG antagonists but they are less selective than SC-19220 (Sanner, 1972; Sanner *et al.*, 1973).

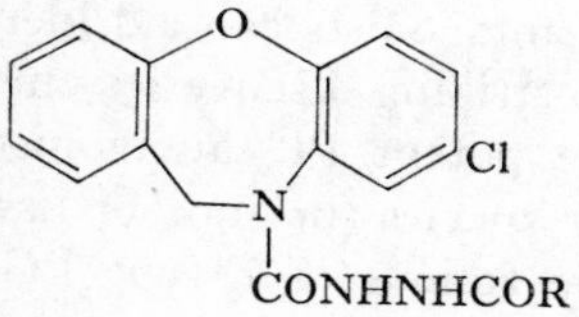

	R
SC-19220	CH_3
SC-18637	$CH_2C_6H_5$
SC-25191	$CH_2CH_2CH_3$
SC-25192	$CH(CH_3)_2$
SC-25038	$(CH_2)_4CH_3$

(3)

Studies of the structure–activity relationships of some dibenzoxazepine derivatives (in which butanoyl, isobutanoyl, and hexanoyl groups replace the acetyl group of SC-19220) show that as the side chain is lengthened potency increases but selectivity decreases (Sanner *et al.*, 1973).

Polyphloretin phosphate (PPP) (4) was synthesized by Diczfaluzy *et al.* (1953) and is a mixture of polyanionic polyesters of phosphoric acid and phloretin. The molecular weight is thought to be less than 5000 (A. B. Leo, private files) but since it is not known exactly, and there are

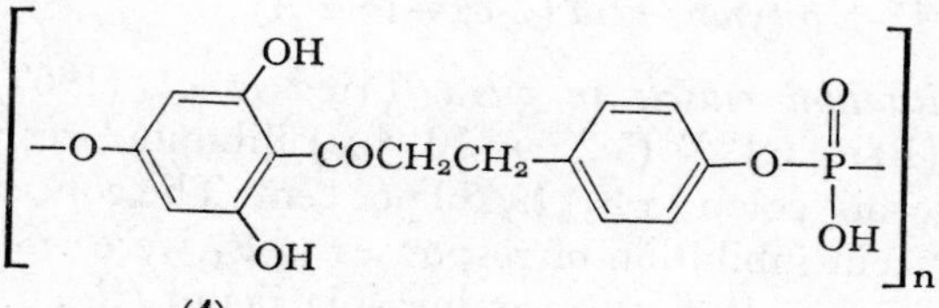

(4)

probably variations between batches, the concentrations can only be given as $\mu g \ ml^{-1}$. The early studies showed it to inhibit various enzymes including hyaluronidase, alkaline phosphatase, and urease. Fries (1956; 1960) found that PPP reduced capillary permeability induced in several tissues, and inhibited the formation of peritoneal adhesions in the rabbit. Other properties, mentioned later, have also been discovered. The first evidence that PPP antagonizes PGs was produced by Beitch and Eakins (1969) in experiments on the rabbit eye, and studies on other tissues followed quickly. It has been shown that the PG antagonist activity resides mainly in the low molecular weight fraction of PPP separated by Sephadex column chromatography, and that diphloretin phosphate (DPP) is more potent than this fraction.

2 Antagonism of prostaglandins on smooth muscle

2.1 GASTROINTESTINAL MUSCLE

Gastrointestinal muscle is discussed first since it has been the subject of many studies and the results obtained are pertinent to the investigation of other tissues. Also, isolated gut tissues are often used for bioassay of extracted PG-like substances, and PG antagonists can aid identification of the biologically active material. Two striking discoveries emerge from these studies: firstly drugs which are potent PG antagonists in one species may not be effective in another species (or another tissue of the same species); secondly, not all of the actions of E-type PGs are antagonized by the compounds presently available so that there may be more than one type of PG receptor. Thus, whereas PGE compounds generally cause *contractions of longitudinal muscle* which can be antagonized, their *inhibition of circular muscle* (Bennett and Fleshler, 1970) is resistant to the antagonists. The PGF compounds cause both muscle layers of the gut to contract, and the effect on both layers can be blocked. The effects of antagonists have been studied only against E and F prostaglandins mainly because A and B prostaglandins have little effect on most tissues and PGC (Jones, 1972) has not been studied widely.

2.1.1 *7-Oxa-13-prostynoic acid (7-oxa-13-PA)*

2.1.1.1 *Longitudinal muscle in vitro.* Fried *et al.* (1969) found that 7-oxa-13-PA ($10 \ \mu g \ ml^{-1}$) (3.25×10^{-5} M) inhibited responses of jird (often called gerbil) colon to $F_{1\alpha}$ by 50 per cent. The concentrations producing 50 per cent inhibition of responses to E_1 were 5.8×10^{-6} M on jird colon and 7.8×10^{-5} M on guinea-pig ileum (Fried, 1970). Flack

(1970) demonstrated that whereas 7-oxa-13-PA 3.25×10^{-5} M antagonized contractions of jird colon to E_1, E_2, $F_{1\alpha}$, and $F_{2\alpha}$ with little or no inhibition of responses to ACh, its effect on guinea-pig ileum and rabbit jejunum were non-selective. Bennett and Posner (1971) confirmed that 7-oxa-13-PA was non-selective: 2 to 8×10^{-5} M solution inhibited responses of the longitudinal muscle of guinea-pig ileum to acetylcholine, nicotine, histamine and E_2; Ehrenpreis et al. (1973) found that 2.6×10^{-5} M blocked electrically induced contractions. At concentrations of 5.5×10^{-5} to 3×10^{-4} M the drug either had little or no effect on responses of human gastric and ileal longitudinal muscle to E_2 and $F_{2\alpha}$, or at higher concentrations it reduced responses to acetylcholine as well as to the PGs. 7-Oxa-13-PA (3×10^{-6} to 8×10^{-5} M) caused dose-dependent *contractions* of the rat fundus, thereby contradicting the view of Fried et al. (1969) that hydroxy group must be present in the molecule for agonist activity. Somova (1973) reported that 7-oxa-13-PA selectively antagonized responses of rat colon and chick rectum to E_2 and $F_{2\alpha}$ but no details were given in this work which was cited as "unpublished data".

2.1.1.2 Circular muscle in vitro.

2.1.1.2 *Circular muscle in vitro*. With few exceptions the circular muscle of the gut is inhibited by E_1 and E_2 (shown by relaxation of tonic preparations or by reduction of drug-induced contractions of atonic muscles) but contracted by $F_{1\alpha}$ and $F_{2\alpha}$. The tone of guinea-pig colon and usually also of human colon was reduced by 7-oxa-13-PA, but that of the circular muscle of the human gastric body was increased. This compound did not affect E_2-induced relaxations (7-oxa-13-PA at least 5.5×10^{-5} M with circular muscle of human gastric body and sigmoid colon, and 2 to 8×10^{-5} M with guinea-pig colon) and showed little selectivity in depressing the contractions to $F_{2\alpha}$ (Bennett and Posner, 1971).

2.1.2 SC-19220 and analogues

2.1.2.1 Longitudinal muscle in vitro

a. Guinea-pig ileum. Sanner (1969) found that SC-19220 3×10^{-6} to 1.5×10^{-4} M (1 to 50 µg ml^{-1}) antagonized contractions of guinea-pig ileum to E_2 (pA$_2$ 5.5) whereas responses to acetylcholine, 5-HT and bradykinin were unaffected below 6×10^{-5} M SC-19220. Concentrations of 7.5×10^{-6} to 3×10^{-5} M caused parallel shifts to the right of the dose–response curve for E_2 without depressing the maximum response, suggesting that the antagonism was competitive. At 6×10^{-5} M and higher, the slope of the curve decreased and the maximum response was reduced, indicating some degree of non-competitive antagonism.

SC-19220 5×10^{-6} to 10^{-5} M antagonized the contractions produced by E_2 (Fig. 1) and $F_{2\alpha}$ on the longitudinal muscle of guinea-pig ileum with similar pA_2 values (5·5 and 5·6 respectively). This indicates that both PGs might be acting at the same receptor site (Bennett and Posner, 1971); somewhat similar pA_2 values were obtained for E_1, E_2, and $F_{1\alpha}$ by Sanner (1972). There is evidence (Bennett *et al.* 1968; Harry, 1968) that receptors for E_1 and E_2 are located mainly on cholinergic nerves in the longitudinal muscle of guinea-pig ileum. It seems that this is true of receptors for $F_{1\alpha}$ and $F_{2\alpha}$ also since their effects are markedly reduced by hyoscine or tetrodotoxin (Bennett *et al.*, 1973b).

Although SC-19220 was initially found to be relatively selective, Sanner (1971) did find substantial depression of responses to 5-HT with

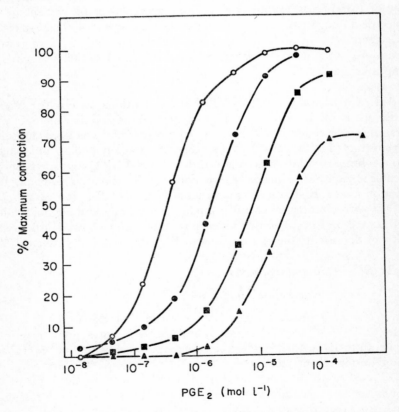

IG. 1. Dose–response curves of PGE_2 on guinea-pig ileum in the presence of SC-19220. $\circ$, Control; $\bullet$, 3×10^{-5}M; $\blacksquare$, 6×10^{-5} M; $\blacktriangle$, $1·2 \times 10^{-4}$ M. (Sanner, 1969.)

9×10^{-5} M SC-19220. The selectivity of SC-19220 was examined further, with a view to using this compound to investigate the role of PGs in peristaltic activity in guinea-pig intestine (Bennett *et al.*, 1973b). As peristalsis depends on the intrinsic innervation, SC-19220 was examined for its effect on responses of guinea-pig isolated ileum to cholinergic nerve stimulation with nicotine and electrical impulses. After SC-19220 (1.5×10^{-5} to 3×10^{-5} M) the contractions to E_2, nicotine, electrical field stimulation and acetylcholine were (per cent $\pm$ SE) 8 ± 5, 36 ± 15, 60 ± 7, and 85 ± 15 per cent respectively of the control responses. Ehrenpreis *et al.* (1973) found that SC-19220 4.5×10^{-5} M blocked electrically induced contractions of guinea-pig ileum. Reduction of responses to electrical stimulation also occurs in guinea-pig trachea (see section 2.2). One possibility is that the drug blocks conduction in nerves, and this would explain why responses to 5-HT are depressed (5-HT acts mainly on cholinergic nerves in guinea-pig ileum; Gaddum and Picarelli, 1957).

The phenylacetyl derivative SC-18637 1.2×10^{-5} M (3) antagonized responses to E_2 with no appreciable effect on contractions to bradykinin or acetylcholine. Its pA_2 was 6.01 and therefore was more potent than SC-19220, but it was not further studied *in vitro* because higher concentrations were less selective than SC-19220 (Sanner, 1972). Structure–activity relationships were studied in three other dibenzoxazepine derivatives by Sanner *et al.* (1973). The butanoyl (SC-25191), and *n*-hexanoyl (SC-25038) derivatives (3) were more potent than SC-19220 whereas the isobutanoyl compound was less potent. Unfortunately, they were all less selective than SC-19220. The authors concluded that lengthening the side chain increases anti-PG potency but decreases selectivity, particularly with regard to 5-HT. Might these drugs also be potent neurone blockers?

b. Rat stomach. (Strips of fundus usually cut parallel to longitudinal muscle.) SC-19220 (5×10^{-6} to 5×10^{-5} M) antagonized responses to E_2 and $F_{2\alpha}$. There was no reduction of contractions to acetylcholine (Bennett and Posner, 1971), and in preparations where the tone was lowered by SC-19220 the responses to acetylcholine even increased. When the tone had been reduced by heavier weighting and frequent dosing with PGs, antagonism occurred without alteration of acetylcholine responses. Splawinski *et al.* (1973) reported that 5×10^{-6} to 10^{-4} M SC-19220 antagonized responses of rat fundus strips to E_2, $F_{2\alpha}$ and their precursor arachidonic acid.

The lowering of tone by SC-19220 might reflect a role of PGs in maintaining tone, since PG synthetase inhibitors also have this effect on the rat fundus. There is also evidence of such a role for PGs in other tissues (Posner, 1970; Ferreira *et al.*, 1972). However, the situation may be more complex because SC-19220 can also reduce contractions to potassium. Another problem with SC-19220 is its low water-solubility, and the solvents (propylene glycol, polyethylene glycol, or ethanol) needed in the initial solubilization can also reduce tissue tone if too much is used. In the studies reported, care has usually been taken not to exceed depressant levels, as shown by control experiments with the solvent alone. No other reports have appeared with SC-19220 on the rat fundus, but the butanoyl, isobutanoyl, and hexanoyl analogues (SC-25191, SC-25192, and SC-25038 (**3**)) have been studied (Sanner *et al.*, 1973). As with guinea-pig ileum discussed previously, lengthening the carbon chain increased anti-PG activity but reduced selectivity for E_2 as shown by depression of responses to acetylcholine and 5-HT.

    c. Jird colon. SC-19220 antagonized E_1 and E_2 with parallel displacement of the dose–response curves and a pA_2 value of 5·45, but $F_{1\alpha}$ and $F_{2\alpha}$ were more difficult to block. At 6×10^{-5} M SC-19220 (the highest possible concentration before a nonselective depressant effect of the polyethylene glycol solvent became apparent) a 20-fold increase in dose of E_2 was required to overcome antagonism whilst the dose-ratio for $F_{1\alpha}$ or $F_{2\alpha}$ was only 2 (Eakins and Miller, 1970, cited by Eakins and Sanner, 1972).

    d. Human gut. Vanasin *et al.* (1970) reported that SC-19220 antagonized contractions of human taenia coli to E_1 and E_2, but the concentration required and the selectivity of blockade were not stated. Bennett and Posner (1971) found that SC-19220 was either ineffective or acted nonselectively on human stomach, ileum or colon. Therefore the lowering of tone by SC-19220 in these tissues would seem to be unrelated to antagonism of E or F compounds, but the possibility cannot be ruled out that other PGs are involved in the maintenance of tone. Its lack of effect on human gut muscle does not necessarily mean that other human tissues will be unaffected: another PG antagonist, polyphoretin phosphate, is active on human gut but not on uterus (Karim, 1973).

    e. Dog colon. SC-19920 antagonized contractions of the longitudinal muscle to E_1 and E_2 but the concentration and selectivity of blockade were not stated (Vanasin *et al.*, 1970).

2.1.2.2 *Circular gut muscle.* SC-19220 10^{-5} M did not antagonize PGE-induced relaxations (guinea-pig colon circular muscle, human circular gastric body), but it antagonized contractions to $F_{2\alpha}$ without inhibiting acetylcholine in guinea-pig colon (Bennett and Posner, 1971). The drug also reduced the tone of both muscle layers and depressed contractions to potassium.

2.1.2.3 *In vivo*. E_2 1 µg injected i.p. in mice causes diarrhoea (Sanner, 1972) which may well be due to stimulation of muscle, although there could be a primary or additional effect on fluid secretion. SC-19220 i.p. 15 minutes before the injection of E_2 prevented the diarrhoea. The dose protecting 50 per cent of the mice (ED50) was approximately 170 mg kg^{-1} when administered as a saline suspension or a solution in polyethylene glycol, but the ED50 was about 17 mg kg^{-1} when 0·1 per cent or 1 per cent polysorbate 80 was used in the saline suspension. Polysorbate also increased the toxicity. The analogue SC-18637 was almost inactive *in vivo*, and even using polysorbate 80 the ED50 was approximately 460 mg kg^{-1}.

2.1.3 *Polyphloretin phosphate (PPP) and its analogues*

2.1.3.1 *Longitudinal muscle in vitro*. PPP has been found to antagonize the effects of E and F prostaglandins on most gastrointestinal muscles studied. Contractions of jird isolated colon to both E and F compounds are inhibited, but the PGEs are less susceptible than the PGFs. The antagonism with PPP 2·5–40 µg ml^{-1} caused parallel shifts of the dose–response curves with little or no depression of the maximum, or of responses to acetylcholine, bradykinin, angiotensin and 5-HT. With 40 µg ml^{-1} PPP, dose-ratios for E_2 and $F_{2\alpha}$ were 128 and 181 respectively (Eakins *et al.*, 1970; Eakins, 1971). The inhibitory action of PPP on jird colon was not due to its ability to inhibit various enzymes, and the parent dihydrochalcone moiety phloretin was inactive. Some other polymeric phosphates with enzyme-inhibitory properties similar to PPP (polyhydroquinone phosphate, polyphloroglucinol phosphate and polyestradiol phosphate) were not PG antagonists. Polystilbol phosphate, however, did antagonize E_2 and $F_{2\alpha}$ on jird colon, but it was less selective than PPP; it antagonized angiotensin and, to a lesser extent acetylcholine; and it was at best only slowly reversible (Eakins *et al.*, 1971).

PPP reversibility antagonizes E_2 and $F_{2\alpha}$ in several other tissues: *rabbit jejunum* (2·5–30 µg ml^{-1}: Eakins *et al.*, 1970) *guinea-pig colon* (50–300 µg ml^{-1}: Bennett and Posner, 1971; Bennett *et al.*, 1973b), *guinea-pig ileum* (20–400 µg ml^{-1}: Bennett *et al.*, 1973a), rat colon (10–20 µg ml^{-1}, $F_{2\alpha}$ blocked more easily than E_2: Gagnon and Sirois, 1972; Somova, 1973), *chick rectum* (Somova, 1973), *human stomach* and *colon* (up to 600 µg ml^{-1}: Bennett and Posner, 1971), *and human foetal intestine* (Hart, 1974). In most cases, however, the selectivity and effectiveness did not approach that seen with jird colon (Eakins *et al.*, 1970; Eakins, 1971). As with 7-oxa-13-PA and SC-19220, PPP reduced responses to nicotine in guinea-pig ileum, but unlike SC-19220 it did not greatly affect electrically-induced contractions. After PPP 40-100

$\mu g \ ml^{-1}$ responses to E_2, nicotine, electrical stimulation and acetylcholine were (per cent $\pm$ SE) 12 ± 4, 12 ± 6, 78 ± 16, and 79 ± 11 per cent of control responses respectively (Bennett et al., 1973b) (see section 2.2). PPP might therefore block nicotinic receptors or nerve conduction proximal to the postganglionic nerve endings. In guinea-pig colon, PPP (like 7-oxa-13-PA and SC-19220) reduced responses to potassium (Bennett and Posner, 1971). Other evidence of nonselectivity is that PPP 20 $\mu g \ ml^{-1}$ inhibited responses of rat colon to low doses of angiotensin I and II (10 ng ml^{-1}) but not to higher doses (Gagnon and Sirois, 1972).

The PG-blocking activity of PPP resides mainly in the low molecular weight material which has little antihyaluronidase activity (Eakins, 1971; Eakins et al., 1973). When PPP was fractionated on Sephadex G-100 with 0·025 N NaOH, the ability to antagonize $F_{1\alpha}$ on the jird colon was most pronounced in the last fractions which contained the low molecular weight material, and the most active principle was the monomer 4-phloretin phosphate. Acid hydrolysis of PPP increased the antagonist activity due to the formation of dimers devoid of primary phosphoric acid ester groups. The dimer di-4-phloretin phosphate (DPP) was a selective and more potent antagonist of $F_{2\alpha}$ on jird colon compared with PPP, but 4'-phloretin monophosphate, and di-4'-phloretin phosphate were less potent.

The effect of PPP on *rat stomach* illustrates another interesting property of this compound. PPP 20–100 $\mu g \ ml^{-1}$ caused small dose-dependent contractions of rat fundus strips but did not greatly affect responses to E_2, $F_{2\alpha}$, and acetylcholine, whereas higher concentrations of PPP (200–2000 $\mu g \ ml^{-1}$) lowered the tone and reduced the effects of all three agonists (Bennett and Posner, 1971). The explanation for the increase in tone with PPP seems to be inhibition of PG-15-hydroxydehydrogenase which converts PGs to the much less active 15-keto derivatives. There is evidence that PG release maintains the tone of the rat fundus, so that inhibition of PG inactivation would cause contraction. Low concentrations of PPP on the rat fundus (0·05–0·8 $\mu g \ ml^{-1}$) caused temporary dose-dependent potentiations of responses to E_2. Higher doses (1–50 μg ml^{-1}) caused either potentiation or some inhibition of E_2, and with concentrations up to 640 $\mu g \ ml^{-1}$ total blockade occurred (Ganesan and Karim, 1973). At no concentration did PPP potentiate the 15-methyl derivative of E_2 which is resistant to breakdown by PG-15-hydroxydehydrogenase, but PPP 50–640 $\mu g \ ml^{-1}$ antagonized its contractile effect. This was probably nonselective since Bennett and Posner (1971) found that PPP 200–2000 $\mu g \ ml^{-1}$ reduced responses to E_2, $F_{2\alpha}$ and acetylcholine. In another study, however, PPP was found to inhibit $F_{2\alpha}$

more than E_2 or acetylcholine (Collier, 1973). DPP seems more satisfactory on this tissue; 1–50 μg ml^{-1} antagonized E_2 and $F_{2\alpha}$ without affecting responses to KCl, although it somewhat reduced those to acetylcholine (Bennett et al., 1973a).

Eakins et al. (1971) had noticed occasional transient contractions or increased pendular movements of rabbit isolated intestine with PPP (100–200 μg ml^{-1}) and this may well have been due to potentiation of intrinsically released PG which is thought to maintain tone in this tissue (Ferreira et al., 1972). Similarly, PPP 20 μg ml^{-1} stimulated longitudinal muscle strips of human jejunum (Ganesan and Karim, 1973), and sometimes transiently increased the tone of guinea-pig colon (Bennett and Posner, 1971). Other evidence relating PPP and its analogues to inhibition of PG-15-hydroxydehydrogenase will be discussed later. This action might explain why PPP often requires a long contact time to exhibit antagonist activity. Lastly, it should be pointed out that in some tissues PPP caused a reduction in tone (human gastric body and colon, guinea-pig colon, rat fundus with high concentrations) but not in the longitudinal muscle of guinea-pig ileum and jird colon which usually have no tone under the conditions used (Bennett and Posner, 1971). This might indicate antagonism of intrinsically released PG.

2.1.3.2 *Circular muscle in vitro.* In common with the other antagonists, PPP did not antagonize the inhibitory effect of E_2 on gut circular muscle (human gastric body and sigmoid colon, PPP 250–1200 μg ml^{-1}; guinea-pig colon, 200–300 μg ml^{-1}). It did, however, antagonize the contractions to $F_{2\alpha}$ in these tissues in addition to the *relaxations* to $F_{2\alpha}$ which sometimes occurred in human ascending colon, and it generally reduced muscle tone (Bennett and Posner, 1971).

2.1.3.3 *In vivo.* PPP 50–200 mg kg^{-1} given i.p. 15 minutes before injecting E_2 i.v. or i.p. in mice prevented the onset of diarrhoea (Eakins and Fairbairn, quoted by Eakins, 1971, and by Eakins and Sanner, 1972). As with SC-19220, it is not clear whether this is an effect on gut muscle or secretion. Initially, PPP 200 mg kg^{-1} i.v. increased the intra-ileal pressure and sometimes increased the stimulant effect of E_2 and $F_{2\alpha}$ i.v. in anaesthetized cats, but subsequently it antagonized the PGs (Villanueva et al., 1972). The initial stimulation could be interpreted as a block of PG-15-hydroxydehydrogenase, followed by antagonism of PG action. PPP 2 g orally did not antagonize the diarrhoea due to E_2 or $F_{2\alpha}$ in human subjects; larger doses (4 g) induced PG-like diarrhoea, again possibly due to inhibition of the dehydrogenase (Karim, 1973).

2.2   BRONCHIAL AND TRACHEAL MUSCLE

2.2.1   *In vitro*

a. Fenamates. Collier and Sweatman (1968) found that sodium meclofenamate (5) and flufenamate (6) 3×10^{-7} to 3×10^{-6} M antagonized contractions of human bronchial muscle to $F_{2\alpha}$. Contractions to slow reacting substance in anaphylaxis (SRS-A) and tissue tone were also reduced but responses to acetylcholine were unaffected. As with circular gut muscle E_1 and E_2 produced relaxations and these were not antagonized by the fenamates.

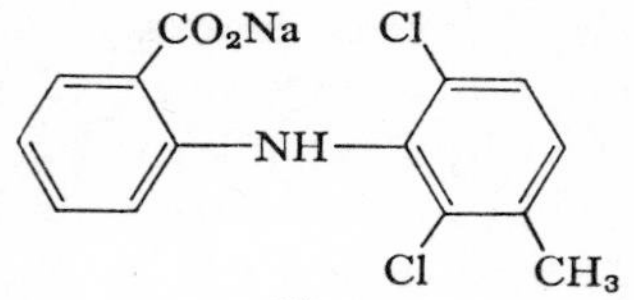

(5)

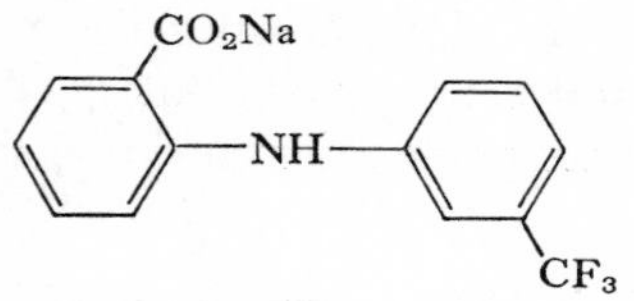

(6)

b. PPP. Concentrations of 10–40 µg ml^{-1} antagonized contractions of *human* isolated bronchial muscle to $F_{2\alpha}$ with a parallel shift of the dose–response curve, but 10–160 µg ml^{-1} did not antagonize relaxations induced by E_1 or E_2. Contractions to acetylcholine or histamine were unaffected at 10–40 µg ml^{-1} PPP but were depressed with 100–160 µg ml^{-1}. PPP caused relaxation, particularly in concentrations above 100 µg ml^{-1} (Mathé *et al.*, 1971). E_1-induced relaxations of *rabbit* isolated tracheal rings were also unaffected by PPP up to 200 µg ml^{-1} (Eakins, 1971). In contrast to human tissue, PPP 300 or 1000 µg ml^{-1} had little or no effect on contractions of *guinea-pig* isolated intact trachea to $F_{2\alpha}$. It reduced the spontaneous activity of the tissue but did not reduce the contraction to transmural stimulation (Coleman, 1973).

As with blockade of SRS-A by fenamates, PPP (12·5–100 µg ml^{-1}) antagonized responses of human bronchial muscle to SRS (an unidentified unsaturated hydroxy fatty acid released from cat paws by compound 48/80) without affecting acetylcholine or histamine (Mathé and Strandberg, 1971). Since no tachyphylaxis occurred they concluded that SRS does not act by releasing PGs, but the data with fenamates and PPP cited above, and the report that SRS-A releases PGs from guinea-pig lung (Piper and Vane, 1969), argue against their view.

c. SC-19220. In *guinea-pig* isolated intact trachea SC-19220 3×10^{-5} M did not affect cumulative dose–response curves to $F_{2\alpha}$, or responses to acetylcholine, histamine, potassium chloride or barium chloride. The maximal responses to these substances increased by 10–50 per cent, but there was no displacement of the dose–response curves to the left if the results were expressed as per cent maximal response. In contrast, the response to co-axial transmural electrical stimulation was virtually abolished (Coleman, 1973), indicating a block of nerve transmission or transmitter release.

Puglisi (1973) obtained results with *guinea-pig* tracheal chains that are contrary to those of everyone else. PPP $0 \cdot 1 \mu g\ ml^{-1}$, SC-19220 3×10^{-7} M and indomethacin $2 \cdot 8 \times 10^{-5}$ M reduced the relaxations produced by E_1 and increased those to $F_{2\alpha}$. The published records do not allow a full interpretation of the results since no constant responses to the PGs were demonstrated before adding the antagonists, and no level of tone was indicated. Thus if the tone were to fall (as happens in the intact isolated guinea-pig trachea with indomethacin, ED50 $1 \cdot 26 \times 10^{-6}$ M; Farmer *et al.*, 1972), the ability to relax to E_1 would decrease and the ability to contract to $F_{2\alpha}$ would increase. Furthermore, the doses of antagonists used are lower than those found to block excitatory responses to the PGs in other tissues.

2.2.2 *In vivo*

a. PPP. Only PPP has been shown to antagonize PGs on the lungs *in vivo.* A dose of 40–80 mg kg^{-1} i.v. inhibited bronchoconstriction caused by $F_{2\alpha}$ in cats and guinea pigs, whereas responses to histamine were either unaffected or even initially increased. PPP (40 mg kg^{-1}) also reduced bronchoconstriction in guinea pigs caused by SRS from cat paws (Mathé *et al.*, 1972). McQueen (1973) found that PPP 40 mg kg^{-1} i.v. in anaesthetized guinea-pigs antagonized bronchoconstriction to $F_{2\alpha}$ without reducing the increase in respiration rate with $F_{2\alpha}$ or E_2, but this dose sometimes caused death due to hypotension. Villanueva *et al.* (1972) used 200 mg kg^{-1} PPP i.v. in cats to block the bronchoconstrictor effect of $F_{2\alpha}$ i.v., and they found this effect harder to block than the increased intra-ileal pressure and hypotension.

b. Fenamates. Although fenamates antagonized $F_{2\alpha}$ on human isolated trachea, they did not antagonize $F_{2\alpha}$-induced bronchoconstriction in anaesthetized guinea-pigs (Collier and Sweatman, 1968).

2.3 BLOOD VESSELS

The effects of PGs may vary with the type of blood vessel, the species, and the vascular bed. Unlike many other tissues, much of the work on blood vessels has been *in vivo* since it is relatively easy to measure changes in blood pressure. However, it is important to remember that *in vivo* measurements may be a composite of several possible factors.

2.3.1 *In vitro*

All the *in vitro* work seems to have been done on helical strips of human umbilical arteries by Park and Dyer (1972: 1973) and Park *et al.* (1972). SC-19220 10^{-4} M slightly antagonized contractions to E_2 but responses to 5-HT were reduced almost as much. PPP 10 μg ml^{-1} antagonized E_2 without affecting 5-HT, but at 100 μg ml^{-1} the shift to the right of dose–response curves for E_2 and 5-HT were 9 and 3·6 respectively. The antagonism of 5-HT is unlikely to be due to block of a nerve-mediated action (see section 2) since the umbilical arteries are thought to be without innervation (Boyd and Hamilton, 1970). 7-Oxa-13-PA $3·25 \times 10^{-7}$ M and above caused the arteries to contract (thus resembling its effect on the rat fundus), but when $3·25 \times 10^{-5}$ M was left in contact with the tissue for 30 minutes the initial contraction was followed by a relaxation to about 10 per cent of the maximal contraction to 5-HT. Under these conditions the dose–response curve for E_2 was shifted to the right about 100-fold without altering responses to 5-HT.

2.3.2 *In vivo*

Vascular responses have been studied in a variety of species *in vivo*, using PPP almost exclusively. The first report showed that PPP 25–200 mg kg^{-1} i.v. in *rabbits* caused a variable antagonism of the fall in blood pressure produced by $F_{2\alpha}$ without altering the hypotensive effects of E_2 or acetylcholine (Eakins *et al.*, 1970). This is another example of an inhibitory effect to PGE compounds which is not blocked by PG antagonists, but the fact that $F_{2\alpha}$ was antagonized indicates that the PGE and F receptors are different. Levy and Lindner (1971) found that PPP in doses up to 94 mg kg^{-1} in 2 rabbits did not significantly inhibit the vasodepressor effect of either $F_{2\alpha}$ or E_1. Apart from the small number of animals studied, the discrepancy in results might be attributable to the fact that the dose was less than half the maximum used by Eakins *et al.* (1970), that batch variations probably occur with PPP, or that relatively low amounts of PPP inhibit PG-15-hydroxydehydrogenase, thus tending to potentiate PG effects with inadequate blocking concentrations. Meclofenamic acid 30 mg kg^{-1} i.v. over 20 minutes antagonized the fall in blood pressure with $F_{2\alpha}$ and even reversed the responses, but did not antagonize the hypotensive effects of E_1 or isoprenaline (Levy and Lindner, 1971).

In guinea-pigs anaesthetized with sodium pentobarbitone PPP 40–80 mg infused i.v. over 5–15 minutes sometimes caused a fall in blood pressure and 2 of the 30 animals died (Mathé et al., 1972). At 80 mg kg^{-1} the rise in blood pressure to $F_{2\alpha}$ was reduced by about 50 per cent. In addition the hypertensive effect of SRS "seemed to be antagonized", but there was not enough material for a quantitative study (PPP also antagonizes the effects of SRS on lung tissue, see sections 2.2.1 and 2.2.2). As stated before, McQueen (1973) also found PPP to be rather toxic in guinea-pigs anaesthetized with sodium pentobarbitone or urethane. PPP 40 mg kg^{-1} caused hypotension but it antagonized the pressor effect of $F_{2\alpha}$. The hypotensive effect of E_2 was not antagonized, although after PPP the blood pressure recovered more rapidly. The meaning of this faster recovery is not clear in view of the lower blood pressure following PPP. In *cats* where $F_{2\alpha}$ is hypotensive, PPP 80 mg kg^{-1} approximately halved the response (Mathé et al., 1971) and PPP 200 mg kg^{-1} caused a transient hypotension, but blocked and sometimes even reversed the response to $F_{2\alpha}$ (Villanueva et al., 1972). The hypotension with $F_{2\alpha}$ in anaesthetized cats seems due to a variable and transient fall in peripheral resistance, a decrease in aortic flow following a rise in pulmonary artery pressure, and delayed bradycardia related to both afferent and efferent vagal excitation (Koss et al., 1973). According to these authors, meclofenamic acid 30 mg kg^{-1} selectively blocked the $F_{2\alpha}$-induced vagal activation, but Al-Jubouri and Paterson (1973) found that the vasodilator effects of $F_{2\alpha}$, E_2, and A_2 in cat limbs perfused at constant pressure were reduced or abolished. The mean fall in systemic blood pressure and the effects of isoprenaline were also somewhat reduced.

In anaesthetized *dogs* dilatation of the femoral artery to E_1, E_2, and A_2, and constriction of the pulmonary artery to $F_{2\alpha}$ were not blocked by prior or simultaneous administration of 7-oxa-13-PA $3 \cdot 25 \times 10^{-7}$ to $6 \cdot 5 \times 10^{-7}$ mol kg^{-1} or $3 \cdot 25 \times 10^{-8}$ mol kg^{-1} min^{-1}; SC-19220 3×10^{-7} to 6×10^{-6} mol kg^{-1}, or PPP 1 to 3 mg kg^{-1} (Nakano et al., 1971; Nakano, 1972). By contrast, White and Pennick (1972) found that PPP 100 mg kg^{-1} i.v. reversed the pressor effect of $F_{2\alpha}$ into a prolonged fall. A smaller dose of 50 mg kg^{-1} produced reversal in some animals but it enhanced the hypotensive effect of E_1 and E_2 and shortened that of A_1 and A_2. This might indicate an enhancement of PGE compounds by inhibition of PG-15-hydroxydehydrogenase, and some antagonism of

PGA compounds which are less susceptible to this enzyme (Änggård and Samuelsson, 1967).

Rosek (1970) (cited by Eakins and Sanner, 1972) found that SC-19220 reduced the vasopressor response to E_2 in *rats*. This is the only report of vasodepressor effect of an E compound being inhibited by a PG antagonist. It remains to be confirmed, and has not been published. The antagonist properties of PPP in the rat have not been studied, but such an investigation would be facilitated by the fact that up to 640 mg kg^{-1} PPP does not lower blood pressure (Mathé *et al.*, 1971).

Epicerebral blood vessels are constricted by E_1 and $F_{2\alpha}$ in the dog and by E_1 in the Macaque monkey, and this is prevented by intracarotid ethanol 0·09–0·5 per cent (Yamamoto *et al.*, 1973). It is interesting that Karim and Sharma (1971) found that excessive uterine stimulation following PG administration on obstetric patients was stopped by ethanol i.v., but whether these are merely nonspecific narcotic effects is not known. It seems unlikely to be due to inhibition of PG synthetase since ethanol 0·2 to 2 per cent did not inhibit synthetase in human gut (Bennett *et al.*, 1973c). Blood vessels are also discussed below in section 3.

3 The eye

As with blood vessels, most of the work has been done *in vivo* with PPP. It has concerned mainly changes in intraocular pressure and vasomotor events.

In vitro

The contractions of bovine sphincter pupillae to E_2 were selectively antagonized by SC-19220 5×10^{-7} to 5×10^{-6} M (Posner, 1971; 1973). Chloride transport in frog corneal epithelium *in vitro* was stimulated by E_1, E_2, and $F_{2\alpha}$; PPP and DPP (concentrations not stated) inhibited the responses to E_1 if added 2 minutes before (Beitch *et al.*, 1973).

In vivo

Except for one study in monkeys, all the *in vivo* experiments have been in rabbits mainly with PPP or its allied substances injected (close-arterially, intravenously, subconjunctivally or intravitreally), or instilled into the conjunctival sac. E_1 and E_2 raise the intraocular pressure (IOP) and protein content of the aqueous humour and cause vasodilatation of the iris vessels. $F_{2\alpha}$ acts similarly but is less potent. In rabbits, PPP 0·5 mg per minute infused close-arterially markedly reduced the rise in

IOP and protein content induced by E_1 1 µg injected intraocularly (Beitch and Eakins, 1969), and rates above 0·25 mg per minute reduced the IOP rise with E_1 i.v. (Starr, 1971). Intravitreal injection of PPP 20–24 h previously inhibited the IOP rise with E_1 i.v., and instead a prolonged fall occurred (PPP ED50 50 µg) (Starr, 1971). It is interesting that Cole (1961) had observed that PPP converted the rise in IOP following irritation by mustine to a fall in IOP. In monkeys, however, PPP 1 mg injected into the anterior chamber had virtually no effect on the rises in IOP or protein content caused by the intraocular injection of E_1, E_2, or $F_{1\alpha}$.

Parenteral injection or application of PPP seems less effective in rabbits than close arterial or intraocular administration. Bethel and Eakins (1971a; 1971b) found that PPP 100 mg kg^{-1} i.v. slightly antagonized responses to $F_{2\alpha}$ but not to E_2 or formaldehyde applied topically; instillation of PPP 10 mg into the eye inhibited the IOP rise with applied $F_{2\alpha}$, slightly reduced the response to formaldehyde, but had no effect on E_2. However, subconjunctival administration of this amount of PPP abolished or greatly reduced the rise in IOP to all three substances, but there was no effect on the conjunctival vasodilatation. They thought that the different results with instillation and subconjunctival administration might be due to either prolonged availability with subconjunctival administration, or differences in penetration across the cornea and conjunctiva. Subconjunctival injection of the low molecular weight fraction of PPP also inhibited the IOP rise with E_2, $F_{2\alpha}$, and formaldehyde. The high molecular weight fraction was active only against formaldehyde, possibly by inhibition of penetration due to its antihyaluronidase activity (Bethel and Eakins, 1971b). Other evidence linking inhibition of hyaluronidase to a reduction of inflammation has been found in rat paws (Fabinyi-Szebehely et al., 1953).

Studies using fluorescein angiography (Whitelocke and Eakins, 1973a; 1973b; Whitelocke et al., 1973) confirmed that PPP instilled into the eye or injected subconjunctivally antagonized E_1- or E_2-induced rise in IOP, the increase of capillary permeability and the vasodilatation of iris vessels (as opposed to dilatation of conjunctival vessels which was unaffected; Bethel and Eakins, 1971a; 1971b). They found that both the high molecular weight fraction of PPP and di-4-phloretin phosphate (DPP) were inactive as PG antagonists, but a later study (Whitelocke and Eakins, 1973b) showed that subconjunctivally injected DPP actually increased the response to applied E_1, probably by inhibiting PG-15-hydroxydehydrogenase (Crutchley and Piper, 1973).

Chiang and Thomas (1972) have studied other antagonists in the rabbit eye in addition to PPP, but they examined only the consensual response (rise in IOP in one eye following intracameral injection of E_1 in the contralateral eye) which was possibly due to transfer of E_1 via the blood circulation. The consensual response was prevented by cross-infusion of PPP into the lingual artery, but not by topically applied SC-19220, and paradoxically it was enhanced by intravitreous PPP, topical PPP and 7-oxa-13-PA or its solvent, probably due to nonspecific irritation.

4   Antagonism in tissues where cAMP has been measured

PGs seem to exert their effects through the adenylate cyclase/cAMP system in many tissues. Measurements of cAMP have been made in adipose tissue, ovary, myometrium, thyroid, anterior pituitary, adrenals, and bladder, following treatment with PGs and their antagonists.

4.1   LIPOLYSIS

Lipolysis in fat cells appears to be regulated partly by cAMP (Butcher and Sutherland, 1967). Illiano and Cuatrecasas (1971) found that adrenaline-induced lipolysis in rat epididymal fat cells was inhibited by E_1 and E_2 and enhanced by 7-oxa-13-PA $3 \cdot 25 \times 10^{-5}$ to $1 \cdot 63 \times 10^{-4}$ M or SC-19220 $3 \cdot 6 \times 10^{-5}$ M. Furthermore, 7-oxa-13-PA greatly antagonized (about 70 per cent at $3 \cdot 25 \times 10^{-5}$ M and 90 per cent at $1 \cdot 63 \times 10^{-4}$ M) the inhibitory effect of E_1, and SC-19220 $7 \cdot 5 \times 10^{-5}$ M abolished the effect of E_2. Different PGs were used with each antagonist, and the relation of this to the degree of block is not clear. They state that Sanner's data (1969; 1971b) shows that SC-19220 is much more potent against E_2 than E_1, but in fact the difference was slight and was not significant at any one concentration of antagonist. Neither 7-oxa-13-PA nor SC-19220 affected basal lipolysis, whereas the PG synthetase inhibitor indomethacin caused an increase. Illiano and Cuatrecasas (1971) therefore suggested that different PGs might be involved in the control of basal and stimulated lipolysis. Radzialowski and Novak (1971; 1973) also found that SC-19220 10^{-6} to 10^{-4} M antagonized the E_2-inhibition of adrenaline-stimulated lipolysis in rat epididymal fat pad cells. A plateau of about 60 per cent inhibition occurred between 10^{-5} and 10^{-4} M. As with the findings of Illiano and Cuatrecasas, SC-19220 did not stimulate basal lipolysis, but in contrast to their data it did not potentiate the effect of adrenaline. Some degree of selectivity for SC-19220 was adduced from the finding that it did not reverse the inhibition of adrenaline-stimulated lipolysis by propranolol or insulin.

The site of PG antagonist binding has been studied with ^{3}H-PGE$_2$ in rat adipocytes. 7-Oxa-13-PA, but not SC-19220, PPP or 15-keto

PGE_1, bound to E_2 receptors (Kuehl and Humes, 1972). They concluded that PPP may act after PG binding has occurred (Kuehl *et al.*, 1971), but the nature of the block with SC-19220 was unexplained (see section 5).

4.2 OVARY AND MYOMETRIUM

These are discussed in conjunction since they have been reported on together by Kuehl and his colleagues.

a. *7-Oxa-13-PA*. Stimulation of cAMP production by E_1 and E_2 in the *mouse* ovary was antagonized by 1·63 to 2·44 × 10^{-4} M 7-oxa-13-PA in a competitive manner (K_i 6 × 10^{-5} M for E_1; 3 × 10^{-5} M for E_2; Lineweaver–Burk plots), and E_1-stimulated secretion of progesterone was blocked. This is the first instance cited where there is antagonism of a response known to be associated with an increase in cAMP. The response to luteinizing hormone (LH) was also antagonized (K_i 5 × 10^{-5} M) but there was no effect on basal cAMP formation (Kuehl *et al.*, 1972). These workers suggested that LH may act through PG release and this is supported by the finding that homogenates of rat ovaries pretreated with LH antiserum have a depressed ability to synthesize E_2 whereas addition of LH increases PG synthetase activity (Chasalow and Pharriss, 1972). However, it is possible that the antagonism was non-selective since the concentrations used have been found to depress guinea-pig ileum nonselectively (Bennett and Posner, 1971), to inhibit protein synthesis (Ahrén and Perklev, 1972) and, when administered with E_2, to cause necrotic changes in monkey cultured granulosa cells (Channing, 1972). Furthermore, the synthetase inhibitor fluoroindomethacin did not inhibit the action of LH on cAMP production in mouse ovary or bovine luteal cells whilst preventing synthesis of PGs from added arachidonic acid (Kuehl *et al.*, 1973).

In *monkey* cultured granulosa cells, 7-oxa-13-PA 1·63 × 10^{-4} M caused slight stimulation of luteinization, but it blocked stimulation by E_2 (Channing, 1972). However, in cultured *porcine* granulosa cells, there was no antagonism of E_2 or LH by 1·63 × 10^{-4} M or 3·25 × 10^{-4} M 7-oxa-13-PA (Kolena and Channing, 1972) and "heroic levels" of 7-oxa-13-PA (6·5 × 10^{-4} M) were required to block PG and LH in *bovine* luteal cells (Kuehl *et al.*, 1973). In trying to explain species differences in sensitivity to 7-oxa-13-PA, Kolena and Channing (1972) point out that the mouse ovaries used by Kuehl and his colleagues are a heterogenous cell system whereas the porcine and bovine tissues are respectively homogenous or almost homogenous.

7-Oxa-13-PA (3·25 × 10^{-5} to 3·25 × 10^{-4} M), LH and E_1 all stimulated *rat* ovarian glycogenolysis, so that here is another example of agonism rather than antagonism with the prostynoic acid derivative. In contrast, E_1 but not 7-oxa-13-PA increased the rate of aminoacid uptake and incorporation into protein. The response to E_1 was unaffected by $3·25 \times 10^{-5}$ M 7-oxa-13-PA but at the rather high concentration of $1·63 \times 10^{-4}$ M uptake and incorporation were reduced without affecting protein synthesis. At $3·25 \times 10^{-4}$ M uptake and incorporation were blocked and protein synthesis was also inhibited (Ahrén and Perklev, 1973).

   b. PPP. Contrary to 7-oxa-13-PA, PPP 200 µg ml^{-1} had little effect on E_1-induced cAMP formation in either mouse ovary or rabbit myometrium, but PPP 150 µg ml^{-1} reduced the stimulation of progesterone formation by E_1 (Kuehl et al., 1971; 1973). However, PPP 150 µg ml^{-1} and low molecular weight PPP 75–200 µg ml^{-1} also reduced the progesterone formation in the ovary by dibutyryl-cAMP (DBcAMP), and displaced ^{3}H-cAMP from its receptors (ratio of 10 000:1 of PPP etc. to cAMP) (Kuehl et al., 1971). The authors suggested that PPP is not a true PG antagonist, and that block of protein kinase would account for the inhibition of PG action; PPP and its high and low molecular weight fractions inhibited this enzyme. However, this explanation is not applicable when PPP antagonizes responses to PGE compounds which are associated with inhibition of adenylate cyclase/cAMP (e.g. possibly contraction in gut muscle and uterus).

   In the isolated prepubertal rat ovary PPP in the high concentration of 5 mg ml^{-1} reduced the stimulation of lactic acid production by PGE_1 and LH, but the inhibition was less than 50 per cent. No experiments were performed to assess selectivity (Perklev and Ahrén, 1971).

4.3   THYROID

4.3.1   Bovine

a. 7-Oxa-13-PA. $1·6 \times 10^{-5}$ M significantly inhibited stimulation of adenylate cyclase by E_2, thyroid stimulating hormone (TSH) and long-acting thyroid stimulator in bovine isolated thyroid cells, without affecting basal activity (Burke and Sato, 1971), and 7-oxa-13-PA $1·6 \times 10^{-5}$ to $4·9 \times 10^{-5}$ M inhibited the stimulation of iodide trapping without affecting the response to dibutyryl-cAMP or NH_4^+ (Burke et al., 1971a). This is the second report cited in which 7-oxa-13-PA antagonized a response to E_2 known to be associated with stimulation of adenylate cyclase. At doses of $8·1 \times 10^{-6}$ to $6·5 \times 10^{-5}$ M, 7-oxa-13-PA showed weak agonism. Sato et al. (1972a) also found that both 7-oxa-13-PA and 7-oxa-15-hydroxy-13-PA (both approximately 8×10^{-6} to $6·5 \times 10^{-5}$ M) had slight agonist properties, but 8×10^{-6} to $1·6 \times$

10^{-5} M 7-oxa-13-PA and $> 1.75 \times 10^{-5}$ M 7-oxa-15-hydroxy-13-PA inhibited stimulation of adenylate cyclase by E_1, E_2, and TSH in isolated bovine thyroid cells. 7-Oxa-13-PA (1.6 to 3.2×10^{-5} M) antagonized E_1- and TSH-induced phagocytosis of latex beads. The picture is even more complicated since ineffective or minimally effective concentrations of E_1 or E_2 reduced adenylate cyclase activation by a maximally effective concentration of TSH, and vice versa with a low concentration of TSH.

b. PPP. As with 7-oxa-13-PA, PPP 5 μg ml^{-1} significantly inhibited stimulation of adenylate cyclase by E_2, TSH and long-acting thyroid stimulator in bovine isolated thyroid cells without affecting basal activity (Burke and Sato, 1971). This is the first report cited of antagonism by PPP of a response to E_2 known to be associated with stimulation of adenylate cyclase. It is confirmed by the findings that PPP 1–25 μg ml^{-1} caused dose-dependent inhibition of TSH- and E_2-stimulation of adenylate cyclase without affecting basal levels, although the curves were not displaced in parallel (Sato *et al.*, 1972b). However, the picture is again complex. At 10–100 μg ml^{-1} an opposite effect occurred: the ability to trap ^{131}I increased, as it did with TSH, dibutyryl-cAMP or E_2 alone. The effect of PPP summated with TSH or dibutyryl-cAMP, but was reduced by E_2. At 25–100 μg ml^{-1} the thyroid cells were stimulated to trap latex beads (again as occurred with TSH, dibutyryl-cAMP or E_2 alone) and, as with iodine-trapping, PPP summated with TSH and dibutyryl-cAMP but was reduced by E_2. In contrast to TSH or dibutyryl-cAMP, E_2 was consistently antagonized by PPP 5 μg ml^{-1}. The low molecular weight fraction of PPP was responsible for antagonism of E_2 and TSH, whereas the high molecular weight fraction was responsible for stimulation of iodide trapping and bead phagocytosis.

4.3.2 Dog

In dog thyroid slices 7-oxa-13-PA antagonized the stimulation of cAMP production (at 2 to 7.5×10^{-4} M) and colloid droplet formation (at 3.5×10^{-4} M) by E_2 and TSH (Sato *et al.*, 1972a). Because these high concentrations of antagonist had no effect on basal cAMP levels, and the effect of dibutyryl-cAMP on colloid formation was unaltered, the authors considered that PG release may be an important part in the action of TSH. Before such a suggestion can be accepted, however, much more rigorous proof of selectivity of action etc. must be produced, particularly since Wolff and Moore (1973) found that indomethacin failed to alter responses to TSH in various thyroid preparations. It should also be noted that they used 10^{-3} to 10^{-6} M concentrations of PGE compounds to produce stimulation, although smaller amounts would presumably have been effective.

4.3.2 *Mouse in vivo*

PPP 0·5 mg per mouse inhibited the release of radio-iodine from the thyroid following TSH or long-acting thyroid stimulator without affecting the response to dibutyryl-cAMP (Burke and Sato, 1971). The effect on response to PGs was not reported.

4.4 ANTERIOR PITUITARY

Vale *et al.* (1971) reported that 7-oxa-13-PA 3×10^{-5} M inhibited the release of TSH *in vitro* by TSH releasing factor in *rat* anterior pituitary, and decreased K^+-induced release. They concluded that PG receptors may be involved, but again no evidence of selectivity was obtained. Although E_1 $2·8 \times 10^{-6}$ to $2·8 \times 10^{-5}$ M stimulated TSH release they did not even study its response in the presence of the antagonist. In contrast, Tal *et al.* (1974) found no effect with 7-oxa-13-PA $3·25 \times 10^{-4}$ M on the increased TSH output with TSH releasing factor in this tissue. Furthermore, E_1 5×10^{-5} M did not release TSH; E_1 caused an increase in cAMP levels which was not affected by 7-oxa-13-PA $3·25 \times 10^{-4}$ M, and this concentration of the drug itself slightly increased cAMP levels.

Hedge (1972) stimulated secretion of ACTH in dexamethasone-pretreated rats by injecting E_1, $F_{1\alpha}$, or $F_{2\alpha}$ into the median eminence of the hypothalamus. 7-Oxa-13-PA $8·1 \times 10^{-9}$ mol injected into this site reduced the response to E_1 by about 40 per cent but had no significant effect on the response to $F_{1\alpha}$. Higher doses could not be used by this route because of solubility, but $8·1 \times 10^{-8}$ to $1·62 \times 10^{-6}$ mol kg^{-1} injected into the tail vein of normal rats had no effect on ACTH secretion stimulated by E_1 i.v. or by stress. PPP 250 µg injected into the median eminence stimulated ACTH secretion and was therefore not studied further.

7-Oxa-13-PA $3·25 \times 10^{-5}$, $1·63 \times 10^{-4}$, and $6·5 \times 10^{-4}$ M *in vitro* inhibited the stimulation of growth hormone (GH) release and cAMP production by E_1 in a dose-dependent manner. It had no effect on basal levels, and at $1·63 \times 10^{-4}$ M there was no effect on GH secretion stimulated by theophylline or dibutyryl-cAMP (Ratner *et al.*, 1973). Thus there might be a PG link in the release of the hormone in response to its releasing factor, but the authors consider that since purified growth hormone releasing factor stimulates cGMP but not cAMP (unpublished data of Peake and Steiner, cited by Ratner *et al.*, 1973), the releasing factor may not act through a PG receptor but on another receptor linked to guanyl cyclase. This makes the assumption that PG receptors are not linked to guanyl cyclase, but such a relation is possible in view of data on rat uterus (Kuehl *et al.*, 1973).

Again, with rat anterior pituitaries *in vitro*, Makino (1973) found that 7-oxa-13-PA (1.6×10^{-5} M) or indomethacin (1.4×10^{-6} M) did not alter basal release of LH, FSH or cAMP. Hormone and cAMP production in response to synthetic gonadotrophin-releasing factor was also unaffected except for a small reduction of LH secretion with 7-oxa-13-PA (1.6×10^{-5} M).

4.5 KIDNEY

Both PGE_1 10^{-7} M and 7-oxa-13-PA 10^{-7} M inhibited the increase in cAMP production induced by vasopressin in crude homogenates of golden hamster kidney (Marumo and Edelman, 1971). Here 7-oxa-13-PA was again clearly acting as an agonist. In rabbit renal medulla E_1, E_2, and $F_{2\alpha}$ inhibited vasopressin-induced cAMP production. SC-19220 (concentration not stated) potentiated the effect of $F_{2\alpha}$ (Kalisker, 1972). The content of prostaglandins in the kidney of hypertensive rats was not altered by pretreatment with PPP 50 mg kg^{-1} i.v. or 7-oxa-13-PA 8.1×10^{-7} mol kg^{-1} (Somova, 1973). This indicates no alteration of PG metabolism whereas both drugs appear to inhibit PG synthetase and PG-15-hydroxydehydrogenase *in vitro* (see sections 5.15 and 5.16).

4.6 TOAD BLADDER

E_1 inhibits water flow in response to antidiuretic hormone (ADH) and theophylline, probably by inhibiting adenylate cyclase. 7-Oxa-13-PA 1.2×10^{-5} M antagonized the effect of E_1 10^{-11} M but not 10^{-10} or 10^{-9} M although the response to E_1 10^{-10} M was submaximal. It also caused a small but significant increase of water flow which was ascribed to stimulation of adenylate cyclase (Ozer and Sharp, 1972). However, another explanation might be that PG released in the tissue was being antagonized. This is supported by their finding that the PG precursor arachidonic acid reduced the effect of ADH and theophylline, and it could also explain why the antagonist enhanced a submaximal response to ADH. On the other hand, 7-oxa-13-PA 1.2×10^{-5} M still slightly increased the rate of water flow to theophylline after pretreatment with indomethacin 2.8×10^{-6} M (Flores and Sharp, 1972), but PG synthesis may not have been completely inhibited by indomethacin.

PPP 50 μg ml^{-1} antagonized the inhibitory effect of E_1 10^{-10} M and 10^{-9} M, but not 10^{-8} M which was supramaximal (Ozer and Sharp, 1972). It did not affect basal flow or the response to dibutyryl-cAMP but it markedly increased the effect of theophylline (which prevents cAMP breakdown) and, as with 7-oxa-13-PA, it enhanced a submaximal reponse to ADH. These effects did not appear to be due to impurities of pyridine in PPP. In contrast SC-19220 (up to 4×10^{-4} M) did not antagonize E_1 or affect responses to ADH and theophylline. None of the antagonists affected sodium transport either in the presence or absence of E_1 10^{-7} M. Ozer and Sharp (1973) claimed that the effects of chloropropamide were identical to those of 7-oxa-13-PA. It antagonized the effect of low doses of E_1 on the toad bladder, but a high concentration of chloropropamide (10^{-3} M) was used and no evidence of selectivity was presented. In rat kidney slices, vasopressin stimulated cAMP production and this was reduced by E_1 10^{-8} M. Pretreatment of the rats with chlorpropanide (dose not stated) prevented the inhibition by E_1 (Bode et al., 1973). These findings are difficult to reconcile with those of Hays and Ingelfinger (1969) who found that chlorpropamide 3×10^{-4} M enhanced the effect of E_1 on toad bladder.

5   Miscellaneous

Included under this heading are actions of the antagonists that do not as yet merit a section of their own. In some instances the effects observed may be independent of their action at PG receptors.

Uterus

PPP 2·5–30 µg ml^{-1} reversibly antagonized the contractions of rabbit isolated uterus to E_2 and $F_{2\alpha}$, but the block was long-lasting. Both PGs were antagonized equally, without affecting contractions to acetylcholine or adrenaline (Eakins et al., 1970). *In vivo*, by contrast, up to 94 mg kg^{-1} PPP or 30 mg kg^{-1} meclofenamic acid did not block stimulation of rabbit uterine and oviduct motility by $F_{2\alpha}$, or inhibition of oviduct motility with E_1 (Levy and Lindner, 1971). However, although there were 6 experiments with meclofenamic acid, there were only 2 with PPP. 7-Oxa-13-PA was reported to be nonselective on rat uterus, but no details were given (Flack, 1970). Johnson et al. (1974) found that 7-oxa-13-PA, $3·25 \times 10^{-5}$ M, blocked responses of this tissue to E_2, but selectivity was not studied. SC-19220 10^{-5} M reversibly reduced responses of guinea-pig isolated uterus to E_2 and $F_{2\alpha}$ without affecting those to acetylcholine (Bennett and Posner, 1972).

Vas deferens

SC-19220 did not block E_2 inhibition of the electrically stimulated guinea-pig vas deferens *in vitro*, but no concentration was stated (Ambache and Zar, 1970). Hedqvist and von Euler (1972) found that in this tissue the response to postganglionic nerve stimulation was reduced by low doses of E_1 or E_2 due to inhibition of transmitter release and increased by high doses, and that E_1 increased the effect of exogenous noradrenaline. SC-19220 10^{-4} M antagonized the potentiating effects of E_1 but not the inhibition. The latter was also unaffected by PPP in the low concentration of 1 µg ml^{-1}.

Capillary permeability

PPP 10 mg applied to the rabbit eye or injected subconjunctivally antagonized the increase in capillary permeability to PGE compounds (Eakins, 1971; Whitelocke and Eakins, 1973a; 1973b).

Inflammation

Eakins and Sanner (1972) reported that SC-19220 had no anti-inflammatory activity, but since there is increasing evidence that PGs are involved in inflammation (Vane, 1971; 1972) Sanner and Aspinal (1973) re-investigated this aspect. They found that SC-19220 34 mg kg^{-1} i.p. inhibited mycoplasma-induced arthritis in mice; and 100 mg kg^{-1} intragastrically (but not 25 mg kg^{-1} s.c. or intragastrically) inhibited granuloma formation around cotton pellet implants in adrenalectomized rats. However, in other experiments in rats there was no effect on adjuvant-induced arthritis (SC-19220 20 mg kg^{-1} s.c.) or carrageenin-induced foot oedema (200 mg kg^{-1} s.c.). Thus with parenteral administration of this low-solubility drug there is a hint of anti-inflammatory activity in some tests but not in others. Topical anti-inflammatory effects were a little more impressive. It had approximately 10 per cent of the ability of hydrocortisone to inhibit croton oil-induced inflammation of rat ears, and in rats injected i.v. with Evans blue, application of 1 per cent solution of SC-19220 in organic solvents reduced the skin blueing induced by chemical irritation or ultraviolet irradiation.

Skin

7-Oxa-13-PA intradermally reduced the erythrema due to ultraviolet irradiation of guinea-pig skin (Snyder and Eaglestein, 1973). Pretreatment of human skin with three intradermal injections of 100 µg PPP at hourly intervals reduced the erythrema but not the wheal formation in response to 1 µg PGE_1 injected at the same site (Søndergaard and Jørgensen, 1973).

Bone resorption

PPP 100 μg ml^{-1} markedly reduced the resorption of mouse calvaria by human dental cyst incubates which contained PG-like material (Harris *et al.*, 1973) and PPP 20 μg ml^{-1} or SC-19220 6 $\times$ 10^{-5} M inhibited PG-induced resorption in rat foetal bone (Goodson, 1973). PPP (100 μg ml^{-1}) also blocked resorption by 25-hydroxycholecalciferol (100 ng ml^{-1}), vitamin A (2 μg ml^{-1}) or parathyroid extract (0.1 u ml^{-1}) in mouse cultured calvarium (Harris *et al.*, 1974).

Calcification

Calcification induced in some rat tissues by dihydrotachysterol was inhibited by daily s.c. injections of PPP 10 mg kg^{-1} (Casey *et al.*, 1972). The authors suggest that this effect might be due to inhibition of phosphatases, to inhibition of calcium phosphate precipitation or to PG antagonism.

Gastric acid secretion

SC-19220 7.5 $\times$ 10^{-7} to 1.5 $\times$ 10^{-6} mol kg^{-1} administered i.p. as a suspension in 0.1 per cent polysorbate 80 to pylorus-ligated rats did not antagonize E$_1$-induced inhibition of gastric acid secretion (Engel *et al.*, 1973).

Histamine, mast cells, and anaphylaxis

Only PPP has been studied in these respects, and its effects did not appear to be due to PG antagonism. At 50–100 μg ml^{-1} it greatly inhibited rat mast cell disruption by compound 48/80 and there was a slight effect at 25 μg ml^{-1} (Högberg and Uvnas, 1957). At a concentration of 200 μg ml^{-1}, it abolished the release of histamine by compound 48/80 from rat lung, and at 100 and 1000 μg ml^{-1} but not 10 μg ml^{-1} it inhibited histamine release from pieces of guinea-pig lung (Chakravarty, 1960). PPP 100 μg ml^{-1} antagonized the anaphylactic release of SRS-A and histamine from guinea-pig minced lungs by about 60 per cent (Fredholm and Strandberg, 1973a). When PPP was dialysed into 4 fractions, all inhibited histamine release by compound 48/80 from rat mast cells. The first three fractions were good PG antagonists but the fourth, which had good antihyaluronidase activity, had no PG antagonist activity. Polyphloroglucinol, which had even higher anti-enzyme activity but no PG antagonist properties, had an even greater inhibitory effect on histamine release. These inhibitions seemed due at least partly to chemical interaction with compound 48/80 (Strandberg, 1973). PPP is also effective *in vivo*, since 20 or 40 mg kg^{-1} i.v. in conscious sensitized guinea-pigs protected against convulsions to aerosols of antigen but not of carbachol (Strandberg *et al.*, 1972; Fredholm and Strandberg, 1973a). However, PPP also prolonged the onset of convulsions to aerosols of histamine in conscious guinea-pigs (Strandberg *et al.*, 1973a) and this is an additional property to that of inhibiting histamine release. In contrast, 40–80 mg kg^{-1} PPP i.v. in anaesthetized cats or guinea-pigs did not antagonize bronchoconstriction induced by histamine i.v. (Mathé *et al.*, 1972).

Red blood cells

PPP in high concentrations (1–3 mg ml^{-1}) inhibits the aggregation of red blood cells. This was thought to be due to the negative electrical charge of PPP (Fries, 1959). 7-Oxa-13-PA 6·5 $\times$ 10^{-4} M modifies the sickling induced by E$_2$ in erythrocytes from patients with sickle cell disease (Rabinowitz, 1973).

Platelets

PPP 30–50 mg kg^{-1} i.v. in dogs inhibited platelet aggregation and the subsequent release of vasoactive substances (Swedenborg, 1973a; 1973b). A protective effect also occurred with rat platelets *in vitro* (Fredholm and Strandberg, 1973b) but not with 7-oxa-13-PA against an unspecified PG (Flack, 1970).

Fertility

PPP 10 mg daily by mouth to rats (approximately 50 mg kg^{-1}) lowered fertility. This was thought to be due to its antihyaluronidase activity (Wohlzogen, 1961).

Adenosine triphosphatase (ATPase) and adenylate kinase

Johnson and Ramwell (1973) found that 7-oxa-13-PA (usually 1·5 to 3 $\times$ 10^{-5} M) activated ATPase from human platelets, human erythrocytes, and rat liver mitochondria. The platelet and erythrocyte adenylate kinases were also activated, but the enzyme from skeletal muscle was inhibited.

Central nervous system

SC-19220 in common with some other dibenzoxazepine derivatives was found to have anticonvulsant and analgesic properties (Coyne and Cusic,

1968). However, CNS effects do not correlate with anti-PG activity (Sanner, 1971b), and the anticonvulsant diphenylhydantoin 0·8 to 2×10^{-5} M did not antagonize E_2 on the rat stomach strip (Bennett *et al.*, 1973d). It is interesting that in the CNS tests with SC-19220 the solvent included polysorbate which is now known to increase the potency of SC-19220 (Sanner, 1972). In the original tests for anti-inflammatory activity, polysorbate was not used and no activity was detected.

Inhibition of PG-synthetase

7-Oxa-13-PA derivatives and especially 5-oxa-13-PA inhibit PG synthetase from bull testes. With $1·5 \times 10^{-4}$ M 7-oxa -13 PA there was about 90 per cent inhibition of E_2 and $F_{2\alpha}$ synthesis from 4×10^{-5} M arachidonate (Fried *et al.*, 1971; McDonald-Gibson *et al.*, 1973). Fredholm and Strandberg (1973a) cited unpublished data of Perkley that PPP inhibits PG synthetase in bovine seminal vesicles.

Inhibition of cholesterol esterification

PPP 0·1–100 µg ml^{-1} inhibited incorporation of cholesterol, palmitate and palmitoyl CoA into cholesteryl esters in mitochondrial and microsomal preparations of pregnant rabbit ovary. E_1 and E_2, $F_{2\alpha}$ acted similarly but were less potent, and the effects of PPP and the PGs were additive. Inhibition of PG 15-hydroxydehydrogenase and of the esterifying enzyme were suggested as explanations of PPP activity (Morin, 1973).

Inhibition of PG 15-hydroxydehydrogenase

Marrazzi and Matschinsky (1972) found that PPP competed with E_1 for the binding site of the dehydrogenase from swine lung. 7-Oxa-13-PA and fatty acids caused noncompetitive inhibition but SC-19220 did not bind. The formation of E_1 from 15-keto-PGE$_1$ was also inhibited by 7-oxa-13-PA $1·57 \times 10^{-4}$ M (Marrazzi *et al.*, 1972). Crutchley and Piper (1973) showed that PPP 1·4 µg ml^{-1} inhibited guinea-pig pulmonary inactivation of E_2, $F_{2\alpha}$, and $F_{2\beta}$ by 50 per cent. At this concentration no PG antagonist activity was detected on various smooth muscles. DPP was even more active against the dehydrogenase (ED50 0·45 µg ml^{-1}) and more than 5 µg ml^{-1} DPP was needed to antagonize PGs. It would therefore appear that PG antagonism by PPP or DPP would tend to be offset by inhibition of any PG 15-hydroxydehydrogenase present. This inhibition of dehydrogenase may well be useful for evaluating the roles of PGs and for treating conditions in which normal output of PGs may be depressed.

Other effects

White and Pennink (1972) reported a variety of negative properties of PPP in dogs. PPP i.v. (presumably 100 mg kg^{-1}) did not block salivation to $F_{2\alpha}$ or writhing and tachypnoea with $F_{2\alpha}$ or A_2. It was not vagolytic, did not cause ganglion- or α-adrenoceptor blockade or interruption of receptors or pathways mediating the response to carotid occlusion. Eakins and Sanner (1972) reported that in rats SC-19220 reduced the chylomicron count following administration of olive oil, and showed weak antiulcer activity. 7-Oxa-13-PA blocked cAMP production by melanocyte stimulating hormone and E_1 in homogenates of mouse Cloudman S-91 melanoma (Kreiner et al., 1972, cited by Kuehl et al., 1973). It had no effect against unspecified PGs on rat adrenal corticosterone production (Flack, 1970). 11,15-Epi-PGE$_2$ 1·4 × 10^{-7} to 2·8 × 10^{-7} M and ent-11,15-epi-PGE$_2$ 2·8 × 10^{-9} to 1·1 × 10^{-8} M contracted at uterus and jird colon, but after washout the tissue sensitivity to E_2 was greatly reduced (Corey et al., 1972).

6   Classification of prostaglandin receptors

PG antagonists provide interesting data with regard to classification of PG receptors. In some tissues different PGs produce opposite effects, only one of which is inhibited by the antagonists (e.g. PGE-induced contraction of the longitudinal muscle of guinea-pig intestine is antagonized by SC-19220 and PPP, but the relaxation of the circular muscle is unaffected: Bennett and Posner, 1971). This suggests the existence of more than one type of PGE receptor. The only evidence for heterogeneity of PGF receptors is that antagonists are effective in some tissues but not others.

Where PGE and F compounds are antagonized similarly (e.g. longitudinal muscle segments of guinea-pig ileum) it is possible that they act at the same receptor. Similar receptors occur in the rat fundus, since $F_{2\alpha}$ and E_1 competed equally with ^{3}H-PGF$_{2\alpha}$ for binding sites (Miller and Magee, 1972). In other tissues (e.g. circular muscle of the gut) where the different PGs have opposite effects, different receptors for E- and F-type compounds seem to be involved. Even when PGE and F compounds produce similar effects, PGF compounds may be preferentially antagonized (e.g. hypotension in the rabbit, contraction of jird colon). In hamster uterus the ability to bind ^{3}H-PGE$_1$ varies throughout the oestrous cycle whilst binding of ^{3}H-PGF$_{2\alpha}$ remains the same. This too could indicate separate PGE and F receptors (Wakeling et al., 1973).

Responses to PGE compounds associated with inhibition of adenylate cyclase-cAMP are usually antagonized by SC-19220 and PPP. They are usually not antagonized where adenylate cyclase is stimulated (e.g. possibly relaxation of gut muscle) (antagonism with PPP in bovine thyroid cells seems to be an exception). 7-Oxa-13-PA in high concentrations of questionable selectivity has been reported in a few instances to antagonize PGE effects known to be associated with an increase in cAMP (mouse ovary, bovine isolated thyroid cells, rat anterior pituitary). This is consistent with the view that 7-oxa-13-PA is the only antagonist which acts at PG receptors (see section 7). It is important to note that other things beside changes in cAMP may be important in responses to PGs: cAMP does not seem to mediate PGE$_1$-induced Na$^+$ movements in human red blood cells (Ramwell and Shaw, 1970); F$_{2\alpha}$ increases levels of cGMP in bovine and canine isolated veins (Dunham et al., 1973) and in rat uterus (Kuehl et al., 1973), a finding which may have wide implications; PGs might also act by modifying other membrane-associated enzymes (Johnson and Ramwell, 1973).

7   The modes of action of the antagonists

All of the three major PG antagonists have been shown to cause parallel shifts to the right of dose-response curves in certain tissues, and with the lower concentrations there is usually no depression of the maximum response. This data is consistent with (but not rigorous proof of) a competitive action at the PG receptor sites. With higher concentrations the maximum response becomes depressed so that a noncompetitive component becomes evident. The drug which most resembles a PG is 7-oxa-13-PA and this compound competes for PGE receptors in rat lipocytes (Kuehl and Humes, 1972; Kuehl et al., 1973), but is only weakly competitive on rat fundus (Miller and Magee, 1973) as indicated by displacement studies with labelled PGs. In these tests SC-19220 (Kuehl et al., 1973) and PPP (Kuehl et al., 1973; Miller and Magee, 1973) did not show competitive displacement and this may indicate a different site of action. Perhaps these drugs alter the responsiveness of the PG receptors by an allosteric mechanism. In the mouse ovary, the antagonism of E$_1$ by PPP might be explained by block of a cAMP-dependent protein kinase (Kuehl et al., 1971), but in situations where there is a decrease in cAMP (as might be the case in contraction of smooth muscle) such a mechanism could not apply. Little is known about the structure of PG recepters but since 7-oxa-13-PA 3×10^{-5} M protects isolated rat uterus against irreversible inhibition of E_2 by 1,4-dithiothreitol, 7-oxa-13-PA might interact with disulphide groups (Johnson *et al.*, 1974).

8 The future

The future of PG antagonists lies in several directions. The fenamates seem worthy of further study, and much remains to be done with other drugs presently available. It is important to know whether the antagonists act on PG receptors, but if they act in a different way this would not necessarily reduce their experimental usefulness or therapeutic potential. Hopefully, we shall find drugs which are more active and more selective, and discover substances which antagonize the actions of PGs so far resistant to blockade. PG antagonists may well have clinical applications in pain, inflammation etc. so they will have to meet the criteria for safe use in man. Interestingly, PPP has already been used in parenteral injections to prolong the action of various drugs in man (e.g. corticotrophin, Hedner, 1963) and it is used to prolong the nasal decongestant action of phenylephrine. However, PPP might not be of great clinical use because of its ability to inhibit PG-15-hydroxydehydrogenase, and Karim (1973) found that PPP given orally to male volunteers caused diarrhoea. Diphloretin phosphate may well suffer from the same problem, but it would be wrong to extrapolate from its effect on guineapig lung to actions in man. On the other hand, this property might be valuable for using DPP as an investigative tool or therapeutically to potentiate the effects of PGs released in physiological processes.

Where will the new antagonists come from? Obviously attempts will continue to modify the structure of PGs and of the antagonists already available, but some PG antagonists might come from natural sources. Ramaswami (1971) reported that quercetin and other flavinoids antagonized the contractions of guinea-pig ileum to PGs, and Murari *et al.* (1972) found that black tea contains material which antagonizes contractions of this tissue to E_2 and $F_{2\alpha}$. Extracts of human and ram semen contain material which antagonizes contractions of rabbit uterus to $F_{2\alpha}$ and vascular permeability induced by E_1 in rat skin (Dineen *et al.*, 1974). Unfortunately the important question of selectivity has not yet been examined in many of these cases. Nutmeg also contains PG-antagonist activity but this is not selective (Bennett *et al.*, 1974).

The future will also see a wider application of antagonists to investigate PGs in physiological and pathological processes. Hopefully, there will be less tendency than in the past to implicate PGs solely on the basis of inhibition with high concentrations of antagonists without adequate proof of selectivity. Such a worthy aim demands a much more rigorous approach. Since the antagonists may block some PGs and not others it is necessary to study the drugs on the PGs which either occur in the tissue concerned or reach it through the bloodstream. Although PGs occur in tissues, they do not necessarily play a part in the physiology or pathology of the aspect studied. Evidence of this should be sought with measurements of PG release and with drugs which prevent PG synthesis or inactivation, in addition to studies with antagonists of PG action.

References

Ahrén, K. and Perklev, T. (1973). *In* "Advances in the Biosciences" (Ed. S. Bergström) vol. 9, p. 717. Pergamon Press, Oxford.

Al-Jubouri, H. and Patterson, G. (1973). Personal communication.

Ambache, N. and Zar, M. A. (1970). *J. Physiol. (London)*, **208**, 30P.

Ambache, N., Verney, J. and Zar, M. A. (1970). *J. Physiol. (London)*, **207**, 761.

Änggård, E. and Samuelsson, B. (1967). *In* "Prostaglandins, Proceedings, 2nd Nobel Symposium" (Eds S. Bergström and B. Samuelsson), p. 97. Almqvist and Wiksell, Stockholm.

Beitch, B. R. and Eakins, K. E. (1969). *Brit. J. Pharmacol.* **37**, 158.

Beitch, B. R., Beitch, I. and Zadunaisky, J. A. (1973). ARVO Meeting, Sarasota, Assoc. for Research and Vision in Ophthalmology. Abstract, p. 53.

Bennett, A. and Fleshler, B. (1970). *Gastroenterology*, **59**, 790.

Bennett, A. and Posner, J. (1971). *Brit. J. Pharmacol.* **42**, 584.

Bennett, A. and Posner, J. (1972). Unpublished data.

Bennett, A., Eley, K. G. and Scholes, G. B. (1968). *Brit. J. Pharmacol.* **34**, 630.

Bennett, A., Charlier, E. and Szechter, A. (1973a). Unpublished data.

Bennett, A., Eley, K. G. and Stockley, H. L. (1973b). Unpublished data.

Bennett, A., Gradidge, C. F. and Stamford, I. F. (1973c). Unpublished data.

Bennett, A., Stamford, I. F. and Unger, W. G. (1973d) *J. Physiol. (London)*, **229**, 349.

Bennett, A., Gradidge, C. F. and Stamford, I. F. (1974). *New England J. Med.* **290**, 110.

Bethel, R. A. and Eakins, K. E. (1971a). *Fed. Proc.* **30**, 626, Abs.

Bethel, R. A. and Eakins, K. E. (1971b). *Exp. Eye Res.* **13**, 83.

Bode, H. H., Meara, P. A., Jones, H. S. and Crawford, J. D. (1973). *Paediatr. Res.* **7**, 385.

Boyd, J. D. and Hamilton, W. J. (1970). *In* "The Human Placenta", p. 216. Heffer, Cambridge.

Burke, G. and Sato, S. (1971). *Life Sci.* **10**, part II, 969.

Burke, G., Kowalski, K. and Babiarz, D. (1971). *Life Sci.* **10**, part II, 513.

Butcher, R. W. and Sutherland, E. W. (1967). *Ann. New York Acad. Sci.* **139**, 849.

Casey, P. A., Casey, G., Fleisch, H. and Russel, R. G. G. (1972). *Experientia*, **28**, 137.

Chiang, T. S. and Thomas, R. P. (1972). *Fed. Proc.* **31**, 546 Abs.

Chakravarty, N. (1960). *Acta Physiol. Scand.* **48**, 146.

Channing, C. P. (1972). *Prostaglandins*, **2**, 351.

Chasalow, F. I. and Pharriss, B. B. (1972). *Prostaglandins*, **1**, 107.

Cole, D. F. (1961). *Brit. J. Ophthalmol.* **45**, 482.

Coleman, R. (1973). Personal communication.

Collier, H. O. J. and Sweatman, W. J. F. (1968). *Nature*, **219**, 864.

Collier, J. B. (1973). Personal communication.
Corey, E. J., Terashima, S., Ramwell, P. W., Jessup, R., Weinshenker, N. M., Floyd, D. M. and Crosby, G. A. (1972). *J. Org. Chem.* **37**, 3043.
Coyne, W. E. and Cusic, J. W. (1968). *J. Med. Chem.* **11**, 1158.
Crutchley, D. J. and Piper, P. J. (1973). *Naunyn-Schmiedebergs Arch. Pharmakol.*, *Suppl.* **279**, 27.
Diczfaluzy, E., Ferno, O., Fex, H., Högberg, B., Linderot, T. and Rosenberg, Th. (1953). *Acta Chem. Scand.* **7**, 913.
Dineen, J. K., Kelly, J. D., Goodrich, B. S. and Smith, I. D. (1974). *Prostaglandins*, **5**, 209.
Dunham, E. W., Haddox, M. K. and Goldberg, N. D. (1973). *Pharmacologist*, **15**, 158.
Eakins, K. E. (1971). *N. Y. Acad. Sci.* **180**, 386.
Eakins, K. E. and Sanner, J. H. (1972). *In* "The Prostaglandins: Progress in Research" (Ed. S. M. M. Karim), p. 261. Medical and Technical Publishing Co., Oxford.
Eakins, K. E., Karim, S. M. M. and Miller, J. D. (1970). *Brit. J. Pharmacol.* **39**, 556.
Eakins, K. E., Miller, J. D. and Karim, S. M. M. (1971). *J. Pharmacol. Exp. Therap.* **176**, 441.
Eakins, K. E., Fex, H., Fredholm, B., Högberg, B. and Veige, S. (1973). "Advances in the Biosciences" (Ed. S. Bergström), vol. 9, p. 135. Pergamon Press, Oxford.
Ehrenpreis, S., Greenberg, J. and Belman, S. (1973). *Nature New Biol.* **245**, 280.
Engel, J. J., Scruggs, W. and Wilson, D. E. (1973). *Prostaglandins*, **4**, 65.
Fabinyi-Szebehely, M., Hahn, L. and Szebehely, J. (1953). *Brit. J. Pharmacol. Chemother.* **8**, 30.
Farmer, J. B., Farrar, D. G. and Wilson, J. (1972). *Brit. J. Pharmacol.* **46**, 536P.
Ferreira, S. A., Herman, A. and Vane, J. R. (1972). *Brit. J. Pharmacol.* **44**, 328P.
Flack, D. J. (1970). *In* "Recent Progress in Hormone Research", vol. 26, p. 174. Academic Press, New York and London.
Flores, A. G. A. and Sharp, G. W. G. (1972). *Amer. J. Physiol.* **223**, 1392.
Fredholm, B. and Strandberg, K. (1973a). *In* "Advances in the Biosciences" (Ed. S. Bergström), vol. 9, p. 447. Pergamon Press, Oxford.
Fredholm, B. and Strandberg, K. (1973b). Personal communication.
Fried, J. (1970). *In* "Recent Progress in Hormone Research" (Ed. P. W. Ramwell and J. E. Shaw), vol. 26, p. 176. Academic Press, New York and London.
Fried, J., Santhanakrishnan, T. S., Himizu, J., Lin, C. H., Ford, S. H., Rubin, B. and Grigas, E. O. (1969), *Nature*, **223**, 208.
Fried, J., Lin, C. H., Mehra, M. M., Kao, W. L. and Dalven, P. (1971). *Ann. New York Acad. Sci.* **180**, 38.
Fries, B. (1956). *Acta Chir. Scand. Suppl.* **217**, 1.
Fries, B. (1959). *Nature*, **184**, 62.
Fries, B. (1960). *Acta Chir. Scand.* **119**, 1.
Gaddum, J. H. and Picarelli, Z. P. (1957). *Brit. J. Pharmacol. Chemother.* **12**, 323.
Gagnon, D. J. and Sirois, P. (1972). *Brit. J. Pharmacol.* **46**, 89.
Ganesan, P. A. and Karim, S. M. M. (1973). *J. Pharm. Pharmacol.* **25**, 229.
Goodson, J. M. (1973). *In* "Prostaglandins and Cyclic AMP" (Eds R. H. Hahn and W. E. M. Lands), p. 215. Academic Press, New York and London.
Harris, M., Jenkins, M. V., Bennett, A. and Wills, M. R. (1973). *Nature*, **245**, 213.
Harris, M., Jenkins, M. V. and Wills, M. R. (1974). Personal communication.

Harry, J. D. (1968). *Brit. J. Pharmacol. Chemother.* **33**, 213P.
Hart, S. L. (1974). *Brit. J. Pharmacol.* **50**, 159.
Hays, R. M. and Ingelfinger, J. R. (1969). *J. Clin. Invest.* **48**, 37a.
Hedge, G. A. (1972). *Endocrinology*, **91**, 925.
Hedner, P. (1963). *Acta Endocrinol.* **43**, 449.
Hedqvist, P. and Euler, U. S. von (1972). *Neuropharmacology*, **11**, 177.
Högberg, B. and Uvnas, B. (1957). *Acta Physiol. Scand.* **41**, 345.
Illiano, G. and Cuatrecasas, P. (1971). *Nature New Biol.* **234**, 72.
Johnson, M. and Ramwell, P. W. (1973). *In* "Advances in the Biosciences" (Ed.
    S. Bergström), vol. 9, p. 205. Pergamon Press, Oxford.
Johnson, M., Jessup, R. and Ramwell, P. W. (1974). *Prostaglandins*, **5**, 125.
Jones, R. L. (1972). *Brit. J. Pharmacol.* **45**, 144P.
Kalisker, A. (1972). Dissertation Abstracts Intern. B **32**, 11,6551.
Karim, S. M. M. (1973). Personal communication.
Karim, S. M. M. and Sharma, S. D. (1971). *J. Obstet. Gynaecol. Brit. Common-
    wealth*, **78**, 251.
Kelly, R. G. M. and Starr, M. S. (1971). *Canad. J. Ophthal.* **6**, 205.
Kolena, J. and Channing, C. P. (1972). *Endocrinology*, **90**, 1543.
Koss, M. C., Rieger, J. A. and Nakano, J. (1973). *Fed. Proc.* **32**, 787 Abs.
Kuehl, F. A. and Humes, J. L. (1972). *Proc. Nat. Acad. Sci. U.S.A.* **69**, 480.
Kuehl, F. A., Humes, J. L., Tarnoff, J., Cirillo, V. J. and Ham, E. A. (1970a).
    Science, **169**, 883.
Kuehl, F. A., Patanelli, D. J., Tarnoff, J. and Humes, J. L. (1970b). *Biol. Reprod.*
    2, 154.
Kuehl, F. A., Humes, J. L., Mandel, L. R., Cirillo, V. J., Zanetti, M. E. and
    Ham, E. A. (1971). *Biochem. Biophys. Res. Commun.* **44**, 1464.
Kuehl, F. A., Humes, J. L., Arillo, V. J. and Ham, E. A. (1972). *In* "Advances in
    Cyclic Nucleotide Research" (Eds. P. Greengard, R. Paoletti and A. G.
    Robinson), vol. 1, p. 493. Raven Press, New York.
Kuehl, F. A., Cirillo, V. J., Ham, E. A. and Humes, J. L. (1973). *In* "Advances in
    the Biosciences" (Ed. S. Bergström), vol. 9, p. 155. Pergamon Press, Oxford.
Levy, B. and Lindner, H. R. (1971). *Brit. J. Pharmacol.* **43**, 236.
Makino, T. (1973). *Amer. J. Obs. Gyn.* **115**, 606.
Marrazzi, M. A. and Matschinsky, F. M. (1972). *Prostaglandins*, **1**, 373.
Marrazzi, M. A., Shaw, J. E., Tao, F. T. and Matschinsky, F. M. (1972). *Prosta-
    glandins*, **1**, 389.
Marumo, F. and Edelman, I. S. (1971). *J. Clin. Invest.* **50**, 1613.
Mathé, A. A. and Strandberg, K. (1971). *Acta Physiol. Scand.* **82**, 460.
Mathé, A. A., Strandberg, K. and Aström, A. (1971). *Nature New Biol.* **230**, 215.
Mathé, A. A., Strandberg, K. and Fredholm, B. (1972). *J. Pharm. Pharmacol.* **24**,
    378.
McDonald-Gibson, R. G., Flack, J. D. and Ramwell, P. W. (1973). *Biochem. J.*
    132, 117.
McQueen, D. S. (1973). *Life Sci.* **12**, 163.
Miller, O. V. and Magee, W. E. (1973). *In* "Advances in the Biosciences" (Ed. S.
    Bergström), vol. 9, p. 83. Pergamon Press, Oxford.
Morin, R. G. (1973). *Res. Commun. Chem. Pathol. Pharmacol.* **6**, 195.
Murari, R., Natarajan, S., Seshadri, T. R. and Ramaswami, A. S. (1972). *Curr. Sci.*
    41, 435.
Nakano, J. (1972). *Brit. J. Pharmacol.* **44**, 63.

Nakano, J., Prancan, A. V. and Moore, S. (1971). *Clin. Res.* **19**, 712.
Ozer, A. and Sharp, G. W. G. (1972). *Amer. J. Physiol.* **222**, 674.
Ozer, A. and Sharp, G. W. G. (1973). *Eur. J. Pharmacol.* **22**, 227.
Park, M. K. and Dyer, D. C. (1972). *Fed. Proc.* **31**, 556 Abs.
Park, M. K. and Dyer, D. C. (1973). *Prostaglandins*, **3**, 913.
Park, M. K., Rishor, C. and Dyer, D. C. (1972). *Canad. J. Physiol. Pharmacol.* **50**, 393.
Perklev, T. and Ahrén, K. (1971). *Life Sci.* **10**, 1387.
Piper, P. and Vane, J. R. (1969). *Nature*, **223**, 29.
Posner, J. (1971). *J. Physiol. (London)*, **217**, 25P.
Posner, J. (1973). *Brit. J. Pharmacol.* **49**, 415.
Puglisi, L. (1973). In "Advances in the Biosciences". (Ed. S. Bergström), vol. 9, p. 219. Pergamon Press, Oxford.
Rabinowitz, I., Johnson, M. and Wolf, P. L. (1973). *Fed. Proc.* **32**, 803.
Radzialowski, F. M. and Novak, L. N. (1971). *Life Sci.* **10**, part I, 1261.
Radzialowski, F. M. and Rosenberg, L. N. (1973). *Life Sci.* **12**, part II, 337.
Ramaswami, A. S. (1971). Abstracts Seventh World Congress Fertility and Sterility, p. 11. Int. Congr. Serv. 234a, Excerpta Medica, Amsterdam.
Ramwell, P. W. and Shaw, J. E. (1970). In "Recent Progress in Hormone Research", vol. 26, p. 139. Academic Press, New York and London.
Ratner, A., Wilson, C. M. and Peake, G. T. (1973). *Prostaglandins*, **3**, 413.
Sanner, J. H. (1969). *Arch. Int. Pharmacodyn. Thér.* **180**, 46.
Sanner, J. H. (1974). *Arch. Intern. Med.* **133**, 133.
Sanner, J. H. (1971). *Ann. New York Acad. Sci.* **180**, 396.
Sanner, J. H. (1972). *Intra-Sci. Chem. Rep.* **6**, 1.
Sanner, J. H. and Aspinal, R. L. (1973). Personal communication.
Sanner, J. H., Meuller, R. A. and Schulze, R. H. (1973). In "Advances in the Biosciences" (Ed. S. Bergström), vol. 9, p. 139. Pergamon Press, Oxford.
Sato, S., Kowalski, K. and Burke, G. (1972a). *Prostaglandins*, **1**, 345.
Sato, S., Szabo, M., Kowalski, K. and Burke, G. (1972b). *Endocrinology*, **90**, 343.
Saunders, L. N. and Moser, C. (1971). *Pharmacologist*, **13**, 292.
Snyder, D. S. and Englestein, W. H. (1973). *J. Invest. Dermatol.* **60**, 110.
Somova, L. (1973). In "Advances in the Biosciences" (Ed. S. Bergström), vol. 9, p. 335. Pergamon Press, Oxford.
Søndergaard, J. and Jørgensen, H. P. (1973). *Brit. J. Dermatol.* **88**, 51.
Splawinski, J. A., Nies, A. S., Bieck, P. R. and Oates, J. A. (1971). *Pharmacologist*, **13**, 291.
Spalwinski, J. A., Nies, A. S., Sweetman, B. and Oates, J. A. (1973). *J. Pharmacol. Exp. Therap.* **187**, 501.
Starr, M. S. (1971). *Exp. Eye Res.* **11**, 170.
Strandberg, K. (1973). *Acta Pharmacol. Toxicol.* **32**, 33.
Strandberg, K., Mathé, A. A. and Fredholm, B. (1972). *Life Sci.* **11**, part I, 701.
Swedenborg, J. (1973a), Fourth Congress of the International Society of Thrombosis and Haemastasis, Vienna.
Swedenborg, J. (1973b). Personal communication.
Tal, E., Szabo, M. and Burke, G. (1974). *Prostaglandins*, **5**, 175.
Vale, W., Rivier, C. and Guillemin, R. (1971). *Fed. Proc.* **30**, 363 Abs.
Vanasin, B., Greenough, W. and Schuster, M. M. (1970). *Clin. Res.* **18**, 682.
Vane, J. R. (1971). *Nature New Biology*, **231**, 232.
Vane, J. R. (1972). In "Inflammation: Mechanisms and Control" (Eds I. H. Lepow and P. A. Ward), p. 261. Academic Press, New York and London.

Villanueva, R., Hinds, L., Katz, R. L. and Eakins, K. E. (1972). *J. Pharmacol. Exp. Ther.* **180**, 78.

Wakeling, A. E., Kirton, K. T. and Wyngarden, L. J. (1973). *Prostaglandins*, **4**, 1.

White, R. P. and Pennink, M. (1972). *Arch. Int. Pharmacodyn, Thér.* **197**, 274.

Whitelocke, R. A. F. and Eakins, K. E. (1973a), *Arch. Ophthalmol.* **89**, 495.

Whitelocke, R. A. F. and Eakins, K. E. (1973b). *Exp. Eye Res.* **17**, 395.

Whitelocke, R. A. F., Eakins, K. E. and Bennett, A. (1973). *Proc. Roy. Soc. Med.* **66**, 429.

Wohlzogen, F. X. (1961). *Acta Endocrinol.* **37**, 298.

Wolff, J. and Moore, W. V. (1973). *Biochem. Biophys. Res.* **51**, 34.

Yamamoto, Y. L., Feindel, W., Wolfe, L. S. and Hodge, C. P. (1973). *In* "Advances in the Biosciences" (Ed. S. Bergström), vol. **9**, p. 359. Pergamon Press, Oxford.

Hypothalamic Amines and the Release of Gonadotrophins and other Anterior Pituitary Hormones

CATHERINE A. WILSON, BPharm, PhD

Physiology Department, The Royal Veterinary College, London, England

1   Introduction

It is generally assumed that chemical transmitters are liberated at nerve terminals in the central nervous system (CNS) in exactly the same way as in the peripheral nervous system. The identity of these transmitters is not as yet absolutely proved, but they are most likely to include noradrenaline, dopamine, 5-hydroxytryptamine (5-HT, serotonin) and acetylcholine. These compounds have an unequal distribution in the brain and their concentration is selectively reduced by lesions in specific pathways in the CNS. For example, lesions in the brain stem reduce the levels of noradrenaline and 5-hydroxytryptamine in the forebrain and spinal cord, while lesions in the nigrostriatal tract lower those of dopamine in the basal ganglia.

For a particular chemical compound to be established as a neurotransmitter in the brain, all the following requirements should be demonstrated:

1. the presence of the compound in brain tissue, accompanied by the appropriate metabolizing enzymes;
2. its location inside neurones of specific nerve tracts;
3. the identity of its physiological effects with those produced by electrical stimulation of the nerve tract within which it is located;
4. the release of the transmitter by stimulation or activation of specific nerve tracts;
5. compounds known to interact with the neurotransmitter in the periphery should interact similarly with the neurotransmitter in the brain, producing the expected effects.

These requirements have been met for noradrenaline and 5-hydroxytryptamine except for (3), and for dopamine except (3) and (4) (Barchas *et al.*, 1972). Other substances which may function as transmitters are histamine, substance P, γ-aminobutyric acid, glycine and various other aminoacids and, possibly, prostaglandins. All these compounds have been shown to be released by stimulation of brain tissue (Vogt, 1969; 1973).

This review is concerned only with putative transmitters in the hypothalamus and their control of the hormones of the anterior pituitary. It is prefaced by an account of the distribution of brain amines and their metabolism. Only the catecholamines, 5-hydroxytryptamine and acetylcholine have been shown to be present in the hypothalamus in significant amounts and hence this review is limited to these substances.

2 Anatomical distribution of brain amines

2.1 5-HYDROXYTRYPTAMINE, NORADRENALINE AND DOPAMINE

Significant amounts of 5-hydroxytryptamine are found in mammalian brain (Twarog and Page, 1953; Pletscher et al., 1956), especially in the mesencephalon (midbrain) and diencephalon (hypothalamus and thalamus), the highest concentration being found in the hypothalamus, the lowest in the cortex and none in the cerebellum (Amin et al., 1954). Noradrenaline has a similar distribution (Vogt, 1954; Kovacs and Faredin, 1960) and dopamine is present in high concentrations in the hypothalamus; Fuxe, 1965 (Laverty and Sharman, 1965 corpus striatum).

Fluorescence histochemistry (Falck et al., 1962) enables the amines to be more precisely located in the CNS. After treatment with formaldehyde 5-hydroxytryptamine gives a yellow fluorescence while noradrenaline and dopamine give a green fluorescence. The latter two can be distinguished either by subsequent acidification, or by prior treatment in vivo with selective depleting agents. The vast body of work which followed the introduction of this technique categorized the levels of noradrenaline, dopamine and 5-hydroxytryptamine in the various areas and nuclei of the brain (Fuxe, 1965). The localization of these amines in the various hypothalamic areas and nuclei, and some associated extrahypothalamic areas, is shown in Fig. 1. Levels of noradrenaline are high in the preoptic area, the supraoptic nucleus, the paraventricular nucleus, the periventricular nucleus, the arcuate nucleus, the retrochiasmatic area and the internal layer of the median eminence (Carlsson, 1959; Carlsson et al., 1962a; 1962b; Dahlstrom and Fuxe, 1964; Fuxe, 1965; Weiner et al., 1972a).

Dopamine is found in high concentrations in the same areas, except in the paraventricular nucleus. It is also present in high concentrations in the dorso-medial nucleus, the zona incerta and the external layer of the median eminence (Fuxe, 1965; Smelik, 1966). Recently using a combination of fluorescence histochemistry and microfluorimetric techniques the presence of dopamine has also been shown in cell bodies in the periventricular nucleus, an area in the dorsal hypothalamus and an area in the posterior hypothalamus extending to the caudal thalamus, as well as in the arcuate nucleus (Bjorkland and Nobin, 1973). Until recently methods for measuring concentrations in small areas of the brain were not sufficiently sensitive, but now Cuello et al. (1973) have devised an

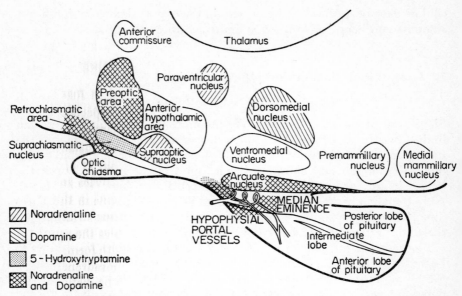

FIG. 1. A sagittal view of the hypothalamus showing the distribution of noradrenaline, dopamine, and 5-hydroxytryptamine in the various hypothalamic nuclei.

assay involving enzymic conversion of the amines to one of their metabolites in the presence of a tritiated aminoacid, so that the metabolite is labelled and therefore can be measured on a radioactivity counter. They have shown that in the rat there are high concentrations of dopamine in the median eminence ($10 \cdot 3$ μg g^{-1}) and the ratio of dopamine to noradrenaline in this area is 2:1. In the arcuate nucleus noradrenaline levels ($1 \cdot 3$ μg g^{-1}) are higher than those of dopamine.

5-Hydroxytryptamine is found in the hypothalamus in high concentrations only in the suprachiasmatic nucleus and in the anterior part of the median eminence (Hamon et al., 1970; Fuxe et al., 1970b).

Outside the hypothalamus, noradrenaline is present in the amygdala, neocortex and spinal cord; dopamine in the substantia nigra and caudate nucleus of the basal ganglia; and 5-hydroxytryptamine in the lower brain stem and spinal cord (Carlsson et al., 1962b; Fuxe, 1965).

Most of the work so far has been carried out on the rat but the distribution in brain areas of the cat, dog and rabbit appear to be similar (see Barchas et al., 1972). More recently species differences in the regional distribution of the amines within the hypothalamus have been found. For example, the levels of dopamine are highest in the median eminence of the rat, mouse, pig and cow, while noradrenaline is at its highest concentration in the medial basal hypothalamus. However, in man, it is noradrenaline which is the predominant amine in the median eminence and it is at its highest concentration in this part of the hypothalamus (Rinne and Sonninen, 1967; 1968). 5-Hydroxytryptamine has been found in significant concentrations in the median eminence of the sheep and ox, as well as in the rat (Piezzi et al., 1970; Wheaton et al., 1972).

It has been possible to map out pathways of 5-hydroxytryptamine, noradrenaline and dopamine in the brain by cutting nerve fibres or making lesions in precisely located areas and noting the fall in fluorescence in other areas, which must therefore be innervated by axons coming from cell bodies in the lesioned area (Ungerstedt, 1971). For example the fluorescence in the median eminence falls after lesions placed in the arcuate nucleus, indicating that axons from cell bodies in the arcuate nucleus terminate in the median eminence (Smith and Fink, 1972). Similarly lesions in the medial forebrain bundle in the lateral hypothalamus cause a fall in 5-hydroxytryptamine in all the more rostral areas in the brain (Harvey et al., 1963; Heller and Moore, 1965; Parent et al., 1969). Confirmation of the pathways can be obtained by stimulating the areas of their origin (i.e. cell bodies) and noting the decrease in fluorescence at the nerve terminals in rats pretreated with amine synthesis inhibitors (Fuxe and Gunne, 1964; Arbuthnott et al., 1970).

A non-adrenergic dorsal pathway starts from the locus coeruleus in the mesencephalon and ends at the cortex. A ventral pathway originates in cell bodies in the reticular formation in the mesencephalon and passes to various hypothalamic nuclei and also to some areas in the limbic system (i.e. in the amygdala). The dopamine pathway starts in the ventral tegmentum in the mesencephalon and passes via the lateral hypothalamus to the basal ganglia and then to the amygdala. There is a separate shorter dopaminergic system originating in the cell bodies of the arcuate nucleus and passing via the dorsal medial nucleus and the lateral border of the periventricular nucleus to the median eminence (Ungerstedt, 1971). The 5-hydroxytrypt amine pathway originates in the cell bodies of the midbrain raphe, passes to the interpeduncular nucleus where it divides, the dorsal branch going to the cortex and the ventral branch travelling anteriorly via the medial forebrain bundle through the lateral hypothalamus. The 5-hydroxytryptamine neurones then separate out to innervate the septum, the cingulum, the amygdala and parts of the hypothalamus (Fuxe et al., 1968a; Parent et al., 1969; Ungerstedt, 1971). The main aminergic pathways are shown in Figs 2 and 3.

Areas concerned with gonadotrophin release, the basal hypothalamus and the median eminence, contain a dopaminergic neural system from cell bodies within the arcuate nucleus area passing to the median emi-

NORADRENALINE

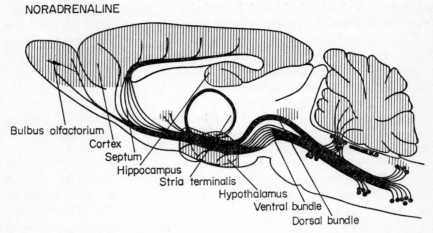

FIG. 2. Sagittal projection of the ascending noradrenaline pathways. The descending pathways are not included. The stripes indicate the major nerve terminal areas. The 5-HT axons follow closely the noradrenaline pathway. (With permission from Ungerstedt, 1971.)

DOPAMINE

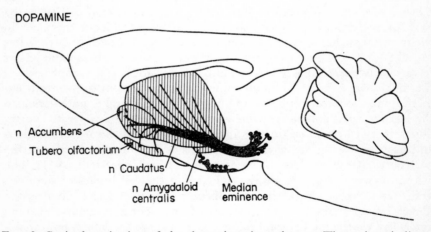

FIG. 3. Sagittal projection of the dopaminergic pathways. The stripes indicate nerve terminal areas. (With permission from Ungerstedt, 1971.)

nence and ending near the capillary loops leading to the hypophyseal portal system. In addition, there is a noradrenergic system originating outside the basal hypothalamic area which passes into the hypothalamus possibly via the medial forebrain bundle and innervates various nuclei which may be concerned with releasing-hormone formation, and gonadotrophin release. These two systems were shown by noting the decrease in fluorescence of hypothalamic noradrenaline, but not dopamine, after deafferentation of the hypothalamus (Jonsson et al., 1972; Smith and Fink, 1972; Weiner et al., 1972a; 1972b).

Electron microscope studies have shown that the amines are in small granular vesicles within the axon, especially at the nerve terminals (Fuxe and Hokfelt, 1969; Kobayashi and Matsui, 1969). The three types of nerve endings in a homogenate of brain tissue can be separated by differential centrifugation of the synaptosome fraction in a sucrose gradient. This has been carried out on homogenates of rat median eminence (Andreoli et al., 1970; Clementi et al., 1970), rat hypothalamus and midbrain and also in other species, i.e. guinea-pig and hamster (Kuhar et al., 1971).

2.2 ADRENALINE

Only about one tenth of the catecholamine content of the whole dog brain is adrenaline (Vogt, 1954). Its presence has been confirmed in the rat, pig (Gunne, 1962) and cat brain (Barchas et al., 1972), although according to Carlsson (1959) it does not appear to be localized in any specific area. Gunne (1962) has shown that there are greater amounts of adrenaline in the avian brain than in the mammalian brain. The enzyme phenylethanol N-methyltransferase (PNMT) (necessary for converting noradrenaline to adrenaline) is present in significant concentrations in the hypothalamus and olfactory bulb. In addition the presence of an inhibitor to N-methyltransferase has been shown to exist in these regions. (Ciaranello et al., 1969; Pohorecky et al., 1969). Recently Hokfelt et al. (1974) in immunohistological studies using antibodies to PNMT showed that this enzyme is present in ascending and descending tracts originating from cell bodies in the midbrain. They suggested that PNMT-containing neurones are adrenergic, that is adrenaline is the neural transmitter. They also showed there are adrenergic nerve terminals in various parts of the brain including the hypothalamus where they are especially dense in the paraventricular nucleus and in lower densities in the dorsomedial nucleus and periventricular area. This has been confirmed by biochemical assay of PNMT in very small portions of brain. In these studies high levels were also noted in the basal hypothalamus, median eminence and arcuate nucleus (Saavedra et al., 1974).

2.3 ACETYLCHOLINE

Cholinergic pathways have been investigated in the central nervous system by detecting cholinesterases in specific areas after lesions in neuronal tracts. The cholinesterase tends to accumulate at the cut end on the cell body side and disappear in the terminal end of the cut axon. Two main cholinesterase-containing pathways exist; the dorsal tegmentum pathway which contains both true and pseudocholinesterase and arises in the dorso-lateral part of the reticular formation in the midbrain. This pathway goes to the thalamus and hippocampus. The second pathway is called the ventral tegmental pathway and arises from the substantia nigra and ventral tegmental area in the midbrain and contains only true cholinesterase. It projects forward to the basal hypothalamus and subthalamic areas lateral to the hypothalamus, to reach the basal forebrain where it synapses in various areas and then continues to the supracortex and the olfactory bulb. It is suggested that this pathway is synonymous with the ascending reticular activating system.

Within the hypothalamus there are large numbers of cholinesterase-containing cell bodies in the mammillary body and in the posterior and lateral hypothalamus. There are also some of these cell bodies in the lateral preoptic area, and both cell bodies and fibres in the dorsal region of the hypothalamus. Cholinergic activity can be seen in the supraoptic and paraventricular nuclei, but there is little or none in the medial preoptic area, the anterior hypothalamus, the suprachiasmatic nucleus and the arcuate nucleus (Shute and Lewis, 1966).

3   Metabolism of the brain amines

3.1   BIOSYNTHESIS

3.1.1   *Catecholamines*

The synthesis of the catecholamines takes place within neurones from tyrosine (Fig. 4). The distribution of tyrosine hydroxylase which converts tyrosine to dopa parallels the distribution of catecholamines in the brain; its concentration is high in the hypothalamus, midbrain, pons and striatum and low in the cortex (McGreer *et al.*, 1967). It is found partially free and partially bound to membranes, the latter form being more active (Costa and Meek, 1974). L-aromatic aminoacid decarboxylase is found only in the soluble fraction of nerve tissue and is present in all parts of the central nervous system (CNS). Dopamine β-hydroxylase which converts dopa to noradrenaline is associated with the synaptic vesicles in which the amines are stored. It is found in high concentrations in the midbrain and hypothalamus, but is low in the striatum (basal ganglia) where dopamine is the main transmitter (Iversen and Glowinski, 1966).

The rate-limiting step for catecholamine synthesis depends on the activity of tyrosine hydroxylase which is under a negative feedback con-

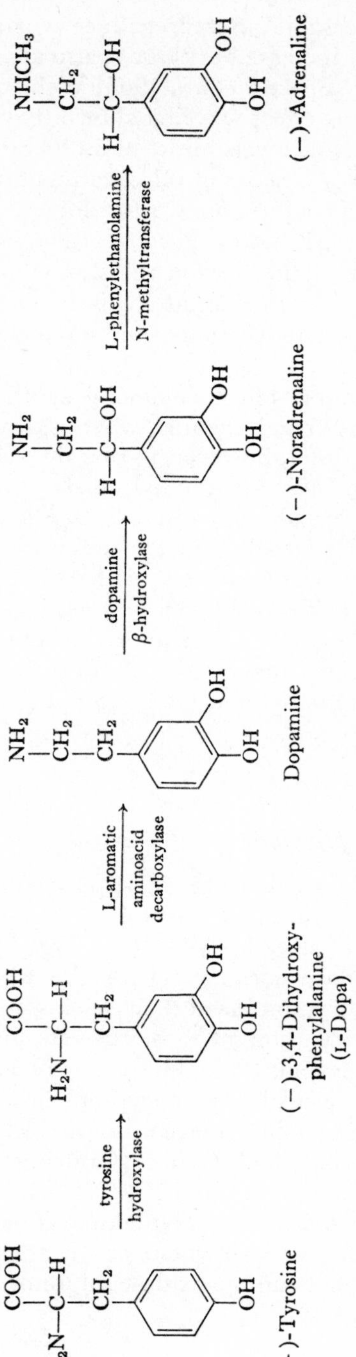

FIG. 4. Biosynthesis of catecholamines.

trol exerted by "releasable" noradrenaline; when this is removed, not only does the activity increase but there is also an increase in synthesis of tyrosine hydroxylase (Spector *et al.*, 1967; Weiner and Rabadjija, 1968). This negative feedback effect was first shown by Costa and Neff (1966); they raised noradrenaline levels in the brain by inhibition of monoamine oxidase and within 1 or 2 hours of this treatment noted a fall in turnover rate. Similar effects have been shown for dopamine (Javoy *et al.*, 1972). Thus it can be expected that the turnover rate will differ in the various areas of the brain, since the sizes of the storage pools are different. For example, the turnover rate for noradrenaline is slowest in the hypothalamus ($t_{\frac{1}{2}}$ = 4 hours), where its storage and uptake is greatest (Iversen and Glowinski, 1966).

The pattern and control of catacholamine synthesis in the brain is very similar to that in the adrenal medulla, where the first investigations were made. The adrenals differ, however, in that they contain high concentrations of phenylethanolamine-N-methyltransferase (PNMT), the enzyme which converts noradrenaline to adrenaline (Axelrod, 1962).

Although levels of adrenaline in the brain are negligible the enzyme PNMT is present especially in the hypothalamus and olfactory bulb. In addition, an inhibitor of PNMT can be found in the same areas, which may explain the low levels of adrenaline in the brain. The presence of the enzyme and its inhibitor suggest that if adrenaline is synthesized in the brain, it is locally regulated and is not stored (Ciarnanello *et al.*, 1969; Pohorecky *et al.*, 1969).

3.1.2   5-*Hydroxytryptamine*

The synthesis of 5-hydroxytryptamine from tryptophan also takes place inside the neurones, under the control of tryptophan hydroxylase and L-aromatic aminoacid decarboxylase (see Fig. 5). The distribution of tryptophan hydroxylase correlates with the distribution of neurones liberating 5-hydroxytryptamine at their synapses (Ichiyama *et al.*, 1970). The hydroxylation was thought to be the rate-limiting step of the synthesis (Moir and Eccleston, 1968), but recent evidence has shown that the rate depends on the availability of tryptophan and its transport across the neuronal membrane since normal brain levels of tryptophan do not saturate the tryptophan hydroxylase (Grahame-Smith, 1971; Tagliomonte *et al.*, 1971b).

Whether the level of 5-hydroxytryptamine at nerve endings can exert a negative feedback effect on its own rate of synthesis is yet to be elucidated. Administration of a monoamine oxidase inhibitor reduces the conversion

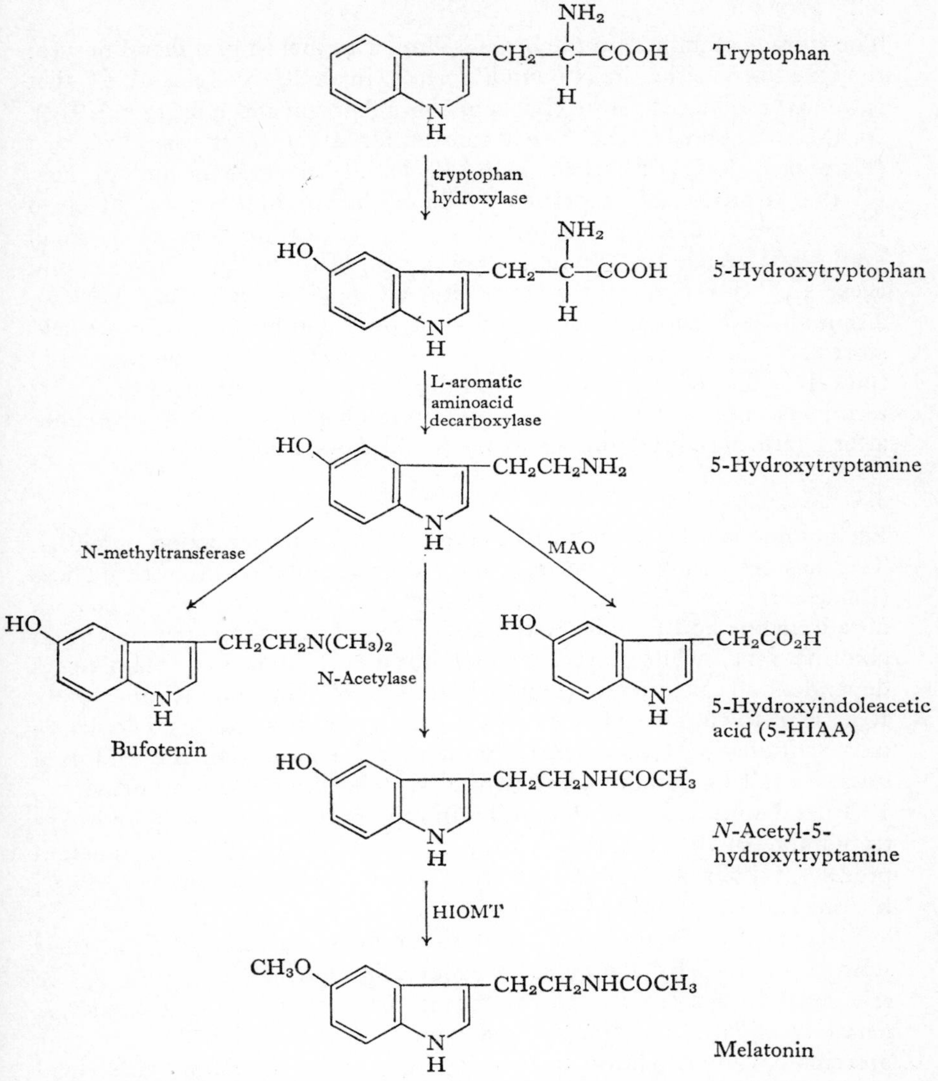

FIG. 5. Biosynthesis and metabolism of 5-hydroxytryptamine.

of ^{3}H-tryptophan to ^{3}H-5-hydroxytryptamine (Macon *et al.*, 1971); however this result has been questioned (Costa and Meek, 1974) since the change in specific activity with time was not taken into account. Indeed Costa has shown that there is no change in turnover rate after increasing 5-hydroxytryptamine brain levels by monoamine oxidase inhibition.

3.2 STORAGE

The storage of amines in the brain is similar to that in peripheral nerves; they are stored either in a "bound" form or in an "easily-releasable", that is to say "functional" store (Iversen, 1967; Aprison and Hurgtgen, 1972). As the most newly synthesized transmitter is the most easily released (Hamon *et al.*, 1970; Farnebo *et al.*, 1971), it seems that the amines must fill the "functional" store before filling the "bound" store. Electron microscope studies have shown that the amines are present in small granulated vesicles in "boutons" (swellings) of the nerve terminals, and these are presumably the storage sites (Kobayashi and Matsui, 1969), although the anatomical distribution of the "bound" and "functional" stores are not known. The storage granules are thought to be formed in the cell bodies of the neurones and to pass down the axon to the nerve terminals. This has been shown by noting changes in histofluorescence after ligaturing noradrenergic axons (Dahlstrom, 1967).

3.3 RELEASE

Each amine is released from its nerve terminal after an action potential. This has been shown to occur *in vitro* after stimulation of cortical slices (Baldessarini and Kopin, 1967; Chase *et al.*, 1967). The release of both noradrenaline and 5-hydroxytryptamine from the brain is dependent on chloride ions, while noradrenaline, but not 5-hydroxytryptamine, is dependent on calcium ions (Goodwin *et al.*, 1969; Katz and Kopin, 1969). Release of the amines after electrical stimulation has also been shown *in vivo*. Stimulation of the ventral noradrenergic bundle in the midbrain causes a fall in noradrenaline in the hypothalamus (Arbuthnott *et al.*, 1970) and stimulation of the midbrain raphe causes a fall in 5-hydroxytryptamine in the forebrain with a concomitant rise in its degradation product, 5-hydroxyindole acetic acid (5-HIAA) (Aghajanian *et al.*, 1967; Sheard and Aghajanian, 1968).

Electron microscopy shows that the amines are released from their storage granules by a process of exocytosis in which the contents are released into the extra-neuronal space; for example, at noradrenergic nerve terminals, noradrenaline, dopamine β-hydroxylase and specific proteins have been shown to be discharged after stimulation (Malamad *et al.*, 1968).

The free or active transmitter after its release acts on the receptor sites of the post-synaptic neurone or organ.

3.4 CATABOLISM

Noradrenaline and dopamine are removed from their site of action mainly by an efficient uptake system back into the nerve terminals, where they are either re-stored or metabolized by the intraneuronal enzyme, mono-amine oxidase, which is found associated with the mitochondria (Schnait-men *et al.*, 1967). Monoamine oxidase has no regional specificity but has its highest concentrations in the hypothalamus (La Motte *et al.*, 1969). The main metabolites produced by this enzyme are shown in Fig. 6. Approximately, 10 per cent of the catecholamines are metabolized extra-neuronally by catechol *O*-methyltransferase (COMT) (Axelrod, 1959) which converts noradrenaline to normetanephrine and dopamine to 3-methoxytryamine (see Fig. 6).

The system is similar for 5-hydroxytryptamine in that there is a specific re-uptake system, so that 5-hydroxytryptamine is either restored or metabolized by monoamine oxidase to 5-hydroxyindoleacetic acid (5-HIAA). There are differences, as COMT does not degrade tryptophan derivatives, but enzymes are found almost exclusively in the pineal gland for converting 5-hydroxytryptamine to melatonin, i.e. *N*-acetylase and hydroxyindole-*O*-methyltransferase (HIOMT) (Wurtman *et al.*, 1968).

More recently two other enzymes that metabolize 5-hydroxytryptamine have been found in the brain. One is an *N*-methyltransferase enzyme (Mandell and Morgan, 1971) which has been identified particularly in the pituitary and the pineal and converts 5-hydroxytryptamine to its methyl derivatives, which may be psychogenic (Himwich, 1971; Brimblecombe, 1974). The other enzyme is 5-hydroxytryptamine sulphotransferase which has been found in the soluble fraction of neuronal tissue and which converts 5-hydroxytryptamine to 5-hydroxytrypt-amine-*O*-sulphate (Hidaka *et al.*, 1969). Figure 5 shows the metabolic pathways for 5-hydroxytryptamine.

3.5 UPTAKE

Uptake mechanisms for inactivation of noradrenaline was first shown in peripheral nerve endings (see Iversen, 1965a; 1965b; 1967), but has since been shown to occur in the brain for noradrenaline, dopamine and 5-hydroxytryptamine. Uptake *in vivo* was demonstrated either by ac-cumulation of radioactively labelled amines at specific sites in the brain after intraventricular injection (Glowinski *et al.*, 1965; Glowinski and Iversen, 1966) or by noting the increase in fluorescence in specific sites after intraperitoneal injection of the amines (Lichtensteiger and Lange-mann, 1966; Lichensteiger *et al.*, 1967; Fuxe *et al.*, 1968b). These sites were usually those which normally contained high endogenous levels of the particular transmitter; for example ^{3}H-noradrenaline uptake was greatest in the hypothalamus and lowest in the cerebellum. *In vitro* uptake of noradrenaline in the brain slices was shown by Dengler *et al.* (1961), and since then uptake into isolated nerve terminals (synaptosomes)

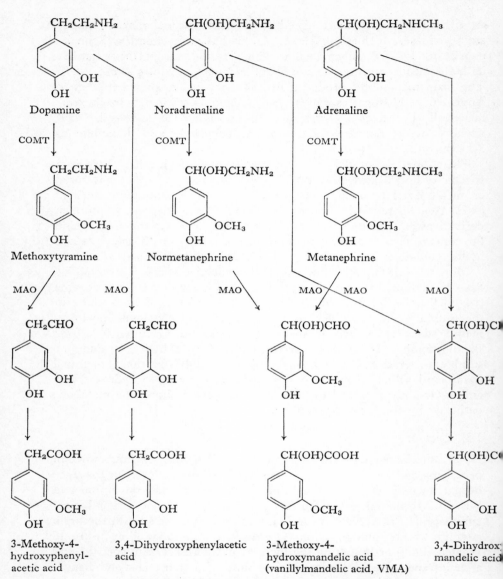

Fig. 6. Metabolic pathways of catecholamines.

of the brain has also been demonstrated (Coyle and Synder, 1969). In the case of noradrenaline 80 per cent of the uptake of exogenous amines occurs into brain nerve terminals, the rest is accumulated by a low affinity mechanism into other brain tissue (Baldessarini and Vogt, 1971).

So far, the extraneuronal Uptake 2 mechanism shown by Iversen (1965a) in the isolated heart, has not been demonstrated in the brain.

The ($-$)-isomer of noradrenaline is taken up preferentially, to the ($+$)-isomer in all areas of the brain, except the corpus striatum where both isomers are accumulated equally (Coyle and Snyder, 1969; Horn et al., 1971), and where the uptake mechanism has a lower affinity for noradrenaline (see Table 1). The K_m for dopamine in the corpus striatum is

TABLE 1

Uptake of amines in the brain

Amine	Area in brain	K_m
($-$)-Noradrenaline	Corpus striatum	2×10^{-6} M
	Rest of brain	4×10^{-7} M
Dopamine	Corpus striatum	4×10^{-7} M
	Rest of brain	0.8×10^{-7} M and 1.4×10^{-6} M
5-Hydroxytryptamine	Whole brain	2×10^{-7} M

4×10^{-7} M, but in most other parts of the brain the uptake can be resolved into two components of $K_m = 0.8 \times 10^{-7}$ M and 1.4×10^{-6} M. The former value is also that of the K_m for the inhibitory effect of dopamine on the uptake of noradrenaline. This indicates that dopamine has (a) a specific uptake system of its own, and (b) more affinity for the noradrenergic system than noradrenaline itself. In fact, exogenous dopamine can be taken up by noradrenergic neurones in the central nervous system and either converted to noradrenaline within 15 to 30 minutes (Glowinski and Axelrod, 1965) or possibly act as a false transmitter (Farnebo et al., 1971).

The uptake of 5-hydroxytryptamine in the brain has been demonstrated in vivo and in vitro (Schanburg, 1963; Robinson et al., 1965; Blackburn et al., 1967). The uptake occurs at two sites: in low concentrations, i.e. below 10^{-7} M, it enters specifically into tryptaminergic nerve endings with a K_m of 2×10^{-7} M, but in higher concentrations it accumulates into catecholaminergic neurones and catecholamines and 5-hydroxytryptamine compete for the same uptake sites (Shaskan and Snyder, 1970; Snyder et al., 1970).

3.6 INTERACTIONS BETWEEN THE AMINES

Other interactions between transmitters have been shown recently in the brain. For example catecholamines can be taken up into tryptaminergic nerve endings (Barrelt and Balch, 1971); administration of L-dopa can cause the release and subsequent depletion of brain 5-hydroxytryptamine, although whether the L-dopa acts directly or after its conversion to dopamine is not known (Goldstein and Frenkel, 1971; Butcher *et al.*, 1972). Dopa also lowers the brain levels of tryptophan and tyrosine and may inhibit their uptake into brain neurones (Karobath *et al.*, 1971). Conversely administration of 5-hydroxytryptophan (5-HTP) can cause the release of dopamine from dopaminergic nerve terminals, in this case it was shown that the 5-HTP was first converted to 5-hydroxytryptamine (Ng *et al.*, 1972). 5-HTP also inhibits the synthesis of noradrenaline from dopa presumably because it competes for the aminoacid decarboxylase necessary for the conversion of both 5-hydroxytryptophan and dopa to 5-hydroxytryptamine and noradrenaline respectively (Feer and Wirz-Justice, 1971). Thus an injection of 5-HTP significantly lowers brain noradrenaline levels (Butcher *et al.*, 1972). 5-Substituted indoles also inhibit the oxidation of dopamine (Hartley and Smith, 1972). These findings show that administration of 5-HTP not only raises 5-hydroxytryptamine levels in the brain, but also alters the metabolism of the brain catecholamines. Care must be taken in judging results after injections of 5-HTP for another reason: after an injection of 5-HTP, it is converted to 5-hydroxytryptamine in all areas of the brain and not just in the serotonergic neurones, so that 5-hydroxytryptamine is present in abnormal sites (Aghajanian and Asher, 1971). In addition, the 5-hydroxytryptamine derived from the 5-HTP does not appear to be stored in the normal manner but is immediatey metabolized (Moir and Eccleston, 1968). Injection of tryptophan raises brain 5-hydroxytryptamine too, but in this case the 5-hydroxytryptamine formed is stored and its distribution in the brain is qualitatively normal, although the levels may be higher than normal.

Figure 7 summarizes the metabolic changes occurring at a noradrenergic nerve terminal. It is assumed that similar changes occur in the dopaminergic and tryptaminergic neurones.

4 Changes in brain amine metabolism

4.1 ONTOGENY OF BRAIN AMINE LEVELS

In rat and mouse brain, amines increase gradually to adult concentrations from a period starting before birth. On the day of birth 5-hydroxytrypt-

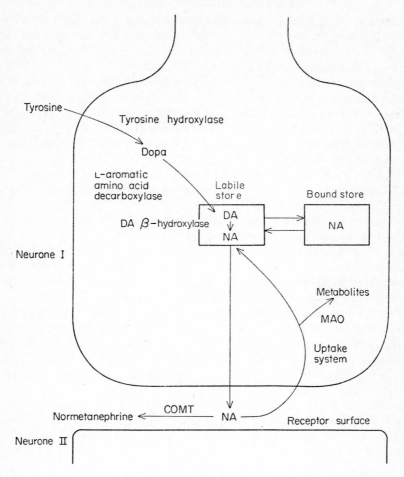

FIG. 7. A model of a noradrenergic neurone. The presynaptic neurone (Neurone I) contains all the synthetic enzymes for producing noradrenaline in the storage granule. The labile and strongly bound stores of noradrenaline are in equilibrium. On release the noradrenaline acts on the postsynaptic receptors on Neurone II and then approximately 10 per cent is destroyed by COMT and 90 per cent is returned to the storage granule by an active uptake mechanism. A small proportion is destroyed by MAO intraneuronally. NA, noradrenaline; DA, dopamine; COMT, catechol-O-methyltransferase; MAO, monoamine oxidase.

amine, noradrenaline and dopamine levels are 30–40, 16–20, and 20–30 per cent respectively of the adult level (Kato, 1960; Nachmais, 1961; Haber and Kamano, 1966; Agrawal *et al.*, 1966; 1968). The 5-hydroxytryptamine adult level is reached before that of the catecholamines and, according to Agrawal *et al.* (1966), well before puberty (i.e. day 25). The low levels of 5-hydroxytryptamine in early life may be due to a reduced capacity in tryptophan hydroxylase (Bennett and Giarman, 1959) or possibly due to the slightly lower 5-hydroxytryptamine-binding capacity of the immature brain compared to the adult brain (Karki *et al.*, 1962), although Haber and Kamano (1966) think this is unlikely. After injection of 5-HTP, a greater proportion enters the brain of 1–4-day-old rats than 21-day-old rats, due to the lower activity of peripheral decarboxylase in the neonate (Kellog and Lundburg, 1972).

The catecholamine levels in the brain rise at a slower rate than those of 5-hydroxytryptamine; noradrenaline reaches adult levels by day 30 in the mouse and day 35 in the rat (Agrawal *et al.*, 1966; 1968). Weiner *et al.* (1969) found that noradrenaline concentrations in the hypothalamus do not reach adult levels until day 50, which suggests that the amines reach adult levels later in the hypothalamus than in the rest of the brain. Dopamine levels take much longer to rise and do not reach adult concentrations until well after puberty, either in the whole brain or the hypothalamus (Agrawal *et al.*, 1966; Weiner *et al.*, 1969).

Parallel with the increase in the brain amines there is an increase in monoamine oxidase concentration (Bennett and Giarman, 1965; Agrawal *et al.*, 1966) especially in the first twenty days of life (Nachmais, 1961) and it reaches adult levels by the 28th day (Baker and Quay, 1969). The uptake mechanisms for the amines into nerve endings and the formation of their storage vesicles also develop slowly and reach the adult state by about day 28 in the rat. The uptake mechanism into nerve endings always develops a few days before the storage granules are completely formed and before the noradrenaline concentrations have reached adult levels (Coyle and Axelrod, 1971).

4.2   CIRCADIAN RHYTHM IN BRAIN AMINE METABOLISM

5-Hydroxytryptamine, noradrenaline and dopamine have all been shown to have a circadian rhythm in the rat brain.

5-Hydroxytryptamine concentrations alter significantly during a 24-hour period, with a rise during the day to peak in the afternoon and then a sudden drop in the evening at the beginning of the dark period (Dixit and Buckley, 1967; Scheving *et al.*, 1968; Friedman and Walker, 1968; Okado, 1971). This circadian rhythm for 5-hydroxytryptamine is observed only in regions of the brain containing the 5-hydroxytryptamine nerve terminals, i.e. the hypothalamus, frontal cortex and the lateral lower brain stem, while there is little daily alteration in the regions where the cell bodies are situated, i.e. medial brain stem and thalamus (Quay, 1968).

The circadian rhythm for 5-hydroxytryptamine develops only after days 35 to 37 of life in the rat, and in fact correlates well with the development of the normal sleep pattern (Okado, 1971). Héry et al. (1972) have shown that the changes in levels during the 24-hour cycle are due to changes in accumulation of precursors in the brain rather than changes in their conversion rate, so that in the light period there is an increase in synthesis of 5-hydroxytryptamine due to increased accumulation of tryptophan. At the same time, using in vitro and in vivo techniques to study the accumulation of ^{3}H-5-hydroxytryptamine and ^{3}H-5-HIAA, Héry et al. (1972) found that there is an increased release of 5-hydroxytryptamine at the beginning of the dark period coinciding with a sudden fall in brain levels. Correlated with this, there is a significant reduction in accumulation of exogenous ^{3}H-5-hydroxytryptamine in the dark period (Endersby and Wilson, 1974). All these changes may be of great physiological importance.

The circadian rhythm for noradrenaline also develops after days 35 to 37 in the rat (Asano, 1971). The brain levels are higher in the dark period with two or three peaks during this time (Friedman and Walker, 1968; Scheving et al., 1968). When separate areas of the brain were examined this rhythm could be seen in the anterior and posterior hypothalamus, but not in the thalamic, striatal or midbrain areas (Manshardt and Wurtman, 1968). Within the hypothalamus there is an increase in the number and density of granulated vesicles in the dark period (Walker and Friedman, 1969). In the light period noradrenaline levels fall reaching a trough in the afternoon. The rhythms are different in the cat where there is a rise in anterior hypothalamic noradrenaline levels throughout the light period to a peak in the early evening (Reis et al., 1968). The dopamine rhythm in the rat has two peaks, one in the morning and one in the night, with a trough during the light period between (Scheving et al., 1968). The rhythm of the catecholamine concentrations may be correlated with the rhythm of their rate of synthesis, which is higher in the late part of the light period than in the late part of the dark period. There is no rhythm in their rate of release (Zigmond et al., 1969; Zigmond and Werkman, 1970). Accumulation of exogenous ^{3}H-catecholamine into hypothalamic slices shows a diurnal rhythm with a significant peak at midday for noradrenaline (Endersby and Wilson, 1974) and a significantly greater accumulation of dopamine in the morning than in the evening (Hackmann et al., 1973).

5   Neuroendocrinology of gonadotrophin release

5.1   OVULATION AND FEEDBACK EFFECTS

The secretion of the gonadotrophins from the anterior pituitary is controlled by hormones from the hypothalamus and from the ovary and an understanding of the relationships between the hypothalamus, pituitary and ovary is essential for investigations on the control of gonadotrophin secretion. Figure 8 shows this interrelationship: the hypothalamus is connected to the pituitary by a blood supply passing from a series of capillary loops in the median eminence down the pituitary stalk in sinusoidal vessels into the anterior pituitary. This is called the hypophysial portal system and in 1948 Harris suggested that substances synthesized in the central nervous system might pass via this system to the pituitary where they stimulated pituitary hormone release. For the next twenty years attempts were made to isolate these releasing factors (also called releasing hormones), and in 1970 Schally's group isolated the releasing factor for thyroid-stimulating hormone (Bowers et al., 1970). The releasing factor for the luteinizing hormone (LH) was isolated and synthesized by the same group in 1971 (Matsuo et al., 1971). It is a decapeptide and can stimulate the release of both LH and follicle stimulating hormone (FSH). Schally maintains that there is only the one releasing factor for both gonadotrophins. However, recently an active principle has been isolated which has predominantly FSH-releasing properties (Johansson et al., 1973).

The site of synthesis of the releasing hormones is not known although they are known to be stored in specific areas in the hypothalamus and may be synthesized in the same areas. On suitable stimulation the releasing hormones are secreted from their storage sites and pass into the capillary loops of the hypophyseal portal system and thence to the pituitary where they stimulate the release of the pituitary hormones. When the gonadotrophins are released from the pituitary they pass via the blood stream to the ovaries where they can stimulate the secretion of oestrogen and progesterone.

The ovarian steroids are capable of exerting a negative feedback effect on the secretion of the gonadotrophins and so control their own secretion. This has been shown by the great increase in plasma gonadotrophin levels after removal of the gonads, and this increase can be abolished or prevented by administration of oestrogen. Progesterone has little effect on its own, but acts synergistically with oestrogen (McCann, 1962; 1963; Gay and Bogdanove, 1969). The main site of the negative feedback action is the hypothalamus; possibly there is some effect at higher CNS centres and at the pituitary level as well (see also section 5.2).

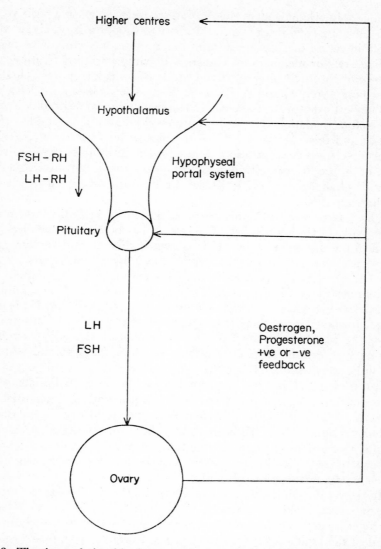

FIG. 8. The interrelationship between the hypothalamic, pituitary and ovarian hormones. LH-releasing hormone (LHRH) from the hypothalamus stimulates the release of the pituitary hormones which then act on the ovary and stimulate the secretion of oestrogen and progesterone. These exert a feedback effect on their own secretion at the hypothalamic and/or pituitary level. The feedback effect can be positive or negative depending on the endocrine condition of the animal.

In certain circumstances the ovarian steroids can exert a positive feed-back effect: a significant rise in both gonadotrophins is obtained when a single injection of either oestradiol or progesterone is given to ovariectomized rats or menopausal women, following a priming treatment with oestradiol to obtain normal blood levels of gonadotrophins (Odell and Swerdloff, 1968; Vande Weile et al., 1970; Caligaris et al., 1968; 1971).

The best example of the positive feedback effect of oestradiol is shown just before ovulation. Ovulation only takes place after a sudden release of LH and this only occurs when the plasma levels of oestradiol rise to a certain critical concentration. The surge can be inhibited by administration of antibodies to oestradiol (Ferin et al., 1969), anti-oestrogen compounds (Labhsetwar, 1970; 1972a), or by critically timed ovariectomy (Schwartz, 1964).

These facts seem to apply to most mammals including the human. The study of the physiology of ovulation has been most detailed in the rat and the sequence of events is shown in Fig. 9, and the changes in hormonal secretion in Fig. 10. Under the influence of FSH (and a low basal level of LH), the ovarian follicles mature and at a certain stage secrete oestradiol (Schwartz, 1969; Ely and Schwartz, 1971). Following a peak level of plasma oestradiol at around midday (Shaikh, 1971) on the day before ovulation, there is a sudden surge of LH, FSH and prolactin from the pituitary in the late afternoon on the day before ovulation, lasting two to four hours (Naftolin et al., 1972; Mahesh and Goldman, 1971; Freeman et al., 1972). The surge of LH (but probably not of FSH or prolactin) is necessary for ovulation to take place. It initiates (1) the secretion of progesterone from the follicles and/or interstitial cells (Leavitt et al., 1971) and (2) changes in the follicle walls so that the follicles rupture about 12 hours later, each follicle releasing an ovum. Luteal tissue then grows to fill the follicles to form corpora lutea which are capable of producing progesterone, although they do not secrete high levels unless fertilization takes place.

In the rat the stimulation of LH release by the rise in plasma oestradiol can only occur during a critical period of two hours during the afternoon of the same day. The exact time is controlled by the time of commencement of the light period for that day. For example, on a fixed regime of 14 hours of light starting at 6.00 hours, the critical period occurs between 14.00 and 16.00 hours (Everett et al., 1949). The actual release of LH into the blood after stimulation occurs between 17.00 and 20.00 hours with a peak at 18.00 hours (see Fig. 10).

The rise in progesterone levels occurring simultaneously, or just after the LH surge, is stimulated by the LH (Barraclough et al., 1971; Piacsek et al., 1971) and only declines slowly over the following dark

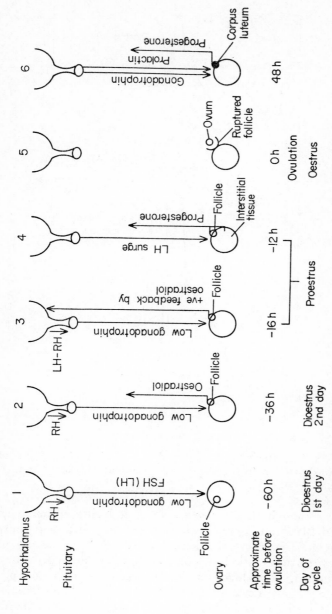

FIG. 9. Diagrammatic representation of the sequence of release of hormones from the hypothalamus, pituitary and ovary which lead to ovulation in the rat.

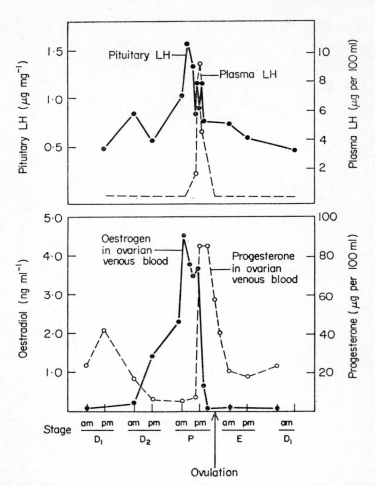

FIG. 10. Cyclic fluctuations of pituitary and plasma LH and oestrogen and pro-gesterone in ovarian venous blood in 4-day cyclic rats. (Adapted from Miyake, 1968.)

period. It is thought to be necessary for inducing sexual receptivity (Boling and Blandeau, 1939) in the rat and may also help control the duration of the LH surge (Kobayashi *et al.*, 1970). In the rat, all these changes occur over a period of 4 or 5 days, called the oestrous cycle.

In the human, an analogous series of changes occur over a period of approximately 28 days called the menstrual cycle, and an example of the plasma hormonal concentrations during this cycle is given in Fig. 11. During the first half of the cycle (or follicular phase) low levels of FSH

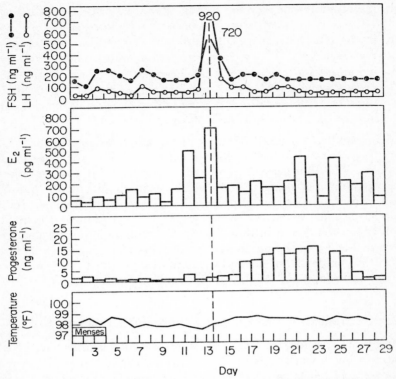

FIG. 11. Simultaneous determinations of plasma LH, FSH, oestradiol, and progesterone and basal body temperature in a woman with normal ovulatory menstrual cycles. (Adapted from Vande Weile *et al.*, 1970.)

and LH stimulate the ovarian follicles to secrete oestrogen which reaches a peak concentration at mid-cycle, and then, either on the same day or one day later, there is a dramatic increase in LH secretion (and to a lesser extent FSH) which lasts 1 or 2 days. This is exactly equivalent to the LH surge in the rat and ovulation takes place at some time towards the end of this mid-cycle period. After ovulation the corpus luteum formed from the ruptured follicle secretes progesterone and also some oestrogen in the second half of the cycle (the luteal phase). If fertilization does not occur the corpus luteum regresses approximately two weeks after its formation and the steroid secretion falls to zero (Ross *et al.*, 1970; Vande Weile *et al.*, 1970). The oestrous and menstrual cycles differ in three main ways:

a. in general only one follicle ruptures in the course of a menstrual cycle, while in the rat an average of 12 ovulations or ruptures occur;

b. the progesterone secreted by the interstitial cells at the time of the LH surge in the rat, does not occur in the human;

c. in the rat, the corpora lutea produce very little progesterone and regress after 2 or 3 days, unless stimulated by coitus or vaginal irritation, in which case they become "functional" and secrete progesterone for 11–14 days before regressing. If this occurs and the rats are not fertilized they are said to be psuedopregnant. In the human the corpus luteum is always functional.

Before puberty ovulation cannot occur spontaneously in the rat, but after day 21 it is possible to induce ovulation with exogenous gonadotrophins. The immature rat induced to ovulate with a single injection of pregnant mares' serum (PMS), which has predominantly FSH properties is a useful experimental preparation. Treatment with PMS initiates exactly the same pattern of events leading to ovulation as described for spontaneous ovulation in the adult animal. Figure 12 shows changes in hormonal levels in the plasma before ovulation in immature rats treated with PMS on day 30 of life and the pattern is similar to that in the adult animal (Wilson *et al.*, 1974b).

5.2   HYPOTHALAMIC SITES OF ACTION OF OVARIAN STEROIDS

The sites of steroidal feedback effects in the hypothalamus have been the object of much work. It is now considered that there is a tonic centre in the arcuate nucleus and median eminence area which controls low tonic secretion of gonadotrophin necessary for maintaining gonadal weight and function. In the female there is an additional centre in the preoptic area, which controls the cyclic release of LH just before ovulation (Gorski, 1966). It is thought that the cyclic centre sends pulses at a regular time each afternoon to stimulate the tonic centre in the median eminence (Tejasen and Everett, 1967; Gorski, 1968), but the latter only responds on the day before ovulation when the oestradiol levels are high. It is suggested that the oestradiol lowers the threshold of stimulation of the median eminence (McDonald and Gilmore, 1971; Sawyer and Hilliard, 1971). Everett (1964) has shown that there is a neural pathway connecting the two centres. Stumpf (1968) demonstrated by autoradiography that oestradiol is taken up in significant quantities in the anterior hypothalamus, especially in the preoptic and median eminence areas, and Kato (1973) showed that there are significantly higher concentrations of oestrogen receptors in these areas. Implants of oestradiol are more effective in inducing gonadotrophin release when placed in the median eminence, although implants in the preoptic are also active in some

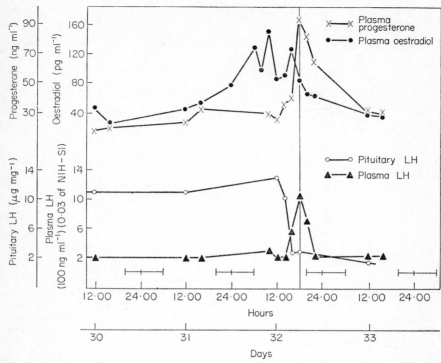

FIG. 12. Fluctuations in pituitary LH and plasma LH, oestradiol, and progesterone in the immature rat treated with 20 i.u. pregnant mares' serum gonadotrophin subcutaneously on day 30 of life. The vertical line indicates the time of the LH peak. The broken lines on the abscissa denote the dark phases of the lighting cycle. (With permission from Wilson et al., 1974b.)

situations (Smith and Davidson, 1967; Davidson, 1969). The site of the negative feedback effect of the steroids also appears to be at the median eminence level (Chowers and McCann, 1967; Smith and Davidson, 1968; Taleisnik et al., 1970). Possibly the steroids have biphasic effect on the threshold of stimulation of the median eminence, first lowering and then raising it (Beyer and Sawyer, 1969). Figure 13 summarizes the hypothalamic control of gonadotrophin release.

The development of the cyclic centre for gonadotrophin release is suppressed in the foetal or neonatal male due to secretion of testosterone from the testes in the last few days of gestation and the first days of life (Harris, 1964). If a female rat is treated with testosterone on any day before day 5 it will not ovulate at maturity, as no cyclic release of LH occurs; these females are said to be androgenized. Conversely castration on day 1

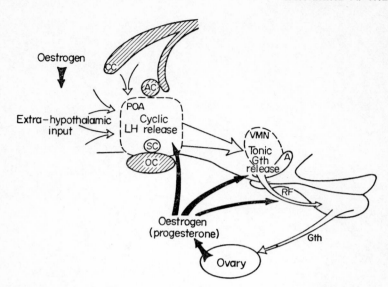

Fig. 13. A model of the localization of the hypothalamic control of the secretion of gonadotrophins in the normal female rat as projected on a schematic midsagittal view of the hypothalamus. A, arcuate nucleus; AC, anterior commisure; CC, corpus callosum; Gth, gonadotrophins; OC, optic chiasma; POA, preoptic area; SC, suprachiasmatic nucleus, VMN, ventromedial nucleus; black arrows represent possible feedback pathways of the ovarian hormones. (With permission from Gorski, 1971.)

of life in the male rat will allow cyclic release to occur and this can be shown by noting ovulation in ovarian grafts in adulthood (Gorski, 1971; Flerko, 1971).

5.3   CONTROL OF PROLACTIN RELEASE

Another pituitary hormone concerned with reproduction is prolactin. In the human, it is known to be necessary for mammary growth and lactation, and other possible physiological activities have not, as yet, been found. However, in the rodent, it has been shown to have additional functions. It is known to be luteotrophic and its secretion is necessary in early pregnancy and pseudopregnancy, in order to stimulate the corpora lutea to produce progesterone (Astwood, 1941; Greenwald and Rothchild, 1968). Freeman and Neill (1972) have suggested that during pseudopregnancy there is a surge of prolactin each night which continues until the condition terminates. Prolactin also appears to be luteolytic in the rat with normal oestrous cycles. There is a rise in plasma prolactin levels on the afternoon of proestrus and this surge causes the regression of the corpora lutea formed in the previous cycle (Billeter and Fluckiger, 1971; Grandison and Meites, 1972).

Oestrogen stimulates the secretion of prolactin, both at the hypothalamic level (Ratner and Meites, 1964) and at the pituitary level (Nicoll and Meites, 1962), and it is clear that the oestrogen secretion on the morning of proestrus in the cyclic rat stimulates the prolactin surge, as well as the LH surge, seen on the afternoon of proestrus (Neill *et al.*, 1971). Prolactin itself can exert a negative feedback effect on its own secretion, probably at the hypothalamic level, since implants of prolactin in the median eminence reduced plasma prolactin levels (Chen *et al.*, 1967; Voogt and Meites, 1971).

The hypothalamus exerts an inhibitory effect on prolactin release from the pituitary. This is clearly shown by the fact that there is an enormous increase in prolactin secretion after sectioning the pituitary stalk (Westman and Jacobsohn, 1938), transplanting the pituitary at a site away from the hypothalamus (Nikitovitch-Winer and Everett, 1958), or lesioning the hypothalamus in the median eminence area (McCann and Friedman, 1960).

An inhibitory principle has been extracted from the hypothalamus called prolactin inhibitory factor (PIF). It has not been isolated, as yet, but is known to have a small molecular weight (Meites *et al.*, 1961; Schally *et al.*, 1967). Substances known to inhibit or stimulate prolactin release at the hypothalamic level have been shown to alter hypothalamic levels of PIF.

Recently, some evidence has been found for the presence of a hypothalamic prolactin releasing factor (PRF). Nicoll *et al.* (1970) have shown that a hypothalamic extract inhibits prolactin release from pituitaries *in vitro* for 4 hours and this is followed by a stimulation of prolactin release. This has been confirmed in other preparations (Mishkinsky *et al.*, 1968; Krulich *et al.*, 1971). In contrast to the rodent, there is no PIF activity present in the avian hypothalamus and therefore no inhibitory effect on prolactin release; on the other hand the presence of PRF has been indicated in hypothalami taken from various avian species (see Meites *et al.*, 1972).

6 The effect of brain amines on the release of gonadotrophins

6.1 THE EFFECT OF CHANGES IN GONADOTROPHIN RELEASE ON HYPOTHALAMIC CATACHOLAMINES

6.1.1 *Changes in hypothalamic catecholamine levels*

One of the first series of experiments showing the correlation between hypothalamic catecholamines and gonadotrophin release was carried out by Donoso and co-workers between 1965 and 1968. They showed that 10 days after castration the level of noradrenaline in the anterior hypothalamus was significantly raised in both male and female rats and could be restored to normal by high doses of oestradiol (5 μg) given together with progesterone (25 mg) for 7 days; the hormones had no effect at lower doses or when given separately (Stefano *et al.*, 1965; Donoso *et al.*, 1966; 1967). At the same time as lowering the noradrenaline levels, the hormone treatment appeared to increase the concentration of hypothalamic dopamine (Donoso and Stefano, 1967). These findings were confirmed by Coppola (1969; 1971) who also found that noradrenaline levels were high in castrated male and female rats, and could be reduced by gonadal steroids. On using physiological doses of the hormones, he was able to demonstrate that oestrogen (1 μg oestrone or 8 μg ethinyl-oestradiol) and progesterone (2 mg) could act separately. Stefano and Donoso (1967) also observed changes in hypothalamic noradrenaline concentration during the oestrous cycle and found the levels were highest on the day of proestrus (i.e. on the day of the gonadotrophin surge), but this fluctuation only took place in the anterior portion of the hypothalamus (Donoso *et al.*, 1966; Stefano and Donoso, 1967).

These findings have not been confirmed by other workers. In fact, Kurachi and Hirota (1969) have obtained exactly opposite results to those of Donoso's group. They found that hypothalamic noradrenaline levels fell 30 days after castration and were brought back to normal by oestradiol (10 μg) treatment. They also found that during the oestrous cycle hypothalamic levels were lowest on the day of proestrus and rose over the rest of the cycle to a peak in late dioestrus. Noradrenaline levels in the cortex and dopamine levels in both the cortex and hypothalamus did not alter in the different endocrine states.

There are many other conflicting results. For instance Sandler (1968) and Weiner *et al.* (1972a) found no change in the anterior hypothalamus on different days of the cycle. Sandler (1968) and Hyyppa and Valavaara (1970) also failed to demonstrate the rise in noradrenaline levels after castration. In addition, Barthwal *et al.* (1971) showed that in ovariectomized rats treatment with a synthetic oestrogen (diethylstilboestrol) increased dopamine levels in the whole brain, while progesterone treatment lowered the content of dopamine. Neither treatment effected noradrenaline or adrenaline.

In all these experiments the amines were extracted from brain tissue and measured by fluoroispectrometric assay. Using the histofluorescence technique of Falck *et al.* (1962), Lichtensteiger and his co-workers (1969) have made a detailed study of changes in the intensity of fluorescence of the cell bodies in the arcuate nucleus. Dopamine is the transmitter in the system originating in the arcuate nucleus and Lichtensteiger (1969) has shown that in the oestrous cycle there is a steady increase in fluorescence from the first day of dioestrus to a maximum at oestrus. After ovariectomy, there is a small but significant rise in fluorescence which is reduced 24–48 hours after treatment with physiological doses of oestradiol (Lichtensteiger *et al.*, 1969) or oestradiol together with progesterone (Lichtensteiger, 1971). Hyyppa and Lorentz (1969) also showed increased fluorescence in cell bodies of the arcuate nucleus after castration in male rats, and at the same time they showed that there was a rise in FSH–RH activity in the hypothalamus. This increase in fluorescence is probably due to dopamine, because castration did not alter the levels of hypothalamic noradrenaline and 5-hydroxytryptamine as measured by spectrofluorescence assay (Hyyppa and Valavaara, 1970). When the castrated rats were treated with testosterone, fluorescence was reduced and this treatment is known to reduce the release of FSH.

Lichtensteiger (1970) has also attempted to correlate changes in fluorescence with gonadotrophin release and showed that when the preoptic area or arcuate nucleus was stimulated there was an increase in fluorescence in the cell bodies of the arcuate, correlated with a rise in plasma LH levels. The increase in fluorescence may be due to an increase in synthesis of dopamine since stimulation in rats pretreated with α-methyltyrosine (an inhibitor of tyrosine hydroxylase) no longer produced the rise in fluorescence (Keller and Lichtensteiger, 1971).

The main body of results seem to show that noradrenaline and dopamine levels are high when gonadotrophin release is enhanced, as after castration or before ovulation, and are low when gonadotrophin release is reduced, as after steroid treatment or in the dioestrous period of the cycle.

6.1.2   *Changes in hypothalamic catacholamine turnover*

Estimation of the concentration of a substance in a particular tissue is not, by itself, a good indication of the activity of that substance; for instance, increased levels may indicate an increase in synthesis or may indicate a decrease in release. A better test of activity is the turnover rate of a substance, which is the balance of the rate of synthesis and the rate of removal, and this can be measured in three ways:

a. by inhibiting synthesis using a tyrosine hydroxylase inhibitor (α-methyl-*p*-tyrosine) or a dopamine β-hydroxylase inhibitor [bis-(4-methyl-1-homopiperazinyl-(thiocarbonyl)disulphide, FLA 63], and then measuring the fall in amine levels either spectrofluorometrically or by histofluorescence;

b. by injecting a labelled amine precursor (e.g. ^{3}H-tyrosine) and measuring the concentration of labelled amine synthesized in a given time;

c. by injecting a labelled amine and noting its disappearance rate.

Each method has its inherent advantages and disadvantages (see Anton-Tay and Wurtman, 1971) and so the discrepancies between the results may be due to the artifacts of the methods. Using all three methods various groups have found that the turnover rate of noradrenaline increases after ovariectomy and the rate is reduced to normal by treatment with ovarian steroids (Donoso et al., 1969; Bapna et al., 1971; Anton-Tay and Wurtman, 1968; Coppola, 1969). In all cases the levels of the amine, whether after injection of labelled amine, amine precursor or synthesis inhibitor, were estimated by first extracting and then spectro-fluorometric assay methods. However, contrary results were obtained by Fuxe and his group using histofluorescence techniques to estimate cata-cholamines. They found no change in turnover of noradrenaline either after synthesis inhibition by α-methyltyrosine or FLA 63, or after injec-tion of ^{3}H-noradrenaline (Fuxe et al., 1970b; Hokfelt and Fuxe, 1972a). The histofluorometric method, however, can be criticized, as it is difficult to quantify.

Fuxe also estimated the turnover rate of dopamine in the ventral hypothalamus by noting changes in fluorescence in the nerve terminals of the median eminence after inhibition of synthesis. He found that dopamine turnover in castrated rats did not fluctuate, as in the rat with normal cycles, but remained at the lower level normally found at oestrus. Treatment with oestradiol, or oestradiol with progesterone, but not pro-gesterone alone or by hydrocortisone, raised the turnover rate significantly (Fuxe et al., 1967; 1969). No other investigator has looked at dopamine turnover because of the difficulty of estimating the hypothalamic levels by any method other than histofluorescence. Fuxe and co-workers have carried out a large amount of work based on this technique and they are confident that it is sufficiently accurate to justify its use to estimate the low concentrations involved. They feel, indeed, that other methods used to investigate noradrenaline are inaccurate due to the low levels of the amines and that the changes noted by Anton-Tay and Wurtman (1968), for instance, are artifacts of the method (Fuxe et al., 1970b).

Turning now to the ovulating animal, turnover rates of noradrenaline rise on the day of the expected LH surge necessary for ovulation. This has been shown in the adult rat with spontaneous ovulation (Donoso and Moyano, 1970) and in the immature rat induced to ovulate (Coppola, 1969). Fuxe's group have shown in adult rats a fall in turnover rate of dopamine on the day of proestrus and early oestrus, compared with the rest of the cycle (Ahren *et al.*, 1971). They have also shown that dopamine turnover falls just at the beginning of the critical period in immature rats induced to ovulate (Fuxe *et al.*, 1972b).

Most workers have found that the level of noradrenaline rises at times when gonadotrophin release is enhanced, i.e. after castration or before ovulation. With the exception of Fuxe's group, most workers have found the turnover rate of noradrenaline also rises when gonadotrophin release is enhanced. Together these findings would indicate that the synthesis rate of noradrenaline is increased at this time.

Dopamine turnover is reduced and levels in the hypothalamus are raised when gonadotrophins are being released. This indicates that there is an inhibition of dopamine release. When gonadotrophin release is inhibited the turnover of dopamine rises with a concomitant fall in levels, suggesting an increase in rate of release, with insufficient increase in synthesis rate to maintain the levels.

It would be interesting in view of these findings to know the changes in the individual mechanisms that go to make up turnover rate; some of these are synthesis rate, release rate, uptake and catabolism. These aspects are discussed in the following paragraphs.

6.1.3 *Changes in catecholamine synthesis rate*

Synthesis rates of noradrenaline *in vivo* has been investigated by either noting the difference in the disappearance rate of an injection of ^{3}H-noradrenaline in control rats and rats pretreated with a synthesis inhibitor (Anton-Tay *et al.*, 1969), or by the rate of conversion of labelled tyrosine to noradrenaline (Bapna *et al.*, 1971). Both methods showed that the synthesis rate was increased in castrated rats, i.e. when gonadotrophin release is enhanced and also on the day of proestrous in cyclic rats (Zschaeck and Wurtman, 1973). The rate-limiting step for catecholamine synthesis is at the stage when tyrosine hydroxylase converts tyrosine to dopa. Tyrosine hydroxylase activity has been shown to increase two- or three-fold after ovariectomy, which would explain the increase in synthesis rate seen at this time. Administration of oestrogen to the ovariectomized rats increased tyrosine hydroxylase activity further, while progesterone reduced its activity. The inhibitory effect of progesterone was enhanced if the animals were primed with oestrogen and could also be demonstrated after *in vitro* application of progesterone to hypothalamic slices (Beattie *et al.*, 1972; Beattie and Soyka, 1973). These results indicate that progesterone may well exert its negative feedback effect on gonadotrophin release by interfering with the synthesis of the catecholamines.

However, in *in vitro* experiments there are some indications that the synthesis rate is lower at proestrus, when gonadotrophin release is high, and increases at oestrus. This was suggested by the results of Hamon *et al.* (see Kordon and Glowinski, 1972) who noted that when hypothalamic slices taken from rats at different stages of the cycle were incubated with ^{3}H-tyrosine the accumulation of ^{3}H-noradrenaline was higher at oestrus than proestrus.

6.1.4   *Changes in catecholamine release rate*

The rate of release of noradrenaline was found to be higher in castrated rats because there were increased concentrations of its extraneuronal metabolite, normetanephrine, in the hypothalami of these animals (Donoso *et al.*, 1969). The presence of oestradiol, on the other hand, has been shown to inhibit the release of noradrenaline after electrical stimulation of brain slices or hypothalamic synaptosomes, *in vitro*. Progesterone acts differently, as it increases the efflux after electrical stimulation of the tissue (Vogel *et al.*, 1970; Janowsky and Davis, 1970).

6.1.5   *Changes in catecholamine uptake*

In vitro experiments on the effect of steroids on uptake have also been carried out and the presence of oestradiol and progesterone in the incubation medium significantly reduces uptake of noradrenaline (Janowsky and Davis, 1970; Endersby and Wilson, 1974). However these experiments are not as physiological as experiments studying uptake of ^{3}H-noradrenaline and ^{3}H-dopamine into the hypothalamic slices from rats pretreated with oestradiol, progesterone or oestradiol together with progesterone (Endersby and Wilson, 1973; 1974). The results of these experiments showed that a physiological dose of oestradiol (1 µg) increased the uptake of ^{3}H-noradrenaline, while progesterone (4 mg) together with a low basal level of oestradiol (0·05 µg) reduced the uptake of dopamine. Progesterone alone had no effect in these experiments. Hackmann *et al.* (1973) confirmed this lack of effect of progesterone on ^{3}H-dopamine uptake.

A particularly interesting finding has been that the uptake of dopamine was significantly increased at the beginning of the critical period and significantly decreased at the end of the period; this was shown in hypothalami taken from immature rats induced to ovulate with PMS (Endersby and Wilson, 1974). This correlates with the findings of Fuxe who showed that the turnover rate of dopamine falls dramatically at the beginning of the critical period in PMS treated rats (Fuxe *et al.*, 1972b). Uptake of noradrenaline was not found to alter at any time on the day before ovulation. It is very hard to interpret these results but it does indicate that the noradrenaline and dopamine activities alter in a different manner with steroid treatment and that dopamine may be involved in the precise timing of the critical period.

6.1.6   Changes in amine catabolism

The effect of steroids on the rate of degradation of the amines has not been studied in an isolated manner, but changes in levels of the enzymes concerned with catabolism have been shown to occur in different hormonal conditions; for instance in castrated rats monoamine oxidases (MAO) in the anterior hypothalamus first fall and then three weeks after castration they rise, and this increase can be reduced to normal by treatment with physiological doses of oestradiol (0·1–1 µg) (Kobayashi et al., 1964; 1966). Histochemical studies in rats 30 days after castration show that the rise in MAO activity occurs in the anterior hypothalamus, i.e. the supraoptic and paraventricular nuclei, while there is a fall in the middle area which includes the dorsomedial, ventromedial and arcuate nuclei (Kurachi and Hirota, 1969).

In the post-menopausal human (when no ovarian secretion occurs) MAO levels in the plasma are high and can be reduced by oestrogen treatment (Klaiber et al., 1971). In the castrated rat administration of oestradiol also reduces MAO levels in the uterus, ovary and adrenals, while progesterone treatment significantly increases MAO levels (Holzbauer and Youdim, 1973). In the human menstrual cycle MAO levels are lower in the first half when oestradiol levels are raised and significantly higher in the second half when progesterone secretion occurs (Briggs and Briggs, 1972).

In the intact rat, the negative correlation between oestrogen and MAO is not so clearly observed, probably because there is a time-lag between increased oestrogen secretion and its effect. Thus at proestrus when oestradiol secretion is high, hypothalamic levels of MAO are also high and remain so during the day of oestrus (Kobayaski et al., 1964; 1966; Zolovick et al., 1966; Salseduc et al., 1966; Kamberi and Danhof, 1968), but the effect of the raised oestradiol levels can be seen on the night of oestrus, when MAO levels fall dramatically (Holzbauer and Youdim, 1973). Kamberi and Kobayashi (1970) have shown a small and transient trough in hypothalamic MAO levels, after the critical period on proestrus followed by a rise of MAO in oestrus. This agrees with histochemical studies which show that MAO activity is high on the day of proestrus in the anterior part of the hypothalamus including the supraoptic and paraventricular nuclei and then is high on the day of oestrus in the middle area, i.e. the ventromedial and arcuate nuclei.

MAO levels in the hypothalamus tend to be lower in early dioestrus and rise during late dioestrus until they reach their peak value on proestrus; this may be a result of increased progesterone secretion by the ovaries and adrenals in early dioestrus (Holzbauer and Youdim, 1973). There may also be a circadian rhythm for brain MAO levels, as it has been shown in the male rat that the levels are low in the hypothalamus and limbic system in the morning, rising in the afternoon to high levels throughout the dark period (Kamberi and Danhof, 1968; Holzbauer and Youdim, 1972): although in a second series of experiments Holzbauer and Youdim (1973) were unable to show any circadian changes.

Catechol-O-methyl transferase (COMT) levels also alter during the oestrous cycle and are lower at oestrus than at dioestrus; proestrus levels were not investigated (Salseduc et al., 1966).

6.1.7 Effect of hormones on the turnover of hypothalamic amines

Returning to the more general measurement of turnover rate, it seems that the steroids exert a negative feedback effect by increasing dopamine activity. Administration of oestradiol or testosterone to the rat raises the turnover rate of dopamine whether it is intact or castrated and even does so when the hypothalamus is isolated from the rest of the brain by deafferentation, indicating that the steroids are acting directly on the hypothalamus and not via some extra-hypothalamic system (Fuxe et al., 1971).

The turnover rate of dopamine is high in the female rat showing persistent oestrus, following constant illumination or neonatal androgenization. This is probably due to the high levels of oestradiol as castration in these animals reduces the turnover rate (Fuxe et al., 1972a). The levels of dopamine in the cell bodies of the arcuate nucleus (as shown by fluorescence) as well as the turnover rate of dopamine in the nerve terminals in the median eminence are high in the pregnant, pseudopregnant and lactating rat (Fuxe et al., 1967). On the other hand, hypophysectomy reduces the turnover rate to a value below that seen after castration or on the day of dioestrus. This indicates that one of the pituitary hormones may control dopamine activity and the findings in the pregnant and lactating rat suggest it is prolactin. In fact, prolactin given to hypophysectomized, castrated and even intact rats will raise the dopamine turnover; growth hormone exerts the same effect in very high doses, but LH, FSH, ACTH, TSH, and vasopressin are all ineffective (Fuxe and Hokfelt, 1970a; Hokfelt and Fuxe, 1972a).

The turnover of noradrenaline has been shown to increase after treatment with FSH, but not LH (Anton-Tay et al., 1969).

6.1.8 *Conclusions*

a. Hypothalamic dopamine activity. Fuxe has proposed that dopamine inhibits gonadotrophin release, and dopaminergic neurones are activated by prolactin. His own experiments provide evidence to support this hypothesis. He further suggests that noradrenaline stimulates gonadotrophin release by first stimulating PIF, which reduces prolactin levels and thus reduces dopamine activity. This removes the inhibitory control on gonadotrophin release and so release can occur. Fuxe suggests this is what happens at the critical period before ovulation and the preoptic stimulation that normally takes place at this time effects gonadotrophin release because (i) the presence of oestrogen lowers the threshold of activation of the median eminence and (ii) the inhibitory action of dopamine has been removed (Fuxe *et al.*, 1970a; 1970b; Fuxe and Hokfelt, 1970a). The fact that Lichtensteiger (1970) found high concentration of dopamine in the hypothalamus at times of enhanced gonadotrophin release suggests that it is the release of dopamine which is inhibited rather than all aspects of dopamine metabolism.

b. Hypothalamic noradrenaline activity. It appears that at times of enhanced gonadotrophin release there is an increase in synthesis and release rate of noradrenaline, as well as raised levels of the amine and MAO, i.e. there is an overall increase in hypothalamic noradrenaline metabolism at this time. These findings are supported by the fact that treatment of the ovariectomized rat with oestradiol inhibits release of noradrenaline, increases uptake and lowers levels of noradrenaline and MAO; also oestradiol together with progesterone reduce tyrosine hydroxylase activity. Thus in circumstances when the steroids inhibit gonadotrophin release they also reduce the general metabolic activity of the amine.

6.2 THE EFFECT OF CHANGING BRAIN CATECHOLAMINE LEVELS ON GONADOTROPHIN RELEASE

The effect of changing levels of hypothalamic catecholamine on the release of gonadotrophins has been studied extensively, either by direct administration of the amines, or by pharmacological agents which alter levels of the amines in the brain. Before 1969, it was not possible to determine changes in levels of gonadotrophins in the peripheral plasma and therefore up to this time indirect methods for noting release of LH were used, such as changes in gonadal weight, onset of puberty, occurrence of ovulation and depletion of ovarian ascorbic acid. This last phenomenon occurs in response to a small concentration of LH and has been used as a biological method for assaying LH (Parlow, 1961). Development of radio-immunoassays for measuring plasma gonadotrophins allowed direct determinations, but it is still important to know whether the changes in gonadotrophin levels after amine administration are physiological and can effect, for instance, the occurrence of ovulation.

6.2.1 *Early experiments*

Adrenaline given subcutaneously inhibited both spontaneous and induced ovulation in mice (Robson, 1931) and rats (Eskin, 1944; Dordoni and Timiras, 1952; Moore, 1959; Jaitley *et al.*, 1967), but this was due to the stressful effect of subcutaneous injection, since agents such as formalin, ether and alloxan also inhibited ovulation (Dordoni and Timiras, 1952; Moore, 1959; Chatterjee, 1967). The stress reaction induced the release of ACTH which inhibited the release of the gonadotrophins and therefore inhibited ovulation (Hagino *et al.*, 1969). However, adrenaline given intravenously had a stimulatory effect on gonadotrophin release. Sawyer and his co-workers showed this effect by inducing ovulation in rabbits pretreated with atropine to protect them against the toxic effects of adrenaline (Markee *et al.*, 1947; 1948; Sawyer *et al.*, 1950a). Adrenaline, by intravenous injection, in doses between 5 and 40 μg also stimulated LH release (as shown by ovarian ascorbic acid depletion) in intact rats and ovariectomized rats treated with ovarian steroids (Guiliani *et al.*, 1960; 1961; Ramirez *et al.*, 1963; Parlow, 1964), but not in hypophysectomized rats (Guiliani *et al.*, 1960). The likelihood of a central site of action was investigated by infusing the adrenaline directly into the pituitary. This treatment did indeed stimulate ovulation (Markee *et al.*, 1947) but this was later proved to be due to the traumatic effect of the infusion (Donovan and Harris, 1956). In some experiments even subcutaneous administration of adrenaline was effective in stimulating gonadotrophin release for instance in rats stressed by under-feeding or in ageing female rats in constant oestrus (Piacsek *et al.*, 1967; Clemens *et al.*, 1969).

The stimulatory effect of adrenaline was confirmed by concomitant experiments in which pharmacological agents were administered in order to alter endogenous levels of the amines or block their receptor sites. These early experiments were carried out by Sawyer and his co-workers (1947; 1949a; 1949b), who showed that the α-adrenergic blocker, dibenamine inhibited ovulation in rabbits and rats, if given before the expected time of the LH surge (Everett *et al.*, 1949). They showed, however, that other adrenergic blockers such as imadozoline and its derivatives were not effective (Sawyer *et al.*, 1950b), and it is possible that the anti-ovulatory effect was due either to stress (Moore, 1961) or an effect at the ovarian level (Ferrando and Nalbandov, 1969).

6.2.2 Recent experiments

In spite of the controversy over the results of early experiments, the basic premise that the catecholamines are necessary for gonadotrophin release has been confirmed many times. Inhibition of catecholamine synthesis by means of α-methyltyrosine has been shown to inhibit spontaneous ovulation in adult mice (Bhargava and Gupta, 1966) and hamsters (Lippmann, 1968); also it inhibited ovulation in immature mice (Brown, 1967b) and decreased ovarian hypertrophy seen after hemicastration in female rats (Donoso and Santolaya, 1969). In addition, depletion of catecholamine stores by reserpine was found to inhibit spontaneous and induced ovulation in rats (Coppola et al., 1966; Meyerson and Sawyer, 1968; Rubinstein and Sawyer, 1970; Ratner and McCann, 1971; Craven and McDonald, 1971b). Coppola studied the effect of a wide range of pharmacological agents known to cause catecholamine depletion and found only those that depleted brain catecholamines inhibited induced ovulation; drugs acting solely as peripheral amine depletors had no effect (Coppola et al., 1966; Lippmann et al., 1967; Coppola, 1968). This proved that the amines were involved with gonadotrophin release at a site within the CNS.

By 1965 the importance of noradrenaline and dopamine as putative transmitters in the CNS was realized and so in subsequent experiments comparisons were made between the effects of adrenaline, noradrenaline and dopamine. Different groups of workers tend to favour different amines as the stimulatory transmitter for gonadotrophin release, and so the account which follows favours each of the three catecholamines in turn.

6.2.3 Dopamine as the transmitter for gonadotrophin release

The results obtained after altering levels of hypothalamic dopamine fall into two categories. The earlier work of McCann and his group suggest that this amine stimulates gonadotrophin release, while there is now accumulating evidence suggesting it inhibits gonadotrophin release.

In 1969 McCann and his co-workers started an extensive investigation into the effects of amines on gonadotrophin release. They incubated rat pituitaries with each of the three amines in turn and found that dopamine had no direct effect on the release of gonadotrophins but that adrenaline enhanced the release of FSH and LH, and noradrenaline that of FSH only (Schneider and McCann, 1969a; Kamberi and McCann, 1969a; 1969b; Van Loon and Kragt, 1970; Quijada *et al.*, 1974). When portions of the stalk-median eminence area of the hypothalamus were added to the incubation, the release of both FSH and LH was enhanced by dopamine even at very low concentrations ($0.5-5$ μg ml^{-1}) while noradrenaline and adrenaline had no effect (Schneider and McCann, 1969b; Kamberi *et al.*, 1970a). Dopamine must have acted in these experiments by stimulating the discharge of LH and FSH-releasing hormone from the hypothalamic fragments since it did not potentiate the action of exogenous LH/FSH releasing hormone added to the incubation mixture. α-Adrenergic and dopaminergic blocking agents (phenoxybenzamine, phentolamine and haloperidol) inhibited the release, and a β-adrenergic blocking agent (proprananol) did not (McCann *et al.*, 1972). The prior addition of oestradiol to the incubation also blocked the releasing effect of dopamine and Schneider and McCann (1970a) suggested that oestradiol exerts its negative feedback effect in physiological conditions by inhibiting the stimulating action of dopamine on LH/FSH-RH release.

The stimulating effect of dopamine has also been shown in *in vivo* experiments. Intraventricular injection of $1-4$ μg of dopamine increased the LH/FSH releasing hormone activity in the plasma taken from the hypophyseal portal system (Kamberi *et al.*, 1969a; 1970b; 1970c; 1971a) as well as the peripheral plasma of hypophysectomized rats (Schneider and McCann, 1970b), and this stimulatory effect was prevented by pretreatment with oestradiol (Schneider and McCann, 1970c). Similarly, dopamine stimulated the release of LH and FSH into the circulating blood of intact male and female rats and in ovariectomized female rats pretreated with ovarian hormones (Schneider and McCann, 1970d; Kamberi *et al.*, 1970a; Porter *et al.*, 1972a). In the intact female rat, dopamine was particularly effective on the second day of dioestrus and on proestrus, and these effects were reversed by α-adrenergic blocking agents (Schneider and McCann, 1970d). Parallel experiments using adrenaline and noradrenaline revealed that both amines given intraventricularly stimulated gonadotrophin release but that slightly higher doses ($2.5-5$ μg) were required and that doses of 100 μg or more were required for the two amines to be effective in intact males (Schneider and McCann, 1970b; 1970c; 1970d; Kamberi *et al.*, 1970b).

When the effective intraventricular dose of dopamine was injected directly into the portal hypophyseal system, release of gonadotrophins was not stimulated, thus demonstrating as in the *in vitro* experiments that dopamine did not act directly on the pituitary (Kamberi *et al.*, 1970b). Dopamine was also inactive when perfused into the arteries supplying the anterior and posterior areas of the median eminence, indicating that the median eminence is probably not the site of action either (Porter *et al.*, 1972a).

Other experiments have confirmed that dopamine is of major importance for the release of gonadotrophins. Kordon and Glowinski (1969; 1970) injected α-methyltyrosine and α-methyldopa into immature rats inducted to superovulate by pretreatment with PMS and HCG. They found that these inhibitors of catecholamine synthesis blocked ovulation when given during the critical period but not if given a few hours before. This is strange as these compounds have an onset of action of 2 or 3 hours and a duration of up to 24 hours. Dopa (which restores the levels of both dopamine and noradrenaline) partially reversed the effect of α-methyltyrosine, and dihydroxyphenylserine (DOPS), which restores noradrenaline levels only), had no effect on the ovulation. These experiments suggest that α-methyltyrosine inhibited ovulation due to a reduction of dopamine synthesis during the critical period. Kordon (1971) also found that an intrahypothalamic implantation of α-methyltyrosine inhibited ovulation, but only when placed in the arcuate nucleus-median eminence region, the site where, in fact, the dopamine neurones terminate. In a separate study pimozide (a DA-receptor blocker) was shown to inhibit the release of LRF in hypophysectomized rats (Corbin and Upton, 1973).

A directly opposite role for dopamine has been suggested by Fuxe and his co-workers. They showed that there was increased dopamine activity in the median eminence at the times when gonadotrophin release was inhibited (see section 6.1.8). It is possible, as has been suggested by Fuxe and Hokfelt (1970a) and even by McCann (Donoso *et al.*, 1971), that dopamine is converted into noradrenaline after intraventricular injection and only appears to be more active than noradrenaline because injected noradrenaline is rapidly metabolized. This idea is supported by the fact that phenoxybenzamine—which blocks α-adrenergic and not dopaminergic receptors (Fuxe and Hokfelt, 1970b)—antagonized the gonadotrophin releasing action of dopamine. Also, dopamine infusions are effective in releasing gonadotrophins only when infused into the ventricles and are not effective when infused into the median eminence where the dopaminergic nerve terminals are situated (Porter *et al.*, 1972a). Porter *et al.* (1972b) has found that intravenous injection of saline can induce gonadotrophin release perhaps due to mechanical stretching of the ventricles. It is possible that the results obtained with dopamine *in vivo* are due to this artifact.

The results supporting the hypothesis that dopamine stimulates the release of the gonadotrophins have been widely published, but in fact all the experiments in which dopamine itself was used, either *in vivo* or *in vitro*, came from McCann's laboratory between 1969 and 1971. In 1974

they repeated their *in vitro* experiments by adding dopamine to incubating pituitaries and hypothalamic fragments and found no effect
on gonadotrophin release: the only difference between this experiment
and the previous ones was that three hypothalamic fragments were used
instead of two (Quijada *et al.*, 1974). In a similar type of experiment in
which pituitaries attached by an intact portal system to a median eminence were superfused, the presence of 2·5 µg ml^{-1} of dopamine inhibited gonadotrophin release (Miyachi *et al.*, 1973). The presence of
oestrogen did not alter this effect.

Some *in vivo* experiments have also shown that dopamine can inhibit
gonadotrophin release. In an acute experiment, 80 µg of dopamine was
infused into the arcuate nucleus during the critical period in cyclic rats
and found to inhibit ovulation (Craven and McDonald, 1973). In another
report implants of dopamine were placed into the median eminence area
(as well as other parts of the hypothalamus) and were shown to have an
inhibitory effect. Uemura and Kobayashi (1971) found that implants of
dopamine in cholesterol (2:1) left for two weeks in the posterior part of
the median eminence (which included part of the arcuate nucleus) appeared to suppress the cyclic release of LH, and both the cyclic and tonic
release, when the proportion was 5 to 1. These two implants were
estimated to release 80 and 100 µg dopamine daily, respectively.

Oral administration of 500 mg L-dopa to humans caused a fall in
plasma LH levels within one hour. The decline was never below the
physiological range, but it was suggested that the ovulatory LH surge
in women may be suppressed (Boden *et al.*, 1972).

In conclusion it seems that dopamine may have some inhibitory function in controlling gonadotrophin release. The earlier work showing its
stimulatory effect cannot, as yet, be ignored and perhaps it has a dual
role depending on endogenous endocrine conditions. Recently Ojeda
and McCann (1973) obtained evidence that dopamine may be involved
with FSH, but not LH, release. They showed that pimozide (a dopamine
receptor blocker) selectively lowered plasma FSH levels in the castrated
rat, while diethyl dithiocarbamate (DDC), which lowers noradrenaline by
inhibiting the conversion of dopamine to noradrenaline, lowered plasma
LH. Correlated with this, Choudrey *et al.* (1973) have shown that activating dopamine receptors with apomorphine stimulated FSH release.

6.2.4   *Noradrenaline as the transmitter for gonadotrophin release*

All the results obtained after altering levels of noradrenaline in the hypothalamus indicate that it is concerned in the tonic and cyclic release of LH
and that it acts as a stimulatory transmitter.

When rats are unilaterally ovariectomized, the remaining ovary undergoes compensatory hypertrophy due to an increase in gonadotrophin release because of the reduction in ovarian secretion and therefore in negative feedback effects. Inhibition of catecholamine synthesis by α-methyltyrosine prevented this compensatory growth in immature rats (Muller *et al.*, 1972a; 1972b) and selective destruction of noradrenergic nerve terminals by 6-hydroxydopamine prevented this growth in adult rats (Zolovick, 1972). The effect of α-methyltyrosine was reversed by both dopa and DOPS. These results indicate that noradrenaline is involved in the tonic release of gonadotrophin after unilateral castration. Similar results were obtained in bilaterally castrated males where administration of either α-methyltyrosine or DDC lowered plasma LH levels. In this preparation their effects were reversed by DOPS but not by dopa (Ojeda and McCann, 1973).

Additional evidence supporting the noradrenergic control of tonic gonadotrophin release was shown in rats in which the hypothalamus was completely deafferented. In these rats there was a fall in hypothalamic noradrenaline levels to 38 per cent of the normal concentration and at the same time plasma and pituitary LH levels fell significantly, while dopamine levels remained normal. When only the anterior portion of the hypothalamus was deafferented there was only a small decrease in hypothalamic noradrenaline and only a slight fall in plasma LH (Blake *et al.*, 1972b; Weiner *et al.*, 1972b).

Noradrenaline may also be concerned with the cyclic release of the gonadotrophins in that Kalra and McCann (1973b) have shown that noradrenaline may be the synaptic transmitter in the pathway between the preoptic area and the median eminence, because the LH surge obtained after stimulation of the preoptic area was reduced by α-methyltyrosine (which lowers noradrenaline and dopamine levels in the hypothalamus) and by dopamine β-hydroxylase inhibitors (which lower noradrenaline levels only). The LH surge in these animals was restored by DOPS, which selectively raises noradrenaline levels but not by a dose of dopa which raises mainly dopamine levels. The LH surge after stimulation of the median eminence was not affected by the synthesis inhibitors (Kalra and McCann, 1973b). This type of experiment was also carried out in ovariectomized rats. When these animals are primed with oestrogen and then treated two days later with a single injection of progesterone or oestrogen there is a surge of LH, which can be prevented by the synthesis inhibitors and can be reversed by selectively raising noradrenaline levels, but not dopamine levels (Taleisnik *et al.*, 1971; Kalra *et al.*, 1971; 1972; Kalra and McCann, 1973a).

Craven and McDonald (1971a) have shown that infusion of noradrenaline, but not of dopamine, into the arcuate nucleus in rats pretreated with a monamine oxidase inhibitor can advance the critical period and therefore the time of the LH surge before ovulation. On the other hand, neither noradrenaline nor dopamine placed in the arcuate nucleus was able to overcome the anti-ovulatory effect of pentobarbitone or reserpine (Craven and McDonald, 1971a; 1971b; 1973). They suggested that noradrenaline may be involved in the changes occurring early on the day of proestrus leading up to the LH surge, rather than in the release of the LH surge itself. In this connection, Kanemastu *et al.* (1972) found that intraventricular administration of noradrenaline stimulated the release of LH in rabbits but with a different onset and duration from that produced by coitus or electrical stimulation, suggesting that while noradrenaline was involved with LH release it was not via the same mechanisms as that producing the ovulatory surge of LH.

6.2.5 *Adrenaline as the transmitter of gonadotrophin release*

While nearly all the early experiments involved administration of adrenaline (Sawyer, *et al.*, 1947; 1950a; 1950b), later work has tended to concentrate on noradrenaline and dopamine, mainly because very little adrenaline is present in the mammalian brain (Gunne, 1962). The enzymes necessary for synthesis of adrenaline have been shown to be present in the CNS and recently particularly high levels have been noted in some of the hypothalamic nuclei, including the arcuate nucleus and the median eminence (Hokfelt *et al.*, 1974; Saavedra *et al.*, 1974). Adrenaline is obviously not stored in any significant concentration and for this reason perhaps no metabolic studies on adrenaline in connection with gonadotrophin release have been carried out.

More recently, the effects of the administration of adrenaline have been compared with those of dopamine and noradrenaline. These experiments cannot, unfortunately, be corroborated by the use of pharmacological agents, for although they can distinguish effects of dopamine and noradrenaline, they cannot do so for noradrenaline and adrenaline. As noradrenaline is the precursor of adrenaline it is quite possible that when noradrenaline has been found to be selectively involved in gonadotrophin release it might actually be adrenaline that is the active transmitter.

In some of the experiments in which adrenaline, noradrenaline and dopamine have been administered intraventricularly, adrenaline was the most active in inducing gonadotrophin release. For instance, when ovulation was blocked by treatment with either reserpine or pentobarbitone given before the critical period, intraventricular administration of the amines was able to overcome the blocking effect. In both experiments adrenaline was the most effective, while dopamine, noradrenaline or dopa had to be given in higher doses (Rubinstein and Sawyer, 1970; Raziano *et al.*, 1971). Inexplicably, adrenaline was ineffective when placed in specific hypothalamic nuclei, just as dopamine and noradrenaline were ineffective when infused into the arcuate nucleus (Rubinstein and Sawyer, 1970; Craven and McDonald, 1971a; 1971b).

Intraventricular administration of adrenaline was also more effective than the other two amines in stimulating hypothalamic multiple unit activity (MUA) in oestrogen-primed ovariectomized rats. The stimulation was followed by a long-lasting depression. In this experiment adrenaline was still effective when placed into the median eminence–arcuate nucleus region where it induced the same biphasic effect (Weiner *et al.*, 1971).

These experiments showed adrenaline to be the most active catecholamine for stimulating the ovulatory LH surge. Unfortunately its effect on tonic gonadotrophin release has not yet been investigated.

In conclusion it is clear that the hypothalamic amines are necessary for both the tonic and cyclic release of gonadotrophins, but it is less clear which of the catecholamines is involved as the active transmitter. Taking into account the variation in hypothalamic amine metabolism with gonadotrophin release and the changes in gonadotrophin release on altering hypothalamic amine levels, it seems the more likely that noradrenaline stimulates gonadotrophin release and that this is balanced by inhibitory dopaminergic activity which must be removed at the critical period.

Electron microscopic studies revealed that intraventricular administration of both dopamine and noradrenaline alter the appearance of the floor of the third ventricle, that is the surface of the median eminence area. They caused the surface to become irregular with bleb-like protrusions which, it is suggested, are indications of increased secretion from the median eminence, possibly of release factors or release-inhibitory factors (Schechter and Weiner, 1972).

6.3   THE EFFECT OF 5-HYDROXYTRYPTAMINE ON THE RELEASE OF
        GONADOTROPHINS

6.3.1   *The inhibitory effect of 5-hydroxytryptamine (5-HT)*

Since the administration of 5-HT caused atrophy of the reproductive organs and delayed puberty in immature mice, Robson and Botros (1961) considered it likely that 5-HT was an inhibitor of gonadotrophin release.

This was supported by the findings of Vaughan *et al.* (1970) who showed that intraperitoneal administration of 5-HT prevented the compensatory ovarian hypertrophy normally seen after unilateral ovariectomy in rats. Subcutaneous or intraperitoneal injections of 5-HT were also found to inhibit ovulation both in adult rats and immature rats induced to ovulate with PMS (O'Steen, 1964; 1965; Endersby *et al.*, 1970; Labhsetwar, 1970; Tima *et al.*, 1973). Similar results were obtained by raising levels of 5-HT in the body, including the brain, by administering monoamine oxidase inhibitors; this was shown in the hamster, rat and immature rat (Alleva *et al.*, 1966; Kordon *et al.*, 1968; Kordon, 1969; Labhetswar, 1970).

The hypothesis that 5-HT inhibits gonadotrophin release, however, does not explain all the results. Most drugs that inhibit ovulation by a central action do so by suppressing the hypothalamic stimulation of the pituitary that occurs during the critical period; they must therefore be given just before this period. However, subcutaneous administration of 5-HT had no effect just before the critical period, but only inhibited ovulation when given after the critical period or in late dioestrus (Endersby *et al.*, 1970; Labhsetwar, 1971a; Wilson and McDonald, 1973; 1974). The timing of these inhibitory effects correlates well with the times in the cycle when ovarian hormones are secreted and Wilson and McDonald (1973; 1974) suggested that the anti-ovulatory effect of the 5-HT is due to a peripheral vasoconstrictor action preventing the passage of the ovarian steroids away from the ovary to the hypothalamus. The main support for this hypothesis is that 5-HT can antagonize the ovulatory action of exogenous LH and that the anti-ovulatory effect of 5-HT on spontaneous ovulation is reversed by a vasodilator (dipyridamole). A vasodilator compound (apresoline) has also been shown to prevent the atrophy of the reproductive organs in male rats caused by 5-HT (Boccabella *et al.*, 1962). The experiments in which monoamine oxidase inhibitors showed an anti-ovulatory effect may be due to raised levels of peripheral 5-HT, although the authors correlate the effect with raised brain levels.

In spite of all these findings there is still much evidence that 5-HT may be a central inhibitory transmitter. Firstly, there is the presence of 5-HT nerve terminals in the hypothalamus, particularly the suprachiasmatic nucleus, retrochiasmatic area and the median eminence; this latter area is capable of synthesizing 5-HT from tryptophan and this is known to occur only in tissues containing tryptaminergic neurones (Anden *et al.*, 1965; Hamon *et al.*, 1970). Secondly there is a tryptaminergic tract from the midbrain to the hypothalamus (see section 2.1) (Ungerstedt, 1971; Fuxe *et al.*, 1968a) and electrochemical stimulation of the ventral tegmentum and raphe in the midbrain, or tracts leading from these areas to the hypothalamus, inhibits spontaneous ovulation in rats and also reduces plasma LH levels. This inhibitory effect can be prevented by lesioning the tracts between the two areas (Carrer and Taleisnik, 1970; 1972).

Changes in 5-HT concentrations and metabolism in the hypothalamus in different endocrine states have been noted, although the work is not as extensive as that on the catecholamines. In the intact ewe, 5-HT levels in the median eminence fall significantly just before the LH surge (Wheaton *et al.*, 1972). When ovarian steroids were administered to castrated rats so that they exerted a negative feedback effect on gonadotrophin release, there was a rise in hypothalamic tryptophan levels (Bapna *et al.*, 1971), and also in 5-HT levels in the midbrain area (which included the hypothalamic area in this particular work) (Tonge and Greengrass, 1971). A single injection of oestradiol either on day one or eleven of life raised 5-HT brain levels in immature males and females (Giulian *et al.*, 1973). Kato (1960) found a similar effect after chronic administration of oestradiol to immature rats. Conversely, ovariectomy of neonatal females reduced brain 5-HT. As well as brain 5-HT being influenced by the steroids, the metabolism of the steroids is altered by 5-HT. Pretreatment with 5-HTP increased the accumulation of ^{3}H-oestradiol in the hypothalamus and pituitary after intravenous injection of the labelled steroid (Kordon *et al.*, 1972). Treatment with progesterone may inhibit the synthesis of 5-HT, because accumulation of ^{3}H-tryptophan was reduced in castrated rats pretreated with progesterone (Kordon and Glowinski, 1972).

Intravenous injection of 5-HT can inhibit ovulation in rabbits if given just before the expected LH surge, indicating a central effect (Currie *et al.*, 1969) and intraventricular administration of 5-HT inhibited LH and FSH release in both intact and castrated male and female rats (Kamberi *et al.*, 1970b; 1971a; Kamberi, 1973; Schneider and McCann, 1970d) and caused atrophy of the gonads in immature rats (Corbin and Schottelius, 1961). 5-HT had no effect at the pituitary level, as injection into the hypophyseal portal vessels had no effect on gonadotrophin release (Kamberi *et al.*, 1970b) and 5-HT only inhibited LH release from pituitaries *in vitro* in the presence of hypothalamic fragments (Moszkowska, 1964) and had no effect on the pituitary itself (Kamberi and McCann, 1969a, 1969b).

Reports on the effect of intraventricular 5-HT on spontaneous ovulation differ. When high doses of 5-HT (50–200 μg per rat) were injected at various times on the day of proestrus, there was no effect on ovulation (Rubinstein and Sawyer, 1970; Schneider and McCann, 1970d; Wilson and McDonald, 1974). However, recently Kamberi (1973) found that

1–5 μg 5-HT injected intraventricularly just before the critical period inhibited ovulation; it was ineffective when given by the intracardiac route, while its precursor, 5-HTP, which passes the blood-brain barrier, was effective. Intraventricular 5-HT also inhibited the facilitatory effect of progesterone on induced ovulation (Zolovick and Labhetswar, 1973). Implants of a monoamine oxidase inhibitor (nialamide) in the median eminence were also effective in blocking ovulation, but this may be due to the compound itself and not the raised 5-HT levels (Kordon and Vassent, 1968).

Recently 5-HT has been injected into the ventrolateral part of the anterior hypothalamus, i.e. in the medial forebrain bundle, and shown to inhibit induced ovulation in immature rats (Wilson, 1974). This suggests that the tracts from the midbrain that Carrer and Taleisnik (1970) showed could inhibit ovulation may be stimulated by the 5-HT injections and this may be the site for inhibition of cyclic release.

In 1957, Brodie and Shore suggested that 5-HT and noradrenaline were transmitters in opposing systems, which were in dynamic balance. Lippmann (1968) suggested that gonadotrophin release was controlled, not by individual levels of the amines, but their relative proportions, so that when 5-HT levels were high compared to noradrenaline, or when noradrenaline levels were low compared to 5-HT, then gonadotrophin release was inhibited. Labhsetwar (1971b) made a similar comment and showed that, when both amines were reduced to the same extent, there was no effect on gonadotrophin release. He also showed that dopamine can reverse the inhibitory effects of 5-HT on ovulation, induced by PMS and progesterone (Zolovick and Labhsetwar, 1973).

5-HT is a precursor of the pineal hormone, melatonin, which has been shown to inhibit gonadotrophin release and activity (Wurtman et al., 1968; Debeljuk et al., 1970; Kamberi et al., 1971a), and also to inhibit ovulation (Longenecker and Gallo, 1971; Ying and Greep, 1973) and delay puberty (Collu et al., 1973). Conversely, removal of the pineal can induce ovulation (Mess et al., 1973). Martini and his co-workers (Martini et al., 1968; Fraschini, 1970) investigated the various pineal principles and noted that they had a selective effect on LH and FSH release. They found that implants of melatonin and 5-hydroxytryptophol in the median eminence of castrated male rats reduced pituitary and plasma LH, but did not effect levels of FSH. On the other hand, 5-HT and 5-methoxytryptophol implants only reduced FSH levels in the pituitary. The pineal principles have a diurnal rhythm: in the dark period melatonin concentration is high and 5-HT low and during the day the levels are reversed. Fraschini (1970) suggest that this pineal rhythm controls the rhythm seen in pituitary gonadotrophins which peak daily in the afternoon. They suggest that the pineal substances travel to the basal hypothalamus via the cerebrospinal fluid and then alter releasing-hormone activity.

6.3.2 The stimulatory effect of 5-HT

Although the majority of the results show that 5-HT acts as an inhibitor of gonadotrophin release, there is also some evidence that 5-HT can stimulate both tonic and cyclic gonadotrophin release. Most of the evidence has been obtained after administration of *p*-chlorophenylalanine (PCPA), a compound known to inhibit synthesis of brain 5-HT by antagonizing the action of tryptophan hydroxylase (Koe and Weissman, 1968). It has been shown that PCPA prevents the onset of puberty (Fajer *et al.*, 1970) and the sudden release of FSH normally seen at puberty (Brown, 1971). It also reduces reproductive organ weights in hemicastrated male mice (Fawke *et al.*, 1972) and reduces testosterone levels in the plasma of intact male rats (Bliss *et al.*, 1972). At the same time PCPA raises pituitary FSH levels in intact and castrated male rats (Brown and Fawke, 1972). All these results indicate that the release of FSH stores in the pituitary is inhibited after PCPA and therefore the gonads are not stimulated to grow or secrete steroids. PCPA also inhibits induced ovulation if given 20 hours before the critical period (Kordon *et al.*, 1972), that is at a time when oestradiol secretion is taking place, in order to eventually stimulate the release of the LH surge. Kordon suggested that 5-HT is necessary for the positive feedback effect of the oestradiol, perhaps by enhancing its uptake into particular hypothalamic sites.

Complete deafferentation of the hypothalamus lowers 5-hydroxytryptamine levels within this area by 70 per cent, as well as significantly lowering noradrenaline. It is possible that the reduction in gonadotrophin release seen after the operation is due to the reduction in tryptaminergic activity (Weiner, 1973).

5-HT itself has been shown to stimulate gonadotrophin release. For instance, chronic subcutaneous administration of 5-HT for 12 weeks increases spermatogenesis in adult male rats (Kinson and Lui, 1973); intraocular or subcutaneous 5-HT induces ovulation in persistent oestrus rats (Takehashi *et al.*, 1973); a single intravenous injection of 5-HT raises plasma LH levels in ovariectomized rats pretreated with ovarian steroids (McCann *et al.*, 1960); intraventricular 5-HT was shown to stimulate a transient release of LH (but not FSH) for approximately two hours in intact male rats (Porter *et al.*, 1971; 1972). This is very strange as exactly opposite results were obtained in 1970 by the same group (Kamberi *et al.*, 1970b; 1971a), when intraventricular 5-HT inhibited LH release. The authors could not explain the difference.

Interesting results have been obtained on the immature animal induced to ovulate with PMS. Brown (1966; 1967a) showed that subcutaneous injections of 5-HT potentiated induced ovulation in immature mice, while anti-5-HT compounds, such as LSD and methysergide, inhibited ovulation. Similar results were obtained in immature rats treated with PMS. Thirty-day old rats underweight for their age did not ovulate after PMS treatment, but if 100 mg kg^{-1} of 5-HT was given, subcutaneously, just before the critical period then 50 per cent ovulated (Jaitley et al., 1967). 1 mg kg^{-1} of 5-HT intraventricularly also stimulated induced ovulation in both immature underweight Wistar and Sprague-Dawley rats. The stimulatory site of action of 5-HT appears to be the paraventricular nucleus, as injections (2 µg per rat) specifically into this nucleus stimulated ovulation in 77 per cent of underweight immature rats; injections into the arcuate nucleus, the suprachiasmatic nucleus and the anterior hypothalamus were ineffective (Wilson et al., 1974a). In adult rats, however, the suprachiasmatic nucleus may be the stimulatory site, as this nucleus contains high levels of 5-HT, and while lesions in this area prevented ovulation (Artunes-Rodriges and McCann, 1967), stimulation of this nucleus induced ovulation (Critchlow, 1958).

As mentioned previously, Fraschini et al. (1971) suggested that the circadian rhythm of gonadotrophin release is controlled by the pineal principles. Quay (1963) has shown 5-HT levels in the pineal are at their highest, daily at midday and higher on the day of proestrus, than on other days. He also showed that hypothalamic levels of 5-HT have a circadian rhythm with a peak each day in the late afternoon, at the expected time of the critical period, and when pituitary levels of the gonadotrophins are at their highest. It is possible, therefore, that 5-HT is involved in the control of the release of the ovulatory surge of LH (Quay, 1968).

A most interesting finding by Ladosky and Gaziri (1970) and recently confirmed by Giulian et al. (1973) is that 5-HT may be involved in sexual differentiation. They found that between days 10–14 of life, there is a rise in brain levels of 5-HT in females which can be prevented by administration of testosterone, or by ovariectomy on day one of life. Hardin (1973a) obtained rather different results in that the 5-HT levels in the females were higher only on day two and not in later life. Injections of oestradiol in the neonatal period can raise 5-HT levels in both male and female rats (Kato, 1960; Giulian et al., 1973). The alteration in 5-HT levels may be due to the effect of the steroids on monoamine oxidase (MAO) activity; for instance, activity on day 12 is reduced by testerostone given on day one of life and raised after castration (Ladosky and Gaziri, 1970; Gaziri and Ladosky, 1973). On the other hand the differences may be due to the higher levels of 5-HTP decarboxylase found in 2-day-old females compared to their male litter mates (Hardin, 1973b).

Conversely, Vaughan *et al.* (1969) have shown that early administration of 5-HT can antagonize the androgenizing effects of neonatal testosterone in the female. This would indicate that the prevention of the cyclic release of gonadotrophins by neonatal androgens, as seen in the normal male or after exogenous administration of testosterone to the female occurs via raising MAO levels and thus reducing 5-HT levels in the brain. These findings can be correlated with some fluorescence studies, which showed that when sexual differentiation is prevented in males by neonatal castration or the administration of an anti-androgen (cyproterone acetate) there was an increase in fluorescence in most hypothalamic nuclei due to raised amine levels (Schiebler and Meinhardt, 1971; Hyyppa and Rinne, 1971).

6.3.3 *Summary*

There appear to be two serotonergic systems involved in gonadotrophin release. There is an inhibitory system which originates in the midbrain and passes via the medial forebrain bundle to the hypothalamus with 5-HT as the transmitter. Meyerson (1964) suggested that one of the actions of progesterone is to suppress the inhibitory impulses coming from the midbrain to the hypothalamus. Kordon and Glowinski (1972) indicated that progesterone antagonizes the conversion of tryptophan to 5-HT, and this may explain the relationship between 5-HT and progesterone. A stimulatory serotonergic system also exists which may terminate in the suprachiasmatic or paraventricular nuclei or perhaps both. Kordon and Glowinski (1973) have suggested that 5-HT is involved in the positive feedback of oestradiol, and perhaps enhances the uptake of oestradiol in the hypothalamus. 5-HT may also be involved in sexual differentiation, as there are higher levels in the brain of immature females than in males which are steroid controlled. It is suggested, therefore, that 5-HT antagonizes the differentiating effect of neonatal testosterone.

6.4 THE EFFECT OF ACETYLCHOLINE ON THE RELEASE OF GONADOTROPHINS

In the search for possible neurotransmitters controlling gonadotrophin secretion, most emphasis is placed on the catecholamines and 5-hydroxytryptamine, but as early as 1950 Sawyer suggested that there was a cholinergic link before the adrenergic stimulation of the release of the LH surge in the rabbit. He showed that atropine (which blocks cholinergic receptors) inhibited ovulation and that, while dibenamine had to be given within five minutes of coitus, atropine was only effective when given within two minutes of coitus (Sawyer *et al.*, 1950a). Atropine also inhibited ovulation when given before the critical period to the adult rat (Everett *et al.*, 1949; Sawyer *et al.*, 1949b) or to the immature rat induced to ovulate with PMS (Quinn and Zarrow, 1964). Later experiments have confirmed the inhibitory effect of subcutaneous atropine: it has been shown to inhibit spontaneous ovulation and also reflex ovulation in oestrogen-primed female rats placed with males (Aron and Asch, 1963; Sala *et al.*, 1971; Kamberi, 1973); it inhibits the increase in FSH activity in the plasma of castrated male and female rats (Swelheim, 1964) and the rise in plasma LH before ovulation or after castration in both male and female rats (Libertun and McCann, 1972; 1973; Kamberi, 1973). This last finding was also observed when 250 μg of atropine was given intraventricularly. Implants of atropine into both the preoptic area and the anterior hypothalamus prevented compensatory hypertrophy in hemicastrated females, which indicates a reduction in plasma gonadotrophin (Sala *et al.*, 1971). These last two experiments prove that atropine has a central site of action, and Libertun and McCann (1973) showed its effect could be reversed by LH-releasing hormone, indicating there was no effect at the pituitary level.

A few experiments have been carried out with the cholinergic transmitter itself, acetylcholine. Intravenous injection of acetylcholine had no effect on LH release in conditions when intravenous adrenaline was active, but perhaps it was destroyed too rapidly to exert an effect (Guiliani *et al.*, 1961). Similarly, intrapituitary infusion of acetylcholine were ineffective, but 5 μg of acetylcholine, in the presence of an anticholinesterase agent, eserine, stimulated LH release in rabbits when injected into the basal hypothalamus (Endroczi and Hilliard, 1965). Meyerson and Palis (1970) also showed a stimulatory effect using the long-acting cholinergic agent, pilocarpine. When this was given subcutaneously it advanced ovulation by 24 hours in rats with 5-day cycles. Motta *et al.* (1972) have confirmed these findings by showing *in vitro* that while acetylcholine has no direct effect on isolated pituitaries when added to a system of pituitaries incubated with hypothalamic fragments, it stimulates the release of both LH and FSH. The effect of acetylcholine can be antagonized by atropine and potentiated by an anticholinesterase agent (Martini, 1973).

There is some metabolic evidence for a cholinergic control of gonadotrophin release. It was shown in both intact and castrated rats that cholinesterase activity in the hypothalamus altered with gonadotrophin secretion. The levels of cholinesterase in the anterior hypothalamus were low during proestrus and oestrus in adult rats, and also during the critical period in immature rats induced to ovulate (Kuwajimi, 1957; Kobayashi et al., 1966; Libertun et al., 1973). In ovariectomized rats cholinesterase activity rose in the first ten days after the operation, then fell and rose again by day 30. These changes cannot be explained as yet, and it is very odd that small doses of oestradiol (0·1–1 μg) which inhibit gonadotrophin release also inhibited these increases in cholinesterase activity, while administration of progesterone alone has no effect on either (Kobayashi et al., 1964; 1965; 1966).

Cholinergic neurones may also be involved in sexual differentiation since the enzymes concerned with synthesis and destruction of acetylcholine were significantly higher in 27-day-old females than in males; in neonatally androgenized females the activity of both enzymes was reduced (Libertun et al., 1973).

7 The effect of brain amines on the release of prolactin

Prolactin (or luteotrophin) can in some ways be considered to be another gonadotrophic hormone in rodents, because it maintains the growth of the corpora lutea in the ovary and stimulates progesterone secretion. In primates it is not luteotrophic, but in both primates and rodents prolactin stimulates mammary growth and lactation. Therefore, in experiments before 1969, i.e. before the use of the radio-immunoassay, pseudopregnancy, mammary growth and lactation were used as indications of prolactin release.

The early experiments on the effect of amines on prolactin release showed that subcutaneous administration of adrenaline, noradrenaline, 5-hydroxytryptamine and acetylcholine induced prolactin release in rabbits and rats; this was observed by noting the occurrence of either pseudopregnancy or mammary growth and lactation in oestrogen-primed animals (Swingle et al., 1951a; Meites et al., 1959; 1960; Meites, 1959; Desclin, 1960). As in the early experiments on the release of gonadotrophins, it was shown that any non-specific stress, for instance injection of foreign protein, formaldehyde, alloxan, or excessive cold, restraint, or starvation effected prolactin release, although in the opposite manner to that of the gonadotrophins. All these stressful stimulations induced a release of prolactin causing either pseudopregnancy or lactation depending on the hormonal state of the animal (Swingle et al., 1951a; 1951b; Nicoll et al., 1960) and it now seems clear that subcutaneously administered amines act via their stressful effect, because when they are given intravenously or intraperitoneally they no longer induce pseudopregnancy or raise plasma prolactin levels (Jacobson et al., 1950; Lu *et al.*, 1970). The stress effect still occurs in adrenalectomized animals (Swingle *et al.*, 1951b) and so does not act via endogenous adrenaline from the adrenals; it may act directly at the hypothalamic level lowering the prolactin inhibitory factor (PIF) concentrations (Mittler and Meites, 1967).

However, the effect of reserpine on inhibiting prolactin release is probably via amine depletion as all compounds depleting central catecholamine stores, but not those depleting only peripheral stores, were found to induce pseudopregnancy in adult rats, and lactation in oestrogen-primed rats (Coppola *et al.*, 1965; Arai *et al.*, 1970). Small implants of reserpine into the hypothalamus also induces pseudopregnancy (Van Maanan and Smelik, 1968). The effect of reserpine can be reversed by pretreatment with monoamine oxidase inhibitors, which prevent amine depletion (Coppola *et al.*, 1965). Ratner *et al.* (1965) showed in *in vitro* experiments that reserpine lowered both the synthesis and release of PIF in the hypothalamus, and had no direct effect on the pituitary.

These results show that one or more of the catecholamines exert an inhibitory control on prolactin release, and it was thought at first that the inhibitory action was a direct one at the pituitary level. In order to investigate this, a series of experiments was carried out on the effect of the amines on pituitaries incubated *in vitro*. The results are conflicting as some showed the amines had no effect (Talwalker *et al.*, 1963; Gala and Reece, 1963), stimulated release (Gala and Reece, 1963; Koch *et al.*, 1970) or inhibited release (Jacobs *et al.*, 1968; MacLeod, 1969; Birge *et al.*, 1970). Meites' group have clarified this situation by showing that in low "physiological" concentrations (10–20 ng ml^{-1}) adrenaline and noradrenaline stimulated prolactin release while dopamine at 20–40 ng ml^{-1} had no effect. Between this low range and 100 ng ml^{-1} none of the amines had any effect and in higher concentrations all inhibited prolactin release (Koch *et al.*, 1970). Most of the results found by different workers can be explained on the basis of the concentration of the amine employed. In the late 1960's purified extracts of hypothalamic PIF were obtained and it was clear that this substance was not an amine. This means that hypothalamic amines must be controlling prolactin release via PIF, or possibly PRF, and not directly.

The earlier work of Barraclough and Sawyer (1959) and Coppola (1968) showing that depletion of the catecholamines within the CNS induces pseudopregnancy has been repeated more recently using a direct estimation of plasma prolactin concentration as the end point (Lu *et al.*, 1970; Donoso *et al.*, 1971). As well as amine depletion with reserpine or α-methyltyrosine, blockers of adrenergic and dopaminergic receptor sites can also increase plasma prolactin in rats (Lu *et al.*, 1970; Meites *et al.*, 1972), sheep (Davis and Borger, 1973) and humans (Frantz, 1973). The converse effect was obtained by raising endogenous levels of the catecholamines by administration of dopa or monoamine oxidase inhibitors, which reduce the levels of plasma prolactin and elevate PIF activity in the plasma (Donoso *et al.*, 1971; Lu and Meites, 1971; Davis and Borger, 1973; Smythe and Lazerus, 1973). Dopa treatment has been applied successfully to women suffering from amenorrhoea and galactorrhoea, presumably by reducing prolactin secretion (Zarate *et al.*, 1973).

The identity of the particular amine exerting the inhibitory control has been investigated in three ways. In the first method endogenous levels of amines were altered by means of pharmacological agents. As shown before, α-methyltyrosine, which reduces both noradrenaline and dopamine levels in the hypothalamus, increases plasma prolactin, but a dopamine β-hydroxylase inhibitor (diethyldithiocarbamate, DDC), which only lowers noradrenaline levels, had no effect. On the other hand, when dopamine levels were raised selectively by treatment with dopa plus DDC, prolactin levels were reduced and when only noradrenaline levels were raised using an injection of DOPS, plasma levels of prolactin were increased (Donoso *et al.*, 1971). This indicates that dopamine may be the inhibitory transmitter in the hypothalamus, controlling prolactin release and, more tentatively, noradrenaline may be the stimulatory transmitter.

In the second method, the changes in aminergic neuronal activity in the hypothalamus and changes in prolactin secretion were investigated (see section 6.1). When prolactin secretion was high as during pregnancy, pseudopregnancy, lactation or after pituitary transplantation under the kidney capsule, dopamine turnover in the nerve terminals in the median eminence was increased and dopamine stores in the cell bodies of the arcuate nucleus were elevated (Fuxe and Hokfelt, 1970b; Hokfelt and Fuxe, 1972b; Olson *et al.*, 1972). Similar effects occurred after injection of exogenous prolactin and very high doses of growth hormone, but with no other pituitary hormone (Hokfelt and Fuxe, 1972a). After hypophysectomy or after treatment with ergocornine or CB154 (2-bromo-α-ergocryptine), which inhibit prolactin release, there was a reduction in dopamine turnover. These results suggest that prolactin exerts a negative feedback effect on its own secretion via a dopaminergic inhibitory control (Olson *et al.*, 1972).

The third method is by direct administration of the various amines found in the hypothalamus and noting their differential effects on prolactin release. Lu *et al.* (1970) found that while adrenaline, noradrenaline, dopamine and 5-hydroxytryptamine had no effect on prolactin release when given by the intracarotid route at 0·25–5·0 mg per rat, the much smaller dose of 10 μg per rat of adrenaline and dopamine caused a small reduction in pituitary prolactin levels, without altering plasma levels, indicating a reduction in prolactin synthesis. Noradrenaline had no effect. After intraventricular injection of the amines, it was found that dopamine (1·25–2·5 μg per rat) raised the PIF activity in hypophyseal portal blood (Kamberi et al., 1971b) and at the same time reduced peripheral plasma prolactin levels all in less than 30 minutes. Adrenaline and noradrenaline were effective only at 100 μg per rat (Porter et al., 1972a).

Thus in all three types of experiments, it seems clear that dopamine is the main inhibitory hypothalamic transmitter controlling prolactin release, probably via stimulation of PIF. It is possible too that noradrenaline stimulates prolactin release. This is indicated by the experiments in which endogenous levels of noradrenaline have been raised and also in the in vitro experiments where physiological concentrations of noradrenaline stimulate the release of prolactin by direct action on the pituitary. Thus noradrenaline may act by inhibiting PIF, stimulating PRF, or by an effect at the pituitary level. When the hypothalamus is deafferented, there is a fall in noradrenaline levels, but dopamine levels remain normal. In this situation the prolactin levels in both the pituitary and plasma are low, while the mechanism for prolactin release remains intact and normal (Blake et al., 1972a). Administration of α-methyltyrosine to this preparation depletes dopamine within the deafferented hypothalamus and at the same time increases plasma prolactin levels (Weiner, 1973).

Weiner (1973) suggests that dopamine acts directly on the secretory granules to stimulate the release of PIF, perhaps by some axo-axonal mechanism. This is supported by the fact that intraventricular dopamine caused morphological changes in the lining of the third ventricle consistent with induction of secretory processes (Schechter and Weiner, 1972), but it did not alter multiple unit activity in the hypothalamus indicating that it does not alter neuronal activity (Weiner et al., 1971).

There is some evidence that 5-HT stimulates the release of prolactin both as a hypothalamic transmitter and also in its role as a pineal hormone precursor. Pinealectomy inhibited the release of prolactin as plasma levels are lower and pituitary levels are higher than in intact rats (Relkin, 1972a). This indicates that one of the pineal principles involved in stimulating prolactin release and correlated with this intraventricular injections of 5-HTP, melatonin (50 μg) and 5-HT (2–50 μg) have been shown to stimulate prolactin release (Kamberi et al., 1971a; Meites et al., 1972; Porter et al., 1972b; Lu and Meites, 1973; Calgaris and Taleisnik, 1974). A prolactin surge can be induced in ovariectomized rats treated with steroids (Caligaris and Taleisnik, 1974) or in lactating rats on resumption of suckling after being deprived of their litters (Kordon *et al.*, 1972). PCPA or methysergide prevented this surge and their effect was reversed by 5-HTP. Very recently Caligaris and Taleisnik have suggested that 5-HT is a transmitter in inhibitory presynaptic nerves which impinge on catecholaminergic neurones stimulating PIF release.

Rats show a circadian rhythm for both pituitary and plasma prolactin with peaks in the late afternoon and late dark period. It has been suggested that this may be controlled by a serotonergic or pineal system, stimulating both synthesis and release (Meites *et al.*, 1972; Rønneklein *et al.*, 1973). Relkin (1972b) has provided some evidence for this by showing that prolactin release is inhibited in rats kept in a constant light (when pineal activity is reduced), while there is enhanced release if they are kept in constant dark (when melatonin secretion is high). This enhancement does not occur in the pinealectomized rat.

There is, as yet, little evidence involving acetylcholine in the control of prolactin release, except that implants of atropine in the basal medial hypothalamus induces pseudopregnancy in rats (Gala *et al.*, 1970). This indicates that possibly acetylcholine has some inhibitory control on prolactin.

In summary there is a large body of evidence showing that hypothalamic dopamine inhibits prolactin release, while 5-hydroxytryptamine, melatonin and possibly noradrenalin appear to stimulate prolactin release. Acetylcholine may have an inhibitory effect.

8   The effect of brain amines on sexual behaviour in the rat

8.1   FEMALE BEHAVIOUR

Sexual receptivity in the female rat can be measured by noting the number of lordosis responses to a given number of mounts by the male. The female must be correctly primed with ovarian steroids before she will respond to the male and this can be induced in the ovariectomized female by treating with oestradiol followed 48 hours later by progesterone; lordosis will then occur 6–8 hours later on stimulation by the male (Boling and Blandau, 1939).

Meyerson (1964) showed that increased levels of 5-hydroxytryptamine in the brain reduced the lordosis response in ovariectomized rats treated with oestrogen and progesterone. (He gave 5-HTP or a monoamine oxidase inhibitor in order to raise 5-hydroxytryptamine levels.) When he gave dopa or DOPS in order to raise catecholamine levels, there was no effect on behaviour. Meyerson also showed that reduction of brain 5-hydroxytryptamine increases sexual behaviour in these steroid-treated ovariectomized rats. He gave reserpine or PCPA and found that these drugs could be given in place of progesterone in order to induce lordosis (Meyerson, 1964; Meyerson and Lewander, 1970). Zemplan *et al.* (1973) confirmed the action of PCPA and also showed the same effect after administration of a 5-hydroxytryptamine receptor blocker, methysergide. They also showed that PCPA and methysergide implants in the preoptic area had a stimulatory effect.

In the intact female PCPA was found to be ineffective (Segal and Whalen, 1970), but this may be because the rats were already performing to their full capacity. When intact females were pretreated with testosterone, PCPA increased their male sexual activity without altering female behaviour (Singer, 1972).

Meyerson suggested that there is an inhibitory serotonergic control on sexual behaviour in the female which is overcome by progesterone. It has been further suggested that the midbrain raphe may be the centre for the inhibitory control because it contains cell bodies with high concentrations of 5-hydroxytryptamine whose axons run via the medial forebrain bundle to the hypothalamus. Implants of progesterone in this midbrain are more effective in stimulating lordosis than those placed in the hypothalamus (Ross *et al.*, 1971). Meyerson also looked at the effect of altering brain amines on sexual motivation (i.e. the degree of interest in the male) rather than lordosis and found that MAOI compounds decreased motivation, while PCPA increased it, but only in the oestrogen-primed animal (Meyerson, 1972).

Cholinergic drugs such as pilocarpine and oxotremorine also inhibit sexual behaviour in the castrated female rat treated with oestrogen and progesterone. This effect occurred half an hour after administration and appeared to be due to their muscurinic action, although after PCPA treatment they were no longer effective, indicating that they act via 5-hydroxytryptamine (Lindstrom and Meyerson, 1966; Lindstrom, 1971). Three hours after administration both cholinergic drugs facilitate the effects of oestrogen and progesterone on lordosis. The facilitatory action does not occur after hypophysectomy or adrenalectomy and Lindstrom suggests that the drugs stimulate ACTH which in turn stimulates progesterone synthesis in the adrenal (Lindstrom, 1973).

The hypothesis that 5-hydroxytryptamine is the inhibitory transmitter has not been confirmed by Ahlenius and his co-workers (1972a, 1972b), who also used oestrogen-primed ovariectomized rats. They found that increased sexual activity occurred when dopamine levels were selectively reduced, and that after PCPA treatment the time course of dopamine depletion and increased activity was similar, while by the time the 5-hydroxytryptamine concentrations had reached their nadir (26 hours) sexual behaviour had returned to normal (Ahlenius *et al.*, 1972a; 1972b).

The results were exactly confirmed in castrated males primed with oestrogen in which lordosis activity was stimulated by α-methyltyrosine and inhibited by dopa treatment that preferentially increased dopamine levels. PCPA had no effect in this experiment (Soderstein and Ahlenius, 1972). Alhenius has suggested that lowering dopamine levels in the hypothalamus increases secretion of ACTH which then stimulates the adrenals to produce progesterone which is necessary for sexual behaviour.

8.2 MALE BEHAVIOUR

In many of the experiments discussed here, male sexual behaviour was observed by noting the number of mounts in a given time in either a male–female or male–male situation. This is a poor criterion because it is hard to show significant differences in mounting between intact and castrated males, even though it is clear that sexual behaviour is reduced in the castrated animal. Significant results are obtained if the rate of ejaculation or the ejaculation latency is measured, or best of all, the refractory period after ejaculation.

When brain amine levels were raised after treatment with monoamine oxidase inhibitors, sexual activity in either intact or castrated rats treated with tesosterone was reduced (Malmnas and Meyerson, 1970; Talgiamonte et al., 1971a; Dewsbury et al., 1972). Meyerson showed that by selectively increasing amine concentrations, the inhibitory effect was due to raised levels of 5-hydroxytryptamine, since increasing catecholamine levels had no effect (Malmnas and Meyerson, 1970).

When 5-hydroxytryptamine brain levels are reduced, or its action inhibited, there was an increase in both homo- and heterosexual activity. This was shown in cats, dogs, rabbits, intact rats and castrated rats treated with testosterone. Brain 5-hydroxytryptamine activity was reduced in a variety of ways: by inhibiting synthesis with PCPA, by destruction of serotonergic nerve terminals with 5,6-dihydroxytryptamine, by depletion with reserpine, or anti-5-hydroxytryptamine compounds such as methysergide (Dewsbury and Davis, 1970; Bertolini, 1971; Perez-Cruent et al., 1971; Soulairac and Soulairac, 1971; Tagliomonte et al., 1971a; Benkerto and Eversmann, 1972; Bond et al., 1972; da Prada et al., 1972; Tagliomonte, 1972). The stimulatory effect could be reversed by raising 5-hydroxytryptamine levels by giving 5-hydroxytryptophan (Perez-Cruent et al., 1971; Soulairac and Soulairac, 1971; da Prada et al., 1972). Some conflicting results were obtained with the compound PCPA, and it seems clear that lowering brain 5-hydroxytryptamine levels with this compound had no effect on animals exhibiting full and presumably maximum sexual behaviour (Whalen and Luttge, 1970; Zitrin et al., 1970). But, if the rats showed a subnormal level of behaviour (as for instance castrated rats treated with subthreshold doses of testo-sterone) then the stimulatory effect of PCPA was seen (Malmnas and Meyerson, 1974, in press).

There is some disagreement on the mode of action of PCPA in castra-ted rats. Gessa *et al.* (1970) claimed that PCPA was inactive in the castrated male and that its action was dependent on the presence of testosterone. However, Shillito (1971) has shown that PCPA can stimu-late homosexual behaviour in the castrated and adrenalectomized prepubertal rat. According to da Prada *et al.* (1972) the effect of changing 5-hydroxytryptamine levels is independent of the catecholamine con-centration and the effects are therefore not due to changes in the ratio of catecholamines and 5-hydroxytryptamine but Tagliomonte (1972) showed that the effects of PCPA were potentiated if catecholamine levels were increased by concomitant dopa treatment, and prevented by pretreatment with α-methyltyrosine. da Prada may, however, be correct since dopa is known to reduce brain 5-hydroxytryptamine and the increase in male homosexual behaviour seen after dopa can be reversed by 5-HTP (da Prada *et al.*, 1973). The effect of PCPA on sexual behaviour may be due to a generalized excitatory effect. It is known that PCPA increases the perception and reactivity to stimuli in rats (Weissman, 1973) and it is known that arousing stimuli are capable of potentiating sexual behaviour (Beach and Fowler, 1959; Barfield and Sachs, 1968).

It has been suggested that sexual behaviour is stimulated when catecholamine levels are increased and 5-hydroxytryptamine levels decreased. This is supported by results showing increased sexual behaviour in rats treated with PCPA, which inhibited 5-hydroxytrypt-amine synthesis, followed by treatment with a monoamine oxidase inhibitor, which raised catecholamine levels by preventing their meta-bolism (Ahlenius *et al.*, 1971). Malmnas (1973) showed that dopamine may be the stimulatory transmitter for heterosexual behaviour in the male rat. In the castrated rat treated with testosterone reduction of both dopamine and noradrenaline levels (using α-methyltyrosine) inhibited sexual behaviour. After selectively reducing noradrenaline, this effect was shown to be due to the reduction in dopamine and not noradrenaline. Administration of apomorphine, which stimulates the dopamine re-ceptors, caused an increase in sexual behaviour, with an increased num-ber of mounts and intromissions and a reduced refractory period after ejaculation. Apomorphine had some stimulatory effects in the intact male also (Butcher *et al.*, 1969). Raising brain dopamine levels by treat-ment with dopa plus a decarboxylase inhibitor had a similar effect in these castrated rats (Malmnas, 1973) but not in intact male rats (Hyyppa *et al.*, 1971). Perhaps stimulatory effects cannot be demonstrated in rats showing maximum sexual behaviour. Noradrenaline does not seem to alter copulatory behaviour such as ejaculatory time or refractory period, but it may be involved in motivation, since increased brain noradrenaline increased mounting activity (Malmnas, 1973).

In summary, in the male 5-hydroxytryptamine may exert an inhibitory control on sexual behaviour and dopamine may be stimulatory. In the female, 5-hydroxytryptamine, dopamine and acetylcholine have all been shown to exert an inhibitory effect on sexual behaviour.

9 The effect of brain amines on the release of growth hormone (GH)

The secretion of GH from the pituitary is under the control of the hypo-thalamic GH-releasing hormone (GRH) and possibly GH-inhibitory factor (GIF). The physiological action of GH is to promote protein synthesis at the expense of carbohydrate and fat and so it tends to pre-vent the incorporation of blood sugar into tissue and thus cause raised levels of blood glucose. This is in opposition to the effect of insulin and the two hormones tend to be physiological antagonists; for instance hypoglycaemia induced by insulin stimulates the release of GH. In addition, most forms of stress, including anaesthesia, induce GH release (Meyer and Knobil, 1967; Werrbach et al., 1970).

The work of Muller and his co-workers suggest that the catechol-amines stimulate GH release. They showed that agents that deplete brain noradrenaline (but not peripheral) prevent the fall in pituitary GH which is normally seen after an injection of insulin, indicating that the release of GH has been inhibited (Muller et al., 1967). Conversely, when the catecholamines (dopamine, noradrenaline and adrenaline) are given intraventricularly they cause both a fall in pituitary GH and in hypo-thalamic GRF, indicating a release of GH from the pituitary has occurred. Noradrenaline is a hundred times more effective, at 0·005 µg per rat, than the other two amines. Intraventricular 5-hydroxytryptamine, acetylcholine, posterior pituitary hormones, histamine, and saline have no effect on GH release (Muller et al., 1968). The fall in hypothalamic GRF has been seen in both intact and hypophysectomized rats and a concomitant rise in plasma GRF could be detected in the hypophysec-tomized animals (Muller et al., 1968, 1970; Muller, 1970).

Kato et al. (1973) agreed that there is an adrenergic stimulatory con-trol in the rat, but they found that β-adrenergic stimulation, as after an injection of isoprenaline, caused a rise in plasma GH, while α-adrenergic stimulation by phenylalanine inhibited GH release and reduced plasma GH levels. Administration of α- and β-adrenergic blockers had the opposite effects on GH release to their respective agonists.

The stimulatory catecholamine effect on GH release has been confirmed in primates, i.e. rhesus monkeys, baboons, and humans. Intravenous or oral administration of dopa and α-adrenergic stimulating agents such as phenylephrine and methoxamine cause a rise in plasma GH. On the other hand, α-adrenergic blockers inhibit GH release normally induced by insulin (Blackard and Heidingsfelder, 1968; Boyd et al., 1971; Imura et al., 1971; Kensal et al., 1972; Massara and Camanni, 1972; Souvatzoglov et al., 1973). Administration of the β-adrenergic blocker, proprananol, increases plasma levels of GH in normal subjects and this can be reversed by isoprenaline, suggesting that while an α-adrenergic system stimulates GH release, there is a β-adrenergic system which acts to inhibit release (Imura et al., 1968, 1971; Werrbach et al., 1970). This is opposite to the effects seen in the rat.

The sites of hypothalamic control of GH are known to be in the supraoptic and ventromedial nuclei and infusion of noradrenaline into the ventromedial nucleus of baboons has been shown to stimulate GH release (Toivola and Gale, 1972), although the release of GH normally seen after electrical stimulation of the ventromedial nucleus in the rat, is not effected by pretreatment with α-methyltyrosine. However, the GH release after stimulation of the hippocampus and amygdala is reduced by lowering brain amine levels with α-methyltyrosine, suggesting there is catecholaminergic connection between the limbic system and hypothalamus controlling GH release (Martin, 1972; Martin et al., 1973).

Some conflicting findings have been published recently: Collu et al. (1972) noted changes in plasma GH levels in anaesthetized male rats after intraventricular injection of dopamine, noradrenaline or 5-hydroxytryptamine (1 μg per rat) and found that dopamine reduced plasma GH levels, noradrenaline had no effect and 5-hydroxytryptamine raised the GH levels. The effect of dopamine was reversed by a β-adrenergic blocker. The authors suggest that the differences between their results and those of Muller are due to the anaesthetic used. They used urethane, which does not affect resting GH levels, while Muller used ether which reduces plasma GH and at the same time raises catecholamine turnover. Administration of exogenous noradrenaline may exert a negative feedback effect on endogenous turnover and so reverse the effect of ether on GH release. Unlike ether, pentobarbitone increases plasma GH and at the same time lowers catecholamine turnover and raises 5-hydroxytryptamine turnover. This fits in with the findings of Collu et al. (1972). Another reason for the difference in the results may be due to the method of assaying GH. Muller used a bioassay, while Collu et al. used a radio-immunoassay, and the two methods are known to yield conflicting results (Ganong, 1972a).

In vitro experiments with rat pituitaries also gave conflicting results. Garay and Martin (1970) found that adrenaline and isoprenaline (10–50 μg ml^{-1}) stimulated GH release while in a similar concentration range Hertelendy *et al.* (1971) found that adrenaline inhibited the GH release normally induced by raising cyclic-AMP levels.

10 The effect of brain amines on the release of adrenocortico-trophin hormone (ACTH)

The current view on the release of ACTH from the pituitary is that it is controlled by corticotrophin release factor (CRF) from the anterior hypothalamus. ACTH then brings about the secretion of corticosteroids from the adrenal cortex and these exert a negative feedback effect at the hypothalamic level, the pituitary level, at higher brain centres, or any combination of the three possibilities. There is a circadian rhythm for plasma corticosteroids, plasma ACTH and hypothalamic CRF with a peak in the dark period (at 20.00 h in rats kept in a fixed lighting system of 14 hours light starting at 6.00 h: 10 hours dark starting at 20.00 h). Superimposed on this normal but changing tonic release, any form of stress due to either physical or emotional disturbances stimulate ACTH secretion in a sudden and striking surge (see Donovan, 1970; Kendall, 1971).

In nearly all the experimental work carried out on the control of ACTH release, the release has been followed indirectly by noting the changes in levels of corticosterone in the plasma. In the very early experiments depletion of adrenal ascorbic acid, or reduction in circulating eosinophils, was taken as an indication of ACTH release. Among the stressful agents found to stimulate ACTH release, were subcutaneous injections of the monoamines (Madison 1950; Recant *et al.*, 1950; Kitay *et al.*, 1959). Their effect could be inhibited by the relevant blockers, but the blocking agents did not effect ACTH release induced by injection of formalin or forced immobilization, which indicated that the peripheral amines were not an integral part of the mechanism of release (Guillemin, 1955).

In recent years evidence has accumulated that the amines are involved in ACTH control at the hypothalamic level. An action at the pituitary level was ruled out when it was shown that none of the catecholamines (adrenaline, noradrenaline or dopamine) could stimulate the release of ACTH from pituitaries *in vitro* (Guillemin *et al.*, 1957; van Loon and Kragt, 1970). Placing noradrenaline and 5-hydroxytryptamine directly onto the pituitary *in vivo* also had no effect, although 10 μg of adrenaline was active in stimulating ACTH release (Hiroshige *et al.*, 1968). This may explain why an injection of adrenaline is more stressful than noradrenaline (Madison, 1950).

So far, it seems likely that the tonic release of ACTH, the response to stress and the circadian rhythm are each controlled by different aminergic transmitters, but which specific amine is involved in each mechanism and whether it is stimulatory or inhibitory is in dispute. The work on each amine will, therefore, be reviewed separately.

10.1 CATECHOLAMINES AS TRANSMITTERS FOR ACTH RELEASE

Ganong and his co-workers carried out a large number of experiments showing that the noradrenergic neurones in the hypothalamus exert an inhibitory effect on both the tonic and stress-induced release of ACTH (van Loon, 1973). They used dogs and rats and in both species they found that agents that raise the brain levels of active noradrenaline (e.g. the monoamine oxidase inhibitors, amphetamine, tyramine and dopa) inhibited stress-induced rises in plasma corticosterone (van Loon and Ganong, 1969; van Loon *et al.*, 1971). The effect of the MAO inhibitors was reversed by α-adrenergic blockers but not by β-blockers (Scapagnini and Preziosi, 1972; 1973). Agents that selectively alter dopamine brain concentrations had no effect on ACTH release after stress. When brain levels of noradrenaline were reduced as after treatment with reserpine, α-methyltyrosine, FLA 63 or when an α-adrenergic blocking agent was administered centrally, there was a rise in tonic levels of plasma corticosterone with a significant negative correlation between noradrenaline levels in the brain and corticosterone levels in the plasma (Ganong, 1971; Scapagnini *et al.*, 1970). Care was taken to use the soluble ester of α-methyltyrosine because the intraperitoneal injections of insoluble substances are known to be stressful and therefore cause non-specific corticosterone raises (Thornburg and Moore, 1971).

The increase in corticosterone levels induced by α-methyltyrosine or by nonspecific stress could be reversed by intravenous dopa (van Loon *et al.*, 1971).

Further evidence was provided by intraventricular injection of the amines themselves, such as noradrenaline, dopamine and isoprenaline which all reduced stress-induced rises of plasma corticosterone (van Loon *et al.*, 1971), as well as tonic levels (Schiaffini *et al.*, 1971). Intravenous injection of the amines had no effect, presumably because they could not pass the blood-brain barrier and this suggests that the site of action must be above the barrier and therefore above the median eminence area (Ganong, 1972a). This is supported by the fact that α-methyltyrosine was active in raising corticosterone levels at 20 mg kg^{-1} intraventricularly, this dose being ineffective peripherally (van Loon et al., 1971). Similarly, guanethidine (a catecholamine depletor that cannot pass the blood-brain barrier) was only effective in raising plasma corticosterone when injected intraventricularly (Scapagnini and Preziosi, 1972).

These experiments suggest that the noradrenergic neurones in the hypothalamus exert an inhibitory control on the release of ACTH. This hypothesis is supported by the work of Marks et al. (1970). They first found that intraventricular injection of saline or any of the amines was stressful and therefore stimulated ACTH release and plasma corticosterone levels; but if they used rats pretreated with reserpine, which raised corticosterone plasma levels, then both noradrenaline and dopamine at 1 µg intraventricularly lowered corticosterone levels, while carbachol at 0·1–0·25 µg raised the levels even more. 5-Hydroxytryptamine had no effect. Microelectrophoretically applied noradrenaline and dopamine inhibited the activity of the single neurones in the hypothalamus that are also inhibited by dexamethasone. Dopamine had a greater effect than noradrenaline (Steiner et al., 1968; 1969). In vitro experiments using incubating hypothalamic slices also confirmed the inhibitory action of noradrenaline. Acetylcholine stimulated CRF release in this preparation and its effect was reversed by noradrenaline (Bradbury et al., 1974).

The inhibitory effect of the catecholamines has not been supported by all workers. For instance, de Schaepdryver et al. (1969) and McKinney et al. (1971) found there was no correlation between changes in brain catecholamines, after treatment with either amine depletors or monoamine oxidase inhibitors, and changes in plasma corticosteroids. Similarly, Kaplanski et al. (1972), while confirming that 250 mg kg^{-1} α-methyltyrosine given as the soluble ester raised corticosterone levels, also found that this was a toxic dose. When the same amount of α-methyltyrosine was given in divided doses at regular intervals over 24 hours, the brain noradrenaline depletion was very similar, but there was no rise in plasma corticosterone (Kaplanski et al., 1972; McKinney et al., 1971).

When adult rats were treated with 6-hydroxydopamine in order to destroy catecholaminergic nerve terminals, there was a fall in plasma corticosterone for about 3 days, but both plasma levels and adrenal corticoid production returned to normal in a further 4 days, in spite of the fact that the brain noradrenaline was still low (Lippa et al., 1973; Kaplanski and Smelik, 1973a). In addition, 6-hydroxydopamine did not affect the circadian rhythm of plasma corticosterone (Ulrick and Yuwiler, 1973). As 6-hydroxydopamine did not affect brain dopamine concentrations for more than a few days, it was suggested that it was dopamine that controlled the tonic levels and the circadian rhythm of ACTH release. However, Kaplanski *et al.* (1974) showed that 6-hydroxy-dopamine in new-born rats significantly lowered both dopamine and noradrenaline in the brain and yet had no effect on plasma corticosterone at adulthood. A positive result, however, was obtained from adult rats treated with 6-hydroxydopamine and left for 11 days, so that the tonic plasma corticosterone levels and brain dopamine had returned to normal. In these animals a stressful injection did not induce the usual rise in plasma corticosterone, indicating that the brain noradrenaline may be necessary for stress-induced ACTH release, but was not involved in the tonic release (Lippa *et al.*, 1973).

This last finding suggests that noradrenaline, in fact, has a stimulatory role in ACTH release and some biochemical changes in brain amines during stress tend to support this. Fuxe *et al.* (1970a) showed that the turnover of noradrenaline in the hypothalamus rose when animals were stressed by immobilization, electric shock or exhaustion. Thus there is an increase in noradrenaline activity when ACTH release is stimulated. Similarly, there is an increase in noradrenaline turnover after adrenal-ectomy and a fall in noradrenaline turnover when ACTH release is inhibited by injections of cortisol. Contrary results were obtained by Versteeg (1973) who found an increase in noradrenaline turnover after injection of ACTH. There is also some conflict over the change in turnover of brain dopamine in stress; Fuxe *et al.* (1970a) found it remained unchanged, while Bliss and Ailion (1971) suggested it rose during stress.

Carbachol, noradrenaline, 5-HT, and GABA each stimulated corticosterone levels when placed in the median eminence but only noradrenaline was active in all parts of the limbic system, i.e. the amygdala, hippocampus, and septal region. The other substances were active in particular parts of the limbic system, while carbachol only acted in the hypothalamus and mamillary bodies (Krieger and Krieger, 1970a; 1970b). Naumenko (1968) also placed noradrenaline and acetylcholine implants into the hypothalamus or midbrain, but showed that their stimulatory effect was probably due to stress because they no longer raised plasma corticosterone after sectioning the midbrain. Recently, intravenous infusion of an α-adrenergic stimulating agent, methoxamine, was shown to raise both plasma ACTH and cortisol in humans. The rise was inhibited by phentolamine, but no propranolol (Nakai *et al.*, 1973).

In summary, it seems that the evidence for either an inhibitory or stimulatory effect of noradrenaline on ACTH release is not substantial, because in many cases the results have been due to the non-specific stress of the techniques used. The most likely role for noradrenaline, so far, seems to be in the stress-induced release of ACTH, although whether it is inhibitory or stimulatory remains to be seen.

10.2   5-HYDROXYTRYPTAMINE AS TRANSMITTER FOR ACTH RELEASE

As early as 1957 it was known that systemic administration of 5-hydroxy-tryptamine stimulated ACTH release as shown by adrenal ascorbic acid depletion (Mousatche and Perreira, 1957). It has also been shown to have an ACTH-like action of its own at the adrenal level stimulating steroido-genesis, especially in the glomerulosa cells (Verdesca et al., 1961; Albano et al., 1974; Mendelsohn and Warren, 1974).

More recently a central action for 5-hydroxytryptamine has been in-dicated. Systemic injection of 5-HTP or intraventricular injection of 5-hydroxytryptamine stimulated ACTH release, as shown by raised plasma corticosteroid levels and this effect was seen even when the hypothalamus was completely separated from the rest of the brain by deafferentation (Ganong, 1971; Popova et al., 1972). Rises in plasma corticosterone were also seen after implantation of 5-hydroxytryptamine into the hypothalamus, ventral hippocampus septal region and midbrain. These results, taken all together, indicate that 5-hydroxytryptamine is a stimulatory transmitter in a pathway leading from the midbrain via the limbic system to the hypothalamus, where the 5-hydroxytryptamine is released. The effect of the hypothalamic implants is not due to non-specific stress because they are still active after sectioning of the midbrain which prevents impulses passing via the spinal cord to the peripheral system (Naumenko, 1968). It should be noted, however, that Hedge and Smelik (1968) did not find 5-hydroxytryptamine implants active in the anterior hypothalamus and Naumenko (1969) found implants in the lateral hypothalamus were ineffective. Naumenko (1969) also found that implants of 5-hydroxytryptamine in the dorsal hippocampus and amyg-dala reduced plasma corticosterone levels, indicating the existence of a second serotonergic pathway with an inhibitory control. Similarly, Berger and Barchas (1972) found that administration of 5-hydroxytrypt-amine precursors (tryptophan and 5-HTP) reduced the normal rise in plasma corticosterone seen after stress, while reducing endogenous 5-hydroxytryptamine levels with PCPA enhanced the stress response. They suggest there is an inhibitory serotonergic control in the hippo-campus and the negative feedback effect of the corticosteroids may be exerted via this system (Vernikos-Danellis et al., 1973).

Lowering the levels of 5-hydroxytryptamine in the brain, either by pharmacological agents such as chloramphetamine or PCPA or by feeding the rats with tryptophan-deficient diet, had no effect on the tonic release of ACTH as plasma corticosteroid levels were not lowered, nor was the response of stress-induced ACTH release altered. Perhaps as both the stimulatory and the inhibitory systems were affected equally by the depletion, the net result was no change in ACTH release (Dixit and Buckley, 1969; McKinney et al., 1971; Dixit, 1971). However, lowering brain 5-hydroxytryptamine with PCPA did appear to abolish the circadian rhythm in plasma corticosteroid levels (Krieger and Rizzo, 1969; Scapagnini et al., 1971; Berger and Barchas, 1972; Van Delft et al., 1974). The diurnal rhythm of brain 5-hydroxytryptamine in the hippocampus and amygdala is similar to that of plasma corticosterone (Scapagnini et al., 1971), and abolition of the rhythm by either lowering brain 5-hydroxytryptamine or raising it (by using an MAOI), seemed to abolish the corticosterone rhythm (Krieger and Rizzo, 1969). These results indicate that 5-hydroxytryptamine may control the circadian rhythm in ACTH release.

When rats were subjected to certain stresses the turnover of brain 5-hydroxytryptamine increased, as shown by rises in brain tryptophan and 5-HIAA, although 5-hydroxytryptamine levels themselves hardly changed after the first 16 hours (Curzon and Green, 1969; Knott et al., 1973). This effect was seen after stress due to immobilization, food deprivation, electric shock and heat stress, indicating that 5-hydroxytryptamine may be involved in stress-induced ACTH release. Adrenalectomy had no effect on brain 5-hydroxytryptamine metabolism, except after 10 days when turnover was reduced; it could be restored by administration of cortisol (Fuxe et al., 1970a). Some of these changes can be explained by changes in circulating levels of glucocorticoids. In rats, adrenalectomy lowered the tryptophan hydroxylase levels in the midbrain by 75 per cent, resulting in a reduced 5-hydroxytryptamine turnover. The enzyme activity could be partially restored by administration of corticosterone (Azmitra and McEwen, 1969) and this may explain the increased turnover seen after stress.

Superimposed on this effect on metabolism within the CNS, Curzon (1969) has shown that raised levels of plasma corticosterone (as after stress or systemic injection) can lower 5-hydroxytryptamine brain levels six hours later for a duration of approximately 10 hours. He has shown this is due to induction by corticosteroids of the liver enzyme tryptophan pyrrolase, which catabolizes tryptophan, the precursor of 5-hydroxytryptamine. The depletion does not take place in animals pretreated with a tryptophan pyrrolase inhibitor (allopurinol), nor in adrenalectomized rats (Curzon and Green, 1969). The corticosteroids may have a quite separate effect on 5-hydroxytryptamine levels within the CNS, since

McEwan (1973) has shown that glucocorticoids stimulate the conversion of tryptophan to 5-hydroxytryptamine.

In summary, the results indicate that 5-hydroxytryptamine may control the circadian rhythm for ACTH release. In addition, there appear to be two opposing serotonergic systems: one in the hypothalamus which stimulates tonic release of ACTH and an inhibitory system in the hippocampus which antagonizes the release of ACTH after stress.

10.3 ACETYLCHOLINE AS A TRANSMITTER FOR ACTH RELEASE

In 1967 Smelik showed that depletion of hypothalamic catecholamines had no effect on the stress-induced release of ACTH, indicating that the catecholamines were not involved in the control of ACTH. It is possible, however, that acetylcholine may be the stimulatory transmitter for ACTH release. The long-acting cholinomimetic compound, carbachol, implanted within the median eminence area (6 μg per rat) or injected intraventricularly (0·1–0·25 μg per rat) was found to activate the pituitary-adrenal system (Krieger and Krieger, 1970a; Marks et al., 1970), although according to Naumenko (1968) this effect may be secondary to the stress effect. Microelectrophoretically delivered acetylcholine-stimulated hypothalamic neurones are also stimulated by ACTH and inhibited by dexamethasone (Steiner et al., 1968).

Systemic and central injections of atropine have also been found to alter plasma corticosterone levels, and response to stress. In 1968, Krieger et al. found that atropine prevented the rise normally seen in plasma corticosterone at the beginning of the dark period. The atropine was only effective over a limited time, just before the expected rise and suggested to them that a critical period for ACTH release may exist, as it does for LH, and that acetylcholine is the stimulatory transmitter. Implants of atropine in the anterior hypothalamus also inhibited ACTH release (Hedges and Smelik, 1968). This result is very specific, in that other amines, e.g. noradrenaline, adrenaline, dopamine, 5-hydroxytryptamine and also MAO inhibitors, had no effect in this region, which is an important site for corticosterone negative feedback effects (Smelik, 1969). Further experiments with implants of atropine in the anterior hypothalamus show that it is effective at 15 μg per rat placed bilaterally in inhibiting stress-induced rises in plasma corticosterone. It is only active in the anterior hypothalamus and this effect is not due to a systemic or non-specific local anaesthetic action. The onset of its effect is very rapid, i.e. about 10 minutes and the duration is 2 hours (Kaplanski and Smelik, 1973b). The specificity of the site is confirmed by the fact that intraventricular atropine had no effect on corticosterone levels (Ganong, 1972b).

In vitro experiments support the stimulatory role of acetylcholine. When 10–100 pg ml^{-1} acetylcholine was added to incubating hypothalamic synaptosomes there was a release of CRF. The effect was blocked by atropine, while noradrenaline had no action in this preparation (Bennet and Edwardson, 1974). Bradbury *et al.* (1974) obtained similar results with acetylcholine in incubating hypothalamic slices.

11 The effect of brain amines on the release of thyroid-stimulating hormone (TSH)

The release of TSH from the pituitary is controlled by thyroid-releasing hormone (TRH) present in the hypothalamus. TSH stimulates the secretion of thyroid hormone and its plasma levels are usually monitored by measuring the changes in circulating labelled iodine. Thyroid hormone exerts a negative feedback effect mainly at the pituitary level but also at the hypothalamic level, and TSH can exert a short positive feedback effect on its own secretion by stimulating TRH release. Stress is known to inhibit TSH release perhaps via ACTH which inhibits TSH release (Donovan, 1970).

Experiments carried out between 1947 and 1965 to elucidate the neural control of TSH release are confused and their results conflict mainly because administration of the amines or pharmacological agents may have been stressful in some experiments and so caused inhibition of TSH release. Thus intravenous, intrapituitary or intrahypothalamic administration of the catecholamines, acetylcholine or MAO inhibitors inhibited either TSH or thyroid hormone secretion in rats, guinea-pigs or rabbits (Harrison, 1961; Lupulescu *et al.*, 1964; Samojlik, 1965). A few studies showed that the amines stimulated TSH release and thyroid activity. Subcutaneous administration of adrenaline to thyroidectomized dogs stimulated TSH release (Soffer *et al.*, 1947), and Soderburg (1958) in a careful study in cats pretreated with TSH showed that all the amines given intravenously stimulated thyroid hormone release in the following order of potency: acetylcholine, 5-hydroxytryptamine, adrenaline and noradrenaline. In addition, depletion of the amines by reserpine inhibited thyroid hormone secretion (Harrison, 1961).

In 1970 the structure of TRH was elucidated (Bowers *et al.*, 1970) and so in recent work the effect of amines directly on TRH secretion at the hypothalamic level has been investigated (Reichlin *et al.*, 1972). They have confirmed that amine depletion by reserpine lowers TSH levels and have also shown that it reduces TRH synthetase in the hypothalamus, suggesting that the synthesis of TRH is under amine control. Kotani *et al.* (1973) have confirmed the effect of reserpine and shown that an α-adrenergic blocker and α-methyltyrosine also inhibit TSH release.

In *in vitro* experiments on mouse hypothalami, the same workers have shown that noradrenaline enhances the release of TRH and that dopamine was also effective but to a lesser extent and ineffective if its conversion to noradrenaline was inhibited. Acetylcholine was ineffective and 5-hydroxytryptamine inhibited TRH release (Grimm and Reichlin, 1973). These results indicate that the synthesis and release of hypothalamic TRH is under the stimulatory control of noradrenaline and inhibitory control of 5-hydroxytryptamine.

REFERENCES

Aghajanian, G. K. and Asher, I. M. (1971). *Science*, **172**, 1159.

Aghajanian, G. K., Rosecrans, J. A. and Sheard, M. H. (1967). *Science*, **156**, 402.

Agrawal, H. C., Glisson, S. N. and Himwich, W. A. (1966). *Biochim. Biophys. Acta*, **130**, 511.

Agrawal, H. C., Glisson, S. N. and Himwich, W. A. (1968). *Int. J. Neuropharmacol.* **7**, 97.

Ahlenius, S., Eriksson, H., Larsson, K., Modigh, K. and Sodersten, P. (1971). *Psychopharmacologia*, **20**, 382.

Ahlenius, S., Engel, J., Eriksson, H. and Sodersten, P. (1972a). *J. Neural Transmission*, **33**, 155.

Ahlenius, S., Engel, J., Eriksson, H., Modigh, K. and Sodersten, P. (1972b). *J. Neural Transmission*, **33**, 247.

Ahren, K., Fuxe, K., Hamberger, L. and Hokfelt, T. (1971). *Endocrinology*, **88**, 1415.

Albano, J. D. M., Brown, B. L., Ekins, R. P., Mee, M., Tait, S. A. S. and Tait, J. F. (1974). *J. Endocrinol*. In press.

Alleva, J. J., Overpeck, J. G. and Umberger, E. J. (1966). *Life Sci.* **5**, 1557.

Amin, A. H., Crawford, T. B. B. and Gaddum, J. H. (1954). *J. Physiol. (London)*, **126**, 596.

Anden, N. E., Dahlstrom, A., Fuxe, K. and Larsson, K. (1965). *Life Sci.* **4**, 1275.

Andreoli, V., Ceccarelli, B., Cerati, E., Demonte, M. L. and Clementi, F. (1970). *Exp. Brain Res.* **11**, 17.

Anton-Tay, F. and Wurtman, R. J. (1968). *Science*, **159**, 1245.

Anton-Tay, F. and Wurtman, R. J. (1969). *In* "Society of Endocrinology Program of 51st meeting". No. 104.

Anton-Tay, F. and Wurtman, R. J. (1971). *In* "Frontiers in Neuroendocrinology 1971" (Eds W. F. Ganong and L. Martini), p. 45. Oxford University Press, New York, London and Toronto.

Anton-Tay, F., Pelham, R. W. and Wurtman, R. J. (1969). *Endocrinology*, **84**, 1489.

Aprison, M. H. and Hurgtgen, J. N. (1972). *Fed. Proc.* **31**, 121.

Arai, Y., Knbokura, A., Suzuki, Y. and Masuda, S. (1970). *Endocrinologia Japonica*, **17**, 441.

Arbuthnott, G. W., Crow, T. J., Fuxe, K., Olson, L. and Ungerstedt, U. (1970). *Brain Res.* **24**, 471.

Aron, C. and Asch, G. (1963). *C.R. Soc. Biol.* **157**, 1055.

Artunes-Rodrigues, J. and McCann, S. M. (1967). *Endocrinology*, **81**, 666.

Asano, Y. (1971). *Life Sci.* **10**, 883.

Astwood, E. B. (1941). *Endocrinology*, **28**, 309.

Axelrod, J. (1959). *Physiol. Rev.* **39**, 751.

Axelrod, J. (1962). *J. Biol. Chem.* **237**, 1657.

Azmitra, E. C. and McEwan, B. S. (1969). *Science*, **166**, 1274.

Baker, P. C. and Quay, W. B. (1969). *Brain Res.* **12**, 273.

Baldessarini, R. J. and Kopin, I. J. (1967). *J. Pharmacol. Exp. Ther.* **156**, 31.

Baldessarini, R. J. and Vogt, M. (1971). *J. Neurochem.* **18**, 2519.

Bapna, J., Neff, N. H. and Costa, E. (1971). *Endocrinology*, **89**, 1345.

Barchas, J. D., Ciaranello, R. D., Stolk, J. M., Brodie, K. H. and Hamburg, D. A. (1972). *In* "Hormones & Behaviour" (Ed. S. Levine), p. 235. Academic Press, New York and London.

Barfield, R. J. and Sachs, B. D. (1968). *Science*, **161**, 392.

Barraclough, C. A. and Sawyer, C. H. (1959). *Endocrinology*, **65**, 563.

Barraclough, C. A., Collu, R., Massa, R. and Martini, L. (1971). *Endocrinology*, **88**, 1437.

Barrelt, R. E. and Balch, T. S. (1971). *Experientia*, **27**, 663.

Barthwal, J. P., Gupta, T. K., Gupta, M. L. and Bhargava, K. P. (1971). *Jap. J. Pharmacol.* **21**, 1.

Beach, F. A. and Fowler, H. (1959). *J. Comp. Physiol. Psychol.* **52**, 245.

Beattie, C. W. and Soyka, L. E. (1973). *Endocrinology*, **93**, 1453.

Beattie, C. W., Rodgers, C. H. and Soyka, L. E. (1972). *Endocrinology*, **91**, 276.

Benkerto, O. and Eversmann, T. (1972). *Experientia*, **28**, 532.

Bennett, G. W. and Edwardson, J. A. (1974). Personal communication.

Bennett, D. S. and Giarman, N. J. (1965). *J. Neurochem.* **12**, 911.

Berger, P. A. and Barchas, J. D. (1972). Proc. 5th Int. Cong. Pharmacol. p. 19.

Bertolini, A. (1971). *Riv. Farm. Ter.* **2**, 73.

Beyer, C. and Sawyer, C. H. (1969). *In* "Frontiers in Neuroendocrinology 1969" (Eds W. E. Ganong and L. Martini), p. 255. Oxford University Press, New York, London, Toronto.

Bhargava, K. P. and Gupta, M. L. (1966). *Brit. J. Pharmacol.* **26**, 601.

Billeter, E. and Fluckiger, E. (1971). *Experentia*, **27**, 464.

Birge, C. A., Jacobs, L. S., Hammer, C. T. and Daughaday, W. H. (1970). *Endocrinology*, **86**, 120.

Bjorkland, A. and Nobin, A. (1973). *Brain Res.* **51**, 193.

Blackard, W. G. and Heidingsfelder, S. A. (1968). *J. Clin. Invest.* **47**, 1407.

Blackburn, K. J., French, P. C. and Merrills, R. J. (1967). *Life Sci.* **6**, 1653.

Blake, C. A., Weiner, R. I. and Sawyer, C. H. (1972a). *Endocrinology*, **90**, 862.

Blake, C. A., Weiner, R. I., Gorski, R. A. and Sawyer, C. H. (1972b). *Endocrinology*, **90**, 855.

Bliss, E. L. and Ailion, J. (1971). *Life Sci.* **10**, 1161.

Bliss, E. L., Frischat, A. and Samuels, L. (1972). *Life Sci.* **11**, 231.

Boccabella, A. V., Salgado, E. D. and Alger, E. A. (1962). *Endocrinology*, **71**, 827.

Boden, G., Lundy, L. E. and Owen, O. E. (1972). *Neuroendocrinology*, **10**, 309.

Boling, J. L. and Blandau, R. J. (1939). *Endocrinology*, **25**, 359.

Bond, V. J., Shillito, E. E. and Vogt, M. (1972). *Brit. J. Pharmacol.* **46**, 46.

Bowers, C. Y., Schally, A. V., Enzmann, F., Bøler, J. and Folkers, K. (1970). *Endocrinology*, **86**, 1143.

Boyd, A. E., Lebovitz, H. E. and Feldman, J. M. (1971). *J. Clin. Endocrinol.* **33**, 829.

Bradbury, M. W. B., Burden, J. C., Hillhouse, E. and Jones, M. T. (1974). *J. Physiol. (London)*, **239**, 269.

Briggs, M. and Briggs, M. (1972). *J. Reprod. Fert.* **29**, 447.

Brimblecombe, R. W. (1973). *In* "Advances in Drug Research" (Ed. A. B. Simmonds), vol. 7, p. 165. Academic Press, London and New York.

Brodie, B. B. and Shore, P. A. (1957). *Ann. N.Y. Acad. Sci.* **66**, 631.

Brown, P. S. (1966). *J. Endocrinol.* **35**, 161.

Brown, P. S. (1967a). *J. Endocrinol.* **37**, 327.

Brown, P. S. (1967b). *Nature*, **214**, 1268.

Brown, P. S. (1971). *Neuroendocrinology*, **7**, 183.

Brown, P. S. and Fawke, L. (1972). *J. Reprod. Fert.* **28**, 167.

Butcher, L. L., Butcher, S. H. and Larrson, K. (1969). *Eur. J. Pharmacol.* **7**, 283.

Butcher, L. L., Engel, J. and Fuxe, K. (1972). *Brain Res.* **41**, 387

Caligaris, L. and Taleisnik, S. (1974). *J. Endocrinol.* **62**, 25.

Caligaris, L., Astrada, J. J. and Taleisnik, S. (1968). *Acta Endocrinol. (Copenhagen)*, **59**, 177.

Caligaris, L., Astrada, J. J. and Taleisnik, S. (1971). *Endocrinology*, **89**, 331.

Carlsson, A. (1959). *Pharmacol. Rev.* **11**, 490.

Carlsson, A., Falck, B., Hillarp, N.-A. and Torp, A. (1962a). *Acta Physiol. Scand.* **54**, 385.

Carlsson, A., Falck, B. and Hillarp, N.-A. (1962b). *Acta Physiol. Scand.* **56**, Suppl. 196, 1.

Carrer, H. F. and Taleisnik, S. (1970). *J. Endocrinol.* **48**, 527.

Carrer, H. F. and Taleisnik, S. (1972). *Brain Res.* **38**, 299.

Chase, T. N., Breese, G. R. and Kopin, I. J. (1967). *Science*, **157**, 1461.

Chatterjee, A. (1967). *Endocrinology*, **80**, 983.

Chen, C. L., Minaguchi, H. and Heites, J. (1967). *Proc. Soc. Exp. Biol. Med.* **126**, 317.

Choudhury, S. A. R., Sharpe, R. M. and Brown, P. S. (1973). *Neuroendocrinology*, **12**, 272.

Chowers, I. and McCann, S. M. (1967). *Proc. Soc. Exp. Biol. Med.* **124**, 260.

Ciaranello, R. D., Barchas, R. E., Byers, G. S., Stemmle, D. W. and Barchas, J. D. (1969). *Nature*, **221**, 368.

Clemens, J. A., Amenomoni, Y., Jenkins, T. and Meites, J. (1969). *Proc. Soc. Exp. Biol. Med.* **132**, 561.

Clementi, F., Ceccarelli, B., Cerati, E., Demonte, M. L., Felici, M., Motta, M. and Pecile, A. (1970). *J. Endocrinol.* **48**, 205

Collu, R., Fraschini, F., Visconti, P. and Martini, L. (1972). *Endocrinology*, **90**, 1231.

Collu, R., Fraschini, F. and Martini, L. (1973). *Recent Progr. Brain Res.* **39**, 290.

Coppola, J. A. (1968). *J. Reprod. Fert. Suppl.* **4**, 35.

Coppola, J. A. (1969). *Neuroendocrinology*, **5**, 75.

Coppola, J. A. (1971). *In* "Frontiers in Neuroendocrinology 1971" (Eds W. F. Ganong and L. Martini), p. 129. Oxford University Press, London.

Coppola, J. A., Leonardi, W., Lippmann, W., Perrine, J. W. and Ringler, I. (1965). *Endocrinology*, **77**, 485.

Coppola, J. A., Leonardi, W. and Lippmann, W. (1966). *Endocrinology*, **78**, 225.

Corbin, A. and Schottelius, B. A. (1961). *Amer. J. Physiol.* **201**, 1176.

Corbin, A. and Upton, V. (1973). *Experientia*, **29**, 1552.

Costa, E. and Meek, J. L. (1974). *Ann. Rev. Pharmac.* **14**, 491.

Costa, E. and Neff, N. H. (1966). *In* "Biochemistry and Pharmacology of Basal Ganglia" (Eds E. Costa, L. Cote and M. D. Yarh). Raven Press, New York.

Coyle, J. T. and Snyder, S. A. (1969). *J. Pharmacol. Exp. Ther.* **170**, 221.

Coyle, J. T. and Axelrod, J. (1971). *J. Neurochem.* **18**, 2061.

Craven, R. P. and McDonald, P. G. (1971a). *Life Sci.* **10**, 1409.

Craven, R. P. and McDonald, P. G. (1971b). *J. Reprod. Fert.* **27**, 480.

Craven, R. P. and McDonald, P. G. (1973). *J. Endocrinol.* **58**, 319.

Critchlow, V. (1958). *Amer. J. Physiol.* **195**, 171.

Cuello, A. C., Horn, A. S., MacKay, A. V. P. and Iversen, L. L. (1973). *Nature*, **243**, 465.

Currie, G. N., Black, D. L., Armstrong, D. T. and Greep, R. O. (1969). *Proc. Soc. Exp. Med. Biol.* **130**, 598.

Curzon, G. (1969). *Brit. J. Psychiat.* **115**, 1367.

Curzon, G. and Green, A. R. (1969). *Brit. J. Pharmacol.* **37**, 689.

Dahlstrom, A. (1967). *Naunyn-Schmiedebergs Arch. Pharmakol. Exp. Pathol.* **257**, 93; see Barchas *et al.* (1972). *In* "Hormones and Behaviour" (Ed. S. Levine), p. 235. Academic Press, New York and London.

Dahlstrom, A. and Fuxe, K. (1964). *Acta Physiol. Scand.* **62**, Suppl. 232.

da Prada, M., Carruba, M., O'Brien, R. A., Sauer, A. and Pletscher, A. (1972). *Eur. J. Pharmacol.* **19**, 288.

da Prada, M., Carruba, M., Sauer, A., O'Brien, R. A. and Pletscher, A. (1973). *Brain Res.* **55**, 383.

Davidson, J. M. (1969). *In* "Frontiers in Neuroendocrinology 1969" (Eds W. F. Ganong and L. Martini), p. 343. Oxford University Press, New York, London, Toronto.

Davis, S. L. and Borger, M. L. (1973). *Endocrinology*, **92**, 303.

de Schaepdryer, A., Preziosi, P. and Scapagnini, U. (1969). *Brit. J. Pharmacol.* **35**, 460.

Debeljuk, L., Feder, V. M. and Paulucci, O. A. (1970). *J. Reprod. Fert.* **21**, 363.

Dengler, H. J., Spiegel, H. E. and Titus, E. O. (1961). *Science*, **133**, 1072.

Desclin, L. (1960). *Anat. Rec.* **136**, 182.

Dewsbury, D. A. and Davis, H. N. (1970). *Physiol. Behav.* **5**, 1331.

Dewsbury, D. A., Davis, H. N. and Jansen, P. E. (1972). *Psychopharmacologia*, **24**, 209.

Dixit, B. N. (1971). *Arch. Int. Pharmacodyn*, **189**, 100.

Dixit, B. N. and Buckley, J. P. (1967). *Life Sci.* **6**, 755.

Dixit, B. N. and Buckley, J. P. (1969). *Neuroendocrinology*, **4**, 32.

Donoso, A. O. and Cuckier, J. O. (1968). *Nature*, **218**, 969.

Donoso, A. O. and Moyano, M. B. de G. (1970). *Proc. Soc. Exp. Biol. Med.* **135**, 633.

Donoso, A. O. and Santolaya, R. C. (1969). *Experientia*, **25**, 855.

Donoso, A. O. and Stefano, F. J. E. (1967). *Experientia*, **23**, 665.

Donoso, A. O., Stefano, F. J. E. and Biscardi, A. M. (1966). *Science*, **154**, 680.

Donoso, A. O., Stefano, F. J. E., Biscardi, A. M. and Cukier, J. (1967). *Amer. J. Physiol.* **212**, 737.

Donoso, A. O., Moyano, M. B. de G. and Santolaya, R. G. (1969). *Neuroendocrinology*, **4**, 12.

Donoso, A. O., Bishop, W., Fawcett, C. P., Krulick, L. and McCann, S. M. (1971). *Endocrinology*, **89**, 774.

Donovan, B. T. (1970). *In* "Mammalian Neuroendocrinology". McGraw-Hill, London.

Donovan, B. T. and Harris, G. W. (1956). *J. Physiol.* **132**, 577.

Dordoni, F. and Timiras, P. S. (1952). *J. Pharmacol. Exp. Ther.* **106**, 381.

Ely, C. A. and Schwartz, N. B. (1971). *Endocrinology*, **89**, 1103.

Endersby, C. A. and Wilson, C. (1973). *Brit. J. Pharmacol.* **47**, 647P.

Endersby, C. A. and Wilson, C. (1974). *Brain Res.* In press.

Endersby, C. A., Robson, J. M., Sullivan, F. M. and Wilson, C. (1970). *J. Endocrinol.* **48**, 13.

Endersby, C. A., Gallagher, M., Horth, C. E., McDonald, P. G. and Wilson, C. (1972). *J. Endocrinol.* **57**, 9.

Endroczi, E. and Hilliard, J. (1965). *Endocrinology*, **77**, 667.

Eskin, I. A. (1944). *Byull. Eksper. Biol. i Med.* **18**, 68.

Everett, J. W. (1964). *In* "Major Problems in Neuroendocrinology" (Eds E. Bajusz and G. Jasmin), p. 346. S. Karger, Basel and New York.

Everett, J. W., Sawyer, C. H. and Markee, J. E. (1949). *Endocrinology*, **44**, 234.

Fajer, A. B., Hoffman, D. and Shillito, E. (1970). *J. Reprod. Fert.* **22**, 379.

Falck, B., Hillarp, N. A., Thieme, G. and Torp, A. (1962). *J. Histochem. Cytochem.* **10**, 348.

Farnebo, L. O., Hamberger, B. and Jonsson, G. (1971). *J. Neurochem.* **18**, 2491.

Fawke, L., Morris, A. and Brown, P. S. (1972). *J. Reprod. Fert.* **28**, 177.

Feer, H. and Wirz-Justice, A. (1971). *Experientia*, **27**, 885.

Ferin, M., Tempone, A., Zimmering, P. A. and Van de Weile, R. L. (1969). *Endocrinology*, **85**, 1070.

Ferrando, G. and Nalbandov, A. V. (1969). *Endocrinology*, **85**, 38.

Flerko, B. (1971). *In* "Current Topics in Experimental Endocrinology" (Eds L. Martini and V. H. T. James), p. 42. Academic Press, New York and London.

Frantz, A. G. (1973). *Recent Progr. Horm. Res.* **39**, 311.

Fraschini, F. (1970). *In* "Neurochemical Aspects of Hypothalamic Function" (Eds L. Martini and J. Meites), p. 141. Academic Press, New York and London.

Fraschini, F., Collu, R. and Martini, L. (1971). *In* "Proc. 3rd Int. Cong. Horm. Ster. (Eds V. H. T. James and L. Martini), p. 830. Excerpta Medica Foundation, Amsterdam. Int. Cong. Series No. 210, 1970.

Freeman, M. E. and Neill, J. D. (1972). *Endocrinology*, **90**, 1292.

Freeman, M. E., Reichert, L. E. and Neill, J. D. (1972). *Endocrinology*, **90**, 232.

Friedman, A. H. and Walker, C. A. (1968). *J. Physiol.* **197**, 77.

Fuxe, K. (1965). *Acta Physiol. Scand.* **64**. Suppl. 247, 37.

Fuxe, K. and Gunne, L.-M. (1964). *Acta Physiol. Scand.* **62**, 493.

Fuxe, K. and Hokfelt, T. (1969). *In* "Frontiers in Neuroendocrinology 1969" (Eds W. F. Ganong and L. Martini), p. 47. Oxford University Press, New York, London, Toronto.

Fuxe, K. and Hokfelt, T. (1970a). *In* "Aspects of Neuroendocrinology" (Eds W. Bargmann and B. Scharrer), p. 192. Springer-Verlag, Berlin.

Fuxe, K. and Hokfelt, T. (1970b). *In* "The hypothalamus" (Eds L. Martini, M. Motta and F. Fraschini), p. 123. Academic Press, New York and London.

Fuxe, K., Hokfelt, T. and Nilsson, O. (1967). *Life Sci.* **6**, 2057.

Fuxe, K., Hokfelt, T. and Ungerstedt, U. (1968a). *Advan. Pharmacol.* **6A**, 235.

Fuxe, K., Hokfelt, T., Ritzen, M. and Ungerstedt, U. (1968b). *Histochemie*, **16**, 186.

Fuxe, K., Hokfelt, T. and Nilsson, O. (1969). *Neuroendocrinology*, **5**, 107.

Fuxe, K., Corrodi, H., Hokfelt, T. and Jonsson, G. (1970a). *Progr. Brain Res.* **32**, 42.

Fuxe, K., Hokfelt, T. and Jonsson, G. (1970b). *In* "Neurochemical Aspects of Hypothalamic Function" (Eds L. Martini and J. Meites), p. 61. Academic Press, London and New York.

Fuxe, K., Hokfelt, T. and Jonsson, G. (1971). *In* "Proc. 3rd Int. Cong. Horm. Ster. 1970" (Eds V. H. T. James and L. Martini), p. 62. Excerpta Medica Foundation, Amsterdam. Int. Cong. Series No. 210, 1970.

Fuxe, K., Hokfelt, T. and Nilsson, O. (1972a). *Acta Endocrinol. (Kbh)*, **69**, 625.

Fuxe, K., Hokfelt, T., Sundstedt, C.-O., Ahren, K. and Hamberger, L. (1972b). *Neuroendocrinology*, **10**, 282.

Gala, R. R. and Reece, R. P. (1963). *Fed. Sci. Progr.* **22**, 506.

Gala, R. R., Markarian, P. B. and O'Neill, M. R. (1970). *Life Sci.* **9**, 1055.

Ganong, W. F. (1971). *In* "Proc. 3rd Int. Cong. Horm. Ster. 1970" (Eds V. H. T. James and L. Martini), p. 61. Excerpta Medica Foundation, Amsterdam. Int. Cong. Series No. 210, 1970.

Ganong, W. F. (1972a). *In* "Brain-Endocrine interaction. Median eminence: structure and function". Int. Sym. Munich 1971, p. 254. Karger, Basel.

Ganong, W. F. (1972b). *Progr. Brain Res.* **38**, 41.

Garay, G. L. and Martin, J. M. (1970). 52nd Proc. of Endocrine Soc. Meeting, p. 46, No. 20.

Gay, V. L. and Bogdanove, E. M. (1969). *Endocrinology*, **84**, 1132.

Gaziri, L. C. J. and Ladosky, W. (1973). *Neuroendocrinology*, **12**, 249.

Gessa, G. L., Tagliomonte, A., Tagliomonte, P. and Brodie, B. B. (1970). *Nature*, **227**, 616.

Giulian, D., Pohorecky, L. A. and McEwen, B. S. (1973). *Endocrinology*, **93**, 1329.

Glowinski, J. and Axelrod, J. (1965). *J. Pharmacol. Exp. Ther.* **149**, 43.

Glowinski, J. and Iversen, L. L. (1966). *J. Neurochem.* **13**, 655.

Glowinski, J., Kopin, I. J. and Axelrod, J. (1965). *J. Neurochem.* **12**, 25.

Goldstein, M. and Frenkel, R. (1971). *Nature*, **233**, 179.

Goodwin, J. S., Katz, R. I. and Kopin, I. J. (1969). *Nature*, **221**, 556.

Gorski, R. A. (1966). *J. Reprod. Fert. Suppl.* **1**, 67.

Gorski, R. A. (1968). *In* "Biology of Gestation" (Ed. N. S. Assali), p. 2. Academic Press, New York and London.

Gorski, R. A. (1971). *In* "Frontiers in Neuroendocrinology 1971" (Eds L. Martini and W. F. Ganong), p. 237. Oxford University Press, New York, London, Toronto.

Grahame-Smith, D. G. (1971). *J. Neurochem.* **18**, 1053.

Grandison, L. and Meites, J. (1972). *Proc. Soc. Exp. Med. Biol.* **140**, 323.

Greenwald, G. S. and Rothchild, I. (1968). *J. Anim. Sci.* **27**, Suppl. 139.

Greer, M. A., Yamada, T. and Iiono, S. (1960). *Ann. N.Y. Acad. Sci.* **86**, 667.

Grimm, Y. and Reichlin, S. (1973). *Endocrinology*, **93**, 626.

Guillemin, R. (1955). *Endocrinology*, **56**, 248.

Guillemin, R., Hearn, W. R., Cheek, W. R. and Housholder, D. E. (1957). *Endocrinology*, **60**, 488.

Guiliani, G., Martini, L., Pecile, A. and Fochi, M. (1960). *Acta Endocrinol. (Kbh),* Suppl. 51, 29.

Guiliani, G., Martini, L., Pecile, A. and Fochi, M. (1961). *Acta Endocrinol. (Kbh),* 38, 1.

Gunne, L. M. (1962). *Acta Physiol. Scand.* 56, 324.

Haber, B. and Kamano, A. (1966). *Nature,* 209, 404.

Hackmann, E., Wirz-Justice, A. and Lichtsteiner, M. (1973). *Psychopharmacologia (Berlin),* 32, 183.

Hagino, N., Watanabe, M. and Goldzieher, J. W. (1969). *Endocrinology,* 84, 308.

Hamon, M., Javoy, F., Kordon, C. and Glowinski, J. (1970). *Life Sci.* 9, 167.

Hardin, C. M. (1973a). *Brain Res.* 62, 286.

Hardin, C. M. (1973b). *Brain Res.* 59, 437.

Harris, G. W. (1948). *Physiol. Rev.* 28, 139.

Harris, G. W. (1964). *Endocrinology,* 75, 627.

Harrison, T. S. (1961). *Endocrinology,* 68, 466.

Hartley, R. and Smith, J. A. (1972). *Biochem. Pharmacol.* 21, 2007.

Harvey, J. A., Heller, A. and Moore, R. Y. (1963). *J. Pharmacol. Exp. Ther.* 140, 103.

Hedges, G. A. and Smelik, P. G. (1968). *Science,* 159, 891.

Heller, A. and Moore, R. Y. (1965). *J. Pharmacol. Exp. Ther.* 150, 1.

Hertelendy, F., Todd, H., Peake, G. T., Machlin, L. J., Johnston, G. and Pounds, G. (1971). *Endocrinology,* 89, 1256.

Héry, F., Rouer, E. and Glowinski, J. (1972). *Brain Res.* 43, 445.

Hidaka, H., Nagatsu, T. and Yagi, K. (1969). *J. Neurochem.* 16, 783.

Himwich, H. E. (1971). *In* "Biochemistry, Schizophrenias and the Affective Illnesses". Williams and Wilkins, Baltimore, Maryland.

Hiroshige, T., Kunita, H., Ogura, C. and Itoh, S. (1968). *Jap. J. Physiol.* 18, 609.

Horn, A. S., Coyle, J. T. and Snyder, S. H. (1971). *Mol. Pharmacol.* 7, 66.

Hokfelt, T. and Fuxe, K. (1972a). *In* "Brain-Endocrine Interaction. International Symposium on Brain-Endocrine" (Eds K. M. Knigge, D. E. Scott and A. Weindle), p. 181. Karger, Munich.

Hokfelt, T. and Fuxe, K. (1972b). *Neuroendocrinology,* 9, 100.

Hokfelt, T., Fuxe, K., Goldstein, M. and Johansson, O. (1974). *Brain Res.* 66, 235.

Holzbauer, M. and Youdim, M. B. H. (1972). *Brit. J. Pharmacol.* 44, 355P.

Holzbauer, M. and Youdim, M. B. H. (1973). *Brit. J. Pharmacol.* 48, 600.

Hyyppa, M. and Lorentz, M. (1969). *Acta Endocrinol. (Kbh)* Suppl. 138, 192.

Hyyppa, M. and Rinne, U. K. (1971). *Acta Endocrinol. (Kbh),* 66, 317.

Hyyppa, M. and Valavaara, M. (1970). *Experientia,* 26, 193.

Hyyppa, M., Lehtinen, P. and Rinne, U. K. (1971). *Brain Res.* 30, 265.

Ichiyama, A., Nakamura, S., Nishizuka, Y. and Hayaishi, O. (1970). *J. Biol. Chem.* 245, 1699.

Imura, H., Kato, Y., Ikeda, M., Morimoto, M., Yawata, M. and Fukase, M. (1968). *J. Clin. Endocrinol.* 28, 1079.

Imura, H., Kato, Y., Ikeda, M., Morimoto, M, and Yawata, M. (1971). *J. Clin. Invest.* 50, 1069.

Iversen, L. L. (1965a). *Brit. J. Pharmacol. Chemother.* 25, 18.

Iversen, L. L. (1965b). *In* "Advances in Drug Research" (Eds N. J. Harper and A. B. Simmonds), vol. 2. Academic Press, London and New York.

Iversen, L. L. (1967). *In* "The Uptake and Storage of Noradrenaline in Sympathetic Nerves". Cambridge University Press, Cambridge.

Iversen, L. L. and Glowinski, J. (1966). *J. Neurochem.* **13**, 671.

Jacob, J., Girault, A. and Peindaries, P. (1972). *Neuropharmacology*, **11**, 1.

Jacobs, L. S., Birge, C. A., Hammer, C. and Daughaday, W. H. (1968). *Clin. Res.* **16**, 441.

Jacobson, A., Salhanick, H. A. and Zarrow, M. X. (1950). *Amer. J. Physiol.* **161**, 522.

Jaitley, K. D., Robson, J. M., Sullivan, F. M. and Wilson, C. (1967). *J. Endocrinol.* **37**, xxxi.

Janowksy, D. S. and Davis, J. M. (1970). *Life Sci.* **9**, 525.

Javoy, F., Agid, Y., Bouvet, D. and Glowinski, J. (1972). *J. Pharmacol. Exp. Ther.* **182**, 454.

Johansson, K. N. G., Currie, B. L., Folkers, K. and Bowers, C. Y. (1973). *Biochim. Biophys. Res. Commun.* **50**, 8.

Jonsson, G., Fuxe, K. and Hokfelt, T. (1972). *Brain Res.* **40**, 271.

Kalra, P. S. and McCann, S. M. (1973a). *Recent Progr. Brain Res.* **39**, 185.

Kalra, P. S. and McCann, S. M. (1973b). *Endocrinology*, **93**, 356.

Kalra, P. S., Krulich, L., Quizada, M., Kalra, S. P., Fawcett, C. P. and McCann, S. M. (1971). *In* "Proc. 3rd Int. Cong. Ster. Horm. 1970" (Eds V. H. T. James and L. Martini), p. 708. Excerpta Medica Foundation, Amsterdam. Int. Cong. Series No. 210.

Kalra, P. S., Kalra, S. P., Krulich, L., Fawcett, C. P. and McCann, S. M. (1972). *Endocrinology*, **90**, 1168.

Kamberi, I. A. (1973). *Recent Progr. Brain Res.* **39**, 261.

Kamberi, I. and Dahof, I. E. (1968). *Fed. Proc.* **27**, 288.

Kamberi, I. and Kobayashi, Y. (1970). *J. Neurochem.* **17**, 261.

Kamberi, I. A. and McCann, S. M. (1969a). *J. Reprod. Fert.* **18**, 153.

Kamberi, I. A. and McCann, S. M. (1969b). *Endocrinology*, **85**, 815.

Kamberi, I. A., Mical, R. S. and Porter, J. C. (1969). *Science*, **166**, 388.

Kamberi, I. A., Mical, R. S. and Porter, J. C. (1970a). *Experientia*, **26**, 1150.

Kamberi, I. A., Mical, R. S. and Porter, J. C. (1970b). *Endocrinology*, **87**, 1.

Kamberi, I. A., Mical, R. S. and Porter, J. C. (1970c). *Nature*, **227**, 714.

Kamberi, I. A., Schneider, H. P. G. and McCann, S. M. (1970d). *Endocrinology*, **86**, 278.

Kamberi, I. A., Mical, R. S. and Porter, J. C. (1971a). *Endocrinology*, **88**, 1288.

Kamberi, I. A., Mical, R. S. and Porter, J. C. (1971b). *Endocrinology*, **89**, 1042.

Kanematsu, S., Scaramuzzi, R. J., Hilliard, J. and Sawyer, C. H. (1972). *Biol. Reprod.* **7**, 110.

Kansal, P. C., Brise, J., Talbert, O. R. and Birse, M. G. (1972). *J. Clin. Endocrinol.* **34**, 99.

Kaplanski, J. and Smelik, P. G. (1973a). *Res. Commun. Chem. Pathol. Pharmacol.* **5**, 263.

Kaplanski, J. and Smelik, P. G. (1973b). *Acta Endocrinol.* (*Kbh*), **73**, 651.

Kaplanski, J., Dorst, W. and Smelik, P. G. (1972). *Eur. J. Pharmacol.* **20**, 238.

Kaplanski, J., Nyakas, C., van Delet, A. M. L. and Smelik, P. (1974). *Neuroendocrinology*. In press.

Karki, N., Kuntzman, R. and Brodie, B. B. (1962). *J. Neurochem.* **9**, 53.

Kato, J. (1973). *Acta Endocrinol.* (*Kbh*), **72**, 663.

Kato, R. (1960). *J. Neurochem.* **5**, 202.

Kato, Y., Dupre, J. and Beck, J. C. (1973). *Endocrinology*, **93**, 135.

Karobath, M., Diaz, J. F. and Huttenen, M. O. (1971). *Eur. J. Pharmacol.* **14**, 393.
Katz, R. I. and Kopin, I. J. (1969). *Biochem. Pharmacol.* **18**, 1935.
Keller, P. J. and Lichtensteiger, W. (1971). *J. Physiol.* **219**, 385.
Kellogg, C. and Lundburg, P. (1972). *Neuropharmacol.* **11**, 363.
Kendell, J. W. (1969). *In* "Frontiers in Neuroendocrinology 1969", p. 177. Oxford University Press, New York and London.
Kinson, G. A. and Lui, C.-C. (1973). *Life Sci.* **12**, 173.
Kitay, J. I., Holub, D. A. and Jailer, J. W. (1959). *Endocrinology*, **65**, 548.
Klaiber, E. L., Kobayashi, Y., Bronerman, D. M. and Hall, F. (1971). *J. Clin. Endocrinol.* **33**, 630.
Knott, P. J., Joseph, M. H. and Curzon, G. (1973). *J. Neurochem.* **20**, 249.
Kobayashi, H. and Matsui, T. (1969). *In* "Frontiers in Neuroendocrinology 1969" (Eds W. F. Ganong and L. Martini), p. 3. Oxford University Press, New York, London and Toronto.
Kobayashi, T., Kobayashi, T., Kato, J. and Minaguchi, H. (1964). *Endocrinol. Jap.* **11**, 283.
Kobayashi, T., Kobayashi, T., Kato, J. and Minaguchi, H. (1965). *Endocrinol. Jap.* **12**, 209.
Kobayashi, T., Kobayashi, T., Kato, J. and Minaguchi, H. (1966). *In* "Steroid Dynamics" (Eds G. Pincus, T. Nakeo and J. Tait), p. 303. Academic Press, New York and London.
Kobayashi, F., Hara, K. and Miyake, T. (1970). *Endocrinol. Jap.* **17**, 149.
Koch, Y., Lu, K. H. and Meites, J. (1970). *Endocrinology*, **87**, 673.
Koe, B. K. and Weissman, A. (1966). *J. Pharmacol. Exp. Ther.* **154**, 499.
Koe, B. K. and Weissman, A. (1968). *Advan. Pharmacol.* **6B**, 29.
Kordon, C. (1969). *Neuroendocrinology*, **4**, 129.
Kordon, C. (1971). *J. Neurovisceral. Rel. Suppl.* **10**, 41.
Kordon, C. and Glowinski, J. (1969). *Endocrinology*, **85**, 924.
Kordon, C. and Glowinski, J. (1970). *In* "Neurochemical Aspects of Hypothalamus Function" (Eds L. Martini and J. Meites), p. 85. Academic Press, New York and London.
Kordon, C. and Glowinski, J. (1972). *Neuropharmacology*, **11**, 153.
Kordon, C. and Vassent, G. (1968). *C.R. Acad. Sci.* **266**, 2473.
Kordon, C., Javoy, F., Vassanj, G. and Glowinski, J. (1968). *Eur. J. Pharmacol.* **4**, 169.
Kordon, C., Gogan, F., Hery, M. and Rotsztejn, W. H. (1971–72). *Horm. Antag. Gynec. Invest.* **2**, 116.
Kotani, M., Onaya, T. and Yamada, T. (1973). *Endocrinology*, **92**, 288.
Kovacs, S. and Faredin, I. (1960). *Acta Neuroveg. Wein.* **22**, 184.
Krieger, H. P. and Krieger, D. T. (1970a). *Amer. J. Physiol.* **218**, 1632.
Krieger, D. T. and Krieger, H. P. (1970b). *Endocrinology*, **87**, 179.
Krieger, D. T. and Rizzo, F. (1969). *Amer. J. Physiol.* **217**, 1703.
Krieger, D. T., Silverberg, A. J., Rizzo, F. and Krieger, H. (1968). *Amer. J. Physiol.* **215**, 959.
Krulich, L., Quijada, M. and Illner, P. (1971). Proc. 53rd Meet. Endocrin. Soc. San Francisco. p. A-83.
Kuhar, M. J., Shaskan, E. G. and Snyder, S. H. (1971). *J. Neurochem.* **18**, 333.
Kurachi, K. and Hirota, K. (1969). *Endocrinol. Jap. Suppl.* **1**, 69.
Kuwajimi, S. (1957). *J. Obstet. Gynaecol. Soc.* **9**, 195.
Labhsetwar, A. P. (1970). *J. Endocrinol.* **47**, 481.
Labhsetwar, A. (1971a). *Nature*, **229**, 203.

Labhsetwar, A. (1971b). *Acta Endocrinol. (Kbh)*, **68**, 334.
Labhsetwar, A. P. (1972a). *Endocrinology*, **90**, 941.
Labhsetwar, A. P. (1972b). *J. Endocrinol*. **54**, 269.
Labhsetwar, A. P. and Zolovick, A. (1973). *Nature (New Biol.)*, **246**, 55.
Ladosky, W. and Gaziri, L. C. J. (1970). *Neuroendocrinology*, **6**, 168.
LaMotte, R. H., Schmidt, D. E. and Ruliffson, W. S. (1969). *J. Neurochem*. **16**, 725.
Laverty, R. and Sharman, D. F. (1965). *Brit. J. Pharmacol*. **24**, 538.
Leavitt, W. W., Bosley, C. G. and Blaha, G. C. (1971). *Nature*, **234**, 283.
Libertun, C. and McCann, S. M. (1972), *Biol. Reprod*. **7**, 110.
Libertun, C. and McCann, S. M. (1973). *Endocrinology*, **92**, 1714.
Libertun, C., Timiras, P. S. and Kragt, C. L. (1973). *Neuroendocrinology*, **12**, 73.
Lichtensteiger, W. (1969). *J. Pharmacol. Exp. Ther*. **165**, 204.
Lichtensteiger, W. (1970). *In* "Neurochemical Aspects of Hypothalamic Function" (Eds L. Martini and J. Meites), p. 101. Academic Press, New York and London.
Lichtensteiger, W. (1971). *J. Physiol*. **218**, 63.
Lichtensteiger, W. and Langemann, H. (1966). *J. Pharmacol. Exp. Ther*. **151**, 400.
Lichtensteiger, W., Mutzner, V. and Langemann, H. (1967). *Neurochem*. **14**, 489.
Lichtensteiger, W., Korpela, K., Langemann, H. and Keller, R. J. (1969). *Brain Res*. **16**, 199.
Lindstrom, L. H. (1971). *Eur. J. Pharmacol*. **15**, 60.
Lindstrom, L. H. (1973). *J. Endocrinol*. **56**, 275.
Lindstrom, L. and Meyerson, B. J. (1966). *Acta Physiol. Scand*. **68**, Suppl. **277**, 121.
Lippa, A. S., Antelman, S. M., Fahringer, E. E. and Redgate, E. S. (1973). *Nature New Biol*. **241**, 24.
Lippmann, W. (1968). *Nature*, **218**, 173.
Lippmann, W., Leonardi, R., Ball, J. and Coppola, J. A. (1967). *J. Pharmacol. Exp. Ther*. **156**, 258.
Longenecker, D. E. and Gallo, D. G. (1971). *Proc. Soc. Expt. Biol. Med*. **137**, 623.
Lu, K.-H. and Meites, J. (1971). *Proc. Soc. Exp. Biol. Med*. **137**, 480.
Lu, K.-H. and Meites, J. (1973). *Endocrinology*, **93**, 152.
Lu, K.-H., Amenomori, Y., Chen, C.-L. and Meites, J. (1970). *Endocrinology*, **87**, 667.
Lupulescu, A., Nicolescu-Catargi, A. and Merculiev, E. (1964). *Acta Neruvegetavia*, **25**, 528.
MacLeod, R. M. (1969). *Endocrinology*, **85**, 916.
Macon, J. B., Sokoloff, L. and Glowinski, J. (1971). *J. Neurochem*. **18**, 323.
Madison, L. (1950). *J. Clin. Invest*. **29**, 789.
Mahesh, V. B. and Goldman, B. D. (1971). *In* "Proc. 3rd Int. Cong. Horm. Ster." (Eds V. H. T. James and L. Martini), p. 662. Excerpta Medica Foundation, Amsterdam. Int. Cong. Series No. 210, 1970.
Malamad, S., Poisner, A. M., Trifaro, J. M. and Douglas, W. W. (1968). *Biochem. Pharmacol*. **17**, 241.
Malmnas, C.-O. (1973). *Acta Physiol. Scand., Suppl*. **395**, 1.
Malmnas, C.-O. and Meyerson, B. J. (1970). *Acta Pharmacol. et Toxicol*. **28**, Suppl. 1, No. 49.
Malmnas, C.-O. and Meyerson, B. J. (1974). In press.
Mandell, A. J. and Morgan, M. (1971). *Nature*, **230**, 85.
Manshardt, J. and Wurtman, R. J. (1968). *Nature*, **217**, 574.
Markee, J. E., Sawyer, C. H. and Hollinshead, W. H. (1947). *Anat. Rec*. **97**, 398.
Markee, J. E., Sawyer, C. H. and Hollinshead, W. H. (1948). *Recent Progr. Horm. Res*. **2**, 117.

Marks, B. H., Hall, M. M. and Bhattacharya, N. (1970). *Progr. Brain Res.* **32**, 57.
Martin, J. B. (1972). *Endocrinology*, **91**, 107.
Martin, J. B., Kontor, J. and Mead, P. (1973). *Endocrinology*, **92**, 1354.
Martini, L. (1973). *J. Endocrinol.* **58**, xxxiii.
Martini, L., Fraschini, F. and Motta, M. (1968). *Recent Progr. Horm. Res.* **24**, 439.
Massara, F. and Camanni, F. (1972). *J. Endocrinol.* **54**, 195.
Matsuo, H., Baba, Y., Nair, R. M. and Schally, A. V. (1971). *Biochem. Biophys. Res. Commun.* **43**, 1334.
McCann, S. M. (1962). *Amer. J. Physiol.* **202**, 601.
McCann, S. M. (1963). *Amer. J. Med.* **34**, 379.
McCann, S. M. and Friedman, H. M. (1960). *Endocrinology*, **67**, 597.
McCann, S. M., Taleisnik, S. and Friedman, H. M. (1960). *Proc. Soc. Exp. Biol. Med.* **104**, 432.
McCann, S. M., Kalra, P. S., Donoso, A. O., Bishop, W., Schneider, H. P. G., Fawcett, C. P. and Krulich, L. (1972). *In* "Brain-Endocrine Interaction. Median Eminence, Structure and Function". International Symposium Munich, 1971. p. 224. Karger, Basel.
McDonald, P. G. and Gilmore, D. P. (1971). *J. Endocrinol.* **49**, 421.
McEwan, B. (1973). *In* "Serotonin and Behavior" (Eds J. Barchas and E. Usdin) in discussion following chapter by Lovenburg, W. *et al.*, p. 49. Academic Press, New York and London.
McGeer, E. G., Gibson, S., Wada, J. A. and McGeer, P. L. (1967). *Can. J. Biochem.* **45**, 1943.
McKinney, W. T., Prange, A. J., Majchowicz, E. and Schlesinger, K. (1971). *Dis. Nerv. Syst.* **32**, 308.
Meites, J. (1959). *Proc. Soc. Exp. Biol. Med.* **100**, 750.
Meites, J., Nicoll, C. S. and Talwalker, P. K. (1959). *Proc. Soc. Exp. Biol. Med.* **101**, 563.
Meites, J., Talwalker, P. K. and Nicoll, C. S. (1960). *Proc. Soc. Exp. Biol. Med.* **104**, 192.
Meites, J., Nicoll, C. S. and Talwalker, P. K. (1961). *Symp. Neuroendocrinol. Miami Flo.*
Meites, J., Lu, K.-H., Wuttke, W., Welsch, C. W., Nagasawa, H. and Quadri, S. K. (1972). *Recent Progr. Horm. Res.* **28**, 471.
Mendelsohn, F. A. and Warren, R. L. (1974). *J. Endocrin.* In press.
Mess, B., Tima, L. and Trentini, G. P. (1973). *Recent. Progr. Brain Res.* **39**, 251.
Meyer, V. and Knobil, E. (1967). *Endocrinology*, **80**, 163.
Meyerson, B. J. (1964). *Acta Physiol. Scand.* **63**, Suppl. 241.
Meyerson, B. J. (1972). *Psychopharmacologia Suppl.* **26**, 132.
Meyerson, B. J. and Lewander, T. (1970). *Life Sci.* **9**, 661.
Meyerson, B. J. and Palis, A. (1970). *Acta Pharm. et Tox.* **28**, Suppl. **1**, 68.
Meyerson, B. and Sawyer, C. H. (1968). *Endocrinology*, **83**, 170.
Mishkinsky, J., Khazen, K. and Sulman, F. G. (1968). *Endocrinology*, **82**, 611.
Mittler, J. C. and Meites, J. (1967). *Proc. Soc. Exp. Biol. Med.* **124**, 310.
Miyachi, Y., Mecklenburg, R. S. and Lipsett, M. B. (1973). *Endocrinology*, **93**, 492.
Miyake, T. (1968). *In* "Integrative Mechanisms of Neuroendocrine Systems" (Ed. S. Ioh), p. 139. Hokkaido University, Sapporo.
Moir, A. T. B. and Eccleston, D. (1968). *J. Neurochem.* **15**, 1093.
Moore, W. W. (1959). *The Physiologist*, **2**, 83.
Moore, W. W. (1961). *Amer. J. Physiol.* **200**, 1293.

Moszkowska, A. (1964). *Ann. Endocr.* (*Paris*), Suppl. **25**, 79.

Motta, M., Simonovic, I., Zanisi, M. and Martini, L. (1972). *Hormones*, **3**, 257.

Moussatche, H. and Perreira, N. A. (1957). *Acta Physiol. Lat. Amer.* **7**, 71.

Muller, E. E. (1970). *In* "Aspects of Neuroendocrinology" (Eds W. Bargmann and B. Scharrer), p. 206. Springer-Verlag, Berlin.

Muller, E. E., Sawano, S., Arimura, A. and Schally, A. (1967). *Endocrinology*, **80**, 471.

Muller, E. E., Pra, P. D. and Pecile, A. (1968). *Endocrinology*, **83**, 893.

Muller, E. E., Pecile, A., Felici, M. and Cocchi, D. (1970). *Endocrinology*, **86**, 1376.

Muller, E. E., Cocchi, D. and Fraschini, F. (1972a). *Biol. Reprod.* **7**, 111.

Muller, E. E., Cocchi, D., Villa, A., Zambotti, F. and Fraschini, F. (1972b). *Endocrinology*, **90**, 1267.

Nachmais, V. T. (1960–61). *J. Neurochem.* **6**, 99.

Naftolin, F., Brown-Grant, K. and Corker, C. S. (1972). *J. Endocrinol.* **53**, 17.

Nakai, Y., Imura, H., Yoshimi, T. and Matsukura, S. (1973). *Acta Endocrinol.* (*Kbh*), **74**, 263.

Naumenko, E. V. (1968). *Brain Res.* **11**, 1.

Naumenko, E. V. (1969). *Neuroendocrinology*, **5**, 81.

Neill, J. D., Freeman, M. E. and Tillson, S. A. (1971). *Endocrinology*, **89**, 1448.

Ng, L. K. J., Chase, T. N., Colburn, R. W. and Kopin, I. J. (1972). *Brain Res.* **45**, 499.

Nicoll, C. S. and Meites, J. (1962). *Endocrinology*, **70**, 272.

Nicoll, C. S., Talwalker, P. K. and Meites, J. (1960). *Amer. J. Physiol.* **198**, 1103.

Nicoll, C. S., Fiorindo, R. P., McKenee, C. T. and Parsons, J. A. (1970). *In* "Hypophysiotropic Hormones of the Hypothalamus" (Ed J. Meites), p. 115. Williams and Wilkins, Baltimore, Maryland.

Nikitovitch-Winer, M. and Everett, J. W. (1958). *Endocrinology*, **62**, 522.

Odell, W. D. and Swerdloff, R. S. (1968). *Proc. Nat. Acad. Sci. U.S.* **61**, 529.

Ojeda, S. R. and McCann, S. M. (1973). *Neuroendocrinology*, **12**, 295.

Okado, F. (1971). *Life Sci.* **10**, 77.

Olson, L., Fuxe, K. and Hokfelt, T. (1972). *Acta Endocrinol.* (*Kbh*), **71**, 233.

O'Steen, W. K. (1964). *Endocrinology*, **74**, 885.

O'Steen, W. K. (1965). *Endocrinology*, **77**, 937.

Parent, A., Saint-Jacques, C. and Poirier, L. S. (1969). *Exp. Neurol.* **23**, 67.

Parlow, A. F. (1961). *In* "Human Pituitary Gonadotrophins" (Ed. A. Albert). Charles C. Thomas, Springfield, Illinois.

Parlow, A. F. (1964). Discussion after Guillemin, R. (1964). *Recent Progr. Horm. Res.* **20**, 89.

Perez-Cruent, J., Tagliomonte, A., Tagliomonte, P. and Gessa, G. L. (1971). *Riv. Farm. Ter.* **11**, 27.

Piacsek, B. E. and Meites, J. (1967). *Endocrinology*, **81**, 535.

Piacsek, B. E., Schneider, T. C. and Gay, U. L. (1971). *Endocrinology*, **89**, 39.

Piezzi, R. S., Larin, F. and Wurtman, R. J. (1970). *Endocrinology*, **86**, 1460.

Pletscher, A., Shore, P. A. and Brodie, B. B. (1956). *J. Pharm. Exp. Ther.* **116**, 84.

Pohorecky, L. A., Zigmund, M., Karten, H. and Wurtman, R. J. (1969). *J. Pharm. Exp. Ther.* **165**, 190.

Popova, N. K., Maslova, L. N. and Naumenko, E. V. (1972). *Brain Res.* **47**, 61.

Porter, J. C., Kamberi, I. A. and Ondo, J. C. (1972a). *In* "Brain-Endocrine Interaction. Median Eminence Structure and Function". International Symposium, Munich, 1971, p. 245. Karger, Basel.

Porter, J. C., Mical, R. S. and Cramer, O. M. (1972b). *Horm. Antag. Gynaecol. Invest.* **2**, 13.
Quay, W. B. (1963). *Gen. Comp. Endocrinol.* **3**, 473.
Quay, W. B. (1968). *Amer. J. Physiol.* **215**, 1448.
Quijada, M., Illner, P., Krulich, L. and McCann, S. M. (1974). *Neuroendocrinology*, **13**, 151.
Quinn, D. L. and Zarrow, M. X. (1964). *Endocrinology*, **74**, 309.
Ramirez, V. D. and McCann, S. M. (1963). *Endocrinology*, **73**, 193.
Ratner, A. and McCann, S. M. (1971). *Proc. Soc. Exp. Biol. Med.* **138**, 763.
Ratner, A. and Meites, J. (1964). *Endocrinology*, **75**, 377.
Ratner, A., Talwalker, P. K. and Meites, J. (1965). *Endocrinology*, **77**, 315.
Raziano, J., Cowchock, S., Ferin, M. and Van de Wiele (1971). *Endocrinology*, **88**, 1516.
Recant, L., Hume, D. M., Forsham, P. H. and Thorn, G. W. (1950). *J. Clin. Endocrinol.* **10**, 187.
Reichlin, S., Martin, J. B., Mitnick, M., Boshans, R. L., Grimm, Y., Bollinger, J., Gordon, J. and Malacara, J. (1972). *Recent Progr. Horm. Res.* **28**, 229.
Reis, D. J., Weinbren, M. and Corvelli, A. (1968). *J. Pharm. Exp. Ther.* **164**, 135.
Relkin, R. (1972a). *J. Endocrinol.* **53**, 179.
Relkin, R. (1972b). *Neuroendocrinology*, **9**, 278.
Rinne, U. K. and Sonninen, V. (1967). *Acta Neurol. Scand.* **43**, Suppl. **31**, 209.
Rinne, U. K. and Sonninen, V. (1968). *Experientia*, **24**, 177.
Robinson, J. D., Anderson, J. H. and Green, J. P. (1965). *J. Pharmacol. Exp. Ther.* **147**, 236.
Robson, J. M. (1931). *Proc. Roy. Soc. Edinburgh*, **LII**, 434.
Robson, J. M. and Botros, M. (1961). *J. Endocrinol.* **22**, 165.
Rønneklein, O. K., Krulick, L. and McCann, S. M. (1973). *Endocrinology*, **92**, 1339.
Ross, G. T., Cargille, C. M., Lipsett, M. B., Rayford, P. L., Marshall, J. R., Strott, C. A. and Rodbard, D. (1970). *Recent Progr. Horm. Res.* **26**, 1.
Ross, J., Claybaugh, C., Clemens, L. G. and Gorski, R. A. (1971). *Endocrinology*, **89**, 32.
Rubinstein, L. and Sawyer, C. H. (1970). *Endocrinology*, **86**, 988.
Saavedra, J. M., Palkovits, M., Brownstein, M. J. and Axelrod, J. (1974). *Nature (London)*, **248**, 695.
Sala, M. A., Otegui, J. T., Benedetti, W. L., Monti, J. M. and Grino, E. (1971). *J. Neurovisceral Rel.* **32**, 241.
Salseduc, M., Jofre, I. J. and Izquirerdo, J. A. (1966). *Med. Pharmacol.* **14**, 113.
Samojlick, E. (1965). *Endokrynologia Polska*, **16**, 617.
Sandler, R. (1968). *Endocrinology*, **83**, 1383.
Sawyer, C. H. and Hilliard, J. (1971). Proc. 3rd Int. Cong. Horm. Ster. (Eds V. H. T. James and L. Martini), p. 716. Excerpta Medica Foundation, Amsterdam. Int. Cong. Series No. 210, 1970.
Sawyer, C. H., Markee, J. E. and Hollinshead, W. H. (1947). *Anat. Rec.* **99**, 597.
Sawyer, C. H., Everett, J. W. and Markee, J. E. (1949a). *Endocrinology*, **44**, 218.
Sawyer, C. H., Markee, J. E. and Everett, J. W. (1949b). *Proc. Soc. Exp. Biol. Med.* **71**, 670
Sawyer, C. H., Markee, J. E. and Everett, J. W. (1950a). *J. Exp. Zool.* **113**, 659.
Sawyer, C. H., Markee, J. E. and Everett, J. W. (1950b). *Endocrinology*, **46**, 536.

Scapagnini, V. and Preziosi, P. (1972). *Arch. Int. Pharmacodyn. Ther.* **196**, (Suppl.), 205.

Scapagnini, V. and Preziosi, P. (1973). *Recent Progr. Brain Res.* **39**, 171.

Scapagnini, V., Van Loon, G. R., Moberg, G. P. and Ganong, W. F. (1970). *Europ. J. Pharmacol.* **11**, 266.

Scapagnini, V., Moberg, G. P., Van Loon, C. R., de Groot, J. and Ganong, W. F. (1971). *Neuroendocrinology*, **7**, 90.

Schally, A. V., Kastin, A. J., Locke, W. and Bower, C. Y. (1967). *In* "Hormones in the Blood" (Eds C. H. Gray and H. L. Bacharach), p. 492. Academic Press, New York and London.

Schanberg, S. M. (1963). *J. Pharmacol. Exp. Ther.* **139**, 191.

Schechter, J. and Weiner, R. (1972). *Anat. Rec.* **172**, 643.

Scheving, L. E., Harrison, W. H., Gordon, P. and Pauly, J. E. (1968). *Amer. J. Physiol.* **214**, 166.

Schiaffino, O., Motta, M., Piva, F. and Martini, L. (1971). *In* "Proc. 3rd Int. Cong. Horm. Ster." (Eds V. H. T. James and L. Martini), p. 822. Excerpta Medica Foundation, Amsterdam. Int. Cong. Series, No. 210, 1970.

Schiebler, T. A. and Meinhardt, P. W. (1971). *J. Neurovisceral Rel. Suppl.* **X**, 384.

Schnaitman, C., Erwin, V. G. and Greenawalt, J. W. (1967). *J. Cell. Biol.* **32**, 719.

Schneider, H. P. G. and McCann, S. M. (1969a). *Endocrinology*, **85**, 121.

Schneider, H. P. G. and McCann, S. M. (1969b). *J. Reprod. Fert.* **18**, 178.

Schneider, H. P. G. and McCann, S. M. (1970a). *Endocrinology*, **87**, 330.

Schneider, H. P. G. and McCann, S. M. (1970b). *J. Endocrinol.* **46**, 401.

Schneider, H. P. G. and McCann, S. M. (1970c). *Endocrinology*, **87**, 249.

Schneider, H. P. G. and McCann, S. M. (1970d). *Endocrinology*, **86**, 1127.

Schwartz, N. B. (1964). *Amer. J. Physiol.* **207**, 1251.

Schwartz, N. B. (1969). *Recent Advan. Horm. Res.* **21**, 1.

Shaikh, A. A. (1971). *Biol. Reprod.* **5**, 297.

Shaskan, E. G. and Snyder, S. H. (1970). *J. Pharmacol. Exp. Ther.* **175**, 404.

Sheard, M. H. and Aghajanian, G. K. (1968). *J. Pharmacol. Exp. Ther.* **163**, 425.

Shillito, E. E. (1971). *Brit. J. Pharmacol.* **41**, 404P.

Shute, C. C. D. and Lewis, P. R. (1966). *Brit. Med. Bull.* **22**, 221.

Singer, J. J. (1972). *Psychological Reports*, **30**, 891.

Snyder, S. H., Kuhar, M. J., Green, A. J., Coyle, J. T. and Shaskan, E. G. (1970). *Int. Rev. Neurobiol.* **13**, 127.

Smelik, P. G. (1966). *Acta Physiol. Pharm. Neerl.* **14**, 92.

Smelik, P. G. (1969). *Acta Physiol. Pharm. Neerl.* **15**, 123.

Smith, E. R. and Davidson, J. M. (1967). *Fed. Proc.* **26**, 366.

Smith, E. R. and Davidson, J. M. (1968). *Endocrinology*, **82**, 100.

Smith, G. C. and Fink, G. (1972). *Brain Res.* **43**, 37.

Smythe, G. A. and Lazarus, L. (1973). *Endocrinology*, **93**, 147.

Soderberg, U. (1958). *Acta Physiol. Scand.* **42**, Suppl. **147**, 5.

Sodersten, P. and Ahlenius, S. (1972). *Horm. Behavior*, **3**, 181.

Soffer, L. J., Volterra, M., Gabrilove, J. L., Pollack, A. and Jacobs, M. (1947). *Proc. Soc. Exp. Med. Biol.* **64**, 446.

Soulairac, A. and Soulairac, M.-L. (1971). *C.R. Acad. Sci. Seanc.* **165**, 253.

Souvatzoglou, A., von Werder, K. and Bottermann, P. (1973). *Acta Endocrinol. (Kbh)*, **73**, 259.

Spector, S., Gordon, R., Sjoerdsma, A. and Udenfriend, S. (1967). *Mol. Pharmacol.* **3**, 549.

Stefano, F. J. E. and Donoso, A. O. (1967). *Endocrinology*, **81**, 1405.

Stefano, F. J. E., Donoso, A. O. and Cukier, J. (1965). *Acta Physiol. Lat. Amer.* **15**, 425.

Steiner, F. A., Pieri, L. and Kaufman, L. (1968). *Experientia*, **24**, 1133.

Steiner, F. A., Ruf, K. and Akert, K. (1969). *Brain Res.* **12**, 74.

Stumpf, W. E. (1968). *Science*, **162**, 1001.

Suzuki, T., Hirai, K., Yoshio, H., Kuroiyi, K.-I. and Hirose, T. (1964). *J. Endocrinol.* **31**, 81.

Swelheim, T. (1964). *Kon. Akad. Wetenschappen Amsterdam*, **67c**, 366.

Swingle, W. W., Seay, P., Perlmutt, J., Collins, E. J., Barlow, G. and Fedor, E. J. (1951a). *Amer. J. Physiol.* **167**, 586.

Swingle, W. W., Fedor. E. J., Barlow, G., Collins, E. J. and Perlmutt, J. (1951b). *Amer. J. Physiol.* **167**, 593.

Tagliomonte, A. (1972). *Psychopharmacologia Suppl.* **26**, 131.

Tagliomonte, A., Tagliomonte, P. and Gessa, G. L. (1971a). *Nature*, **230**, 244.

Tagliomonte, A., Tagliomonte, P., Forn, J., Perez-Cruent, J., Krishna, G. and Gessa, G. L. (1971b). *J. Neurochem.* **18**, 1191.

Takahashi, M., Homma, K. and Suzuki, Y. (1973). *Endocrinol. Jap.* **20**, 271.

Taleisnik, S., Velasco, M. E. and Astrada, J. J. (1970). *J. Endocrinol.* **46**, 1.

Taleisnik, S., Caligaris, L. and Astrada, J. J. (1971). *In* "Proc. 3rd Int. Cong. Horm. Steroids 1970" (Eds V. H. T. James and L. Martini), p. 699. Excerpta Medica Foundation, Amsterdam. Int. Cong. Series, No. 210, 1970.

Talwalker, P. K., Ratner, A. and Meites, J. (1963). *Amer. J. Physiol.* **205**, 213.

Tejasen, T. and Everett, J. W. (1967). *Endocrinology*, **81**, 1387.

Thornburg, J. E. and Moore, K. E. (1971). *Arch. Int. Pharmacodyn.* **194**, 158.

Tima, L., Trentini, G. P. and Mess, B. (1973). *Neuroendocrinology*, **12**, 149.

Toivola, P. T. K. and Gale, C. C. (1972). *Endocrinology*, **90**, 895.

Tonge, S. R. and Greengrass, P. M. (1971). *Psychopharmacologica*, **21**, 374.

Twarog, B. M. and Page, I. H. (1953). *Amer. J. Physiol.* **175**, 157.

Uemura, H. and Kobayashi, H. (1971). *Endocrinol. Jap.* **18**, 91.

Ulrich, R. S. and Yuwiler, A. (1973). *Endocrinology*, **92**, 611.

Ungerstedt, U. (1971). *Acta Physiol. Scand. Suppl.* **367**, 1.

Van Delft, A. M. L., Kaplanski, J. and Smelik, P. G. (1973). *J. Endocrinol.* **59**, 465.

Van Loon, G. (1973). *In* "Frontiers in Neuroendocrinology 1973" (Eds L. Martini and W. F. Ganong), p. 209. Oxford University Press, London.

Van Loon, G. R. and Ganong, W. F. (1969). *The Physiologist*, **12**, 381.

Van Loon, G. R. and Kragt, C. L. (1970). *Proc. Soc. Exp. Biol. Med.* **133**, 1137.

Van Loon, G. R., Scapagnini, U., Cohen, R. and Ganong, W. F. (1971). *Neuroendocrinology*, **8**, 257.

Van Maanen, J. H. and Smelik, P. G. (1968). *Neuroendocrinology*, **3**. 177.

VandeWeile, R. L., Bogumil, J., Dyrenforth, I., Ferin, M., Jewelewicz, R., Warren, M., Rizkalcah, T. and Mikhail, G. (1970). *Recent Progr. Horm. Res.* **26**, 63.

Vaughan, M. K., Vaughan, G. M. and O'Steen, W. K. (1969). *J. Endocrinol.* **45**, 141.

Vaughan, M. K., Benson, B. and Norris, J. T. (1970). *J. Endocrinol.* **47**, 397.

Verdesca, A. S., Westermann, C. D., Crampton, R. S., Black, W. C., Nedeljkovic, R. I. and Hilton, J. G. (1961). *Amer. J. Physiol.* **201**, 1065.

Vernikos-Danellis, J., Berger, P. and Barchas, J. D. (1973). *Recent Progr. Brain Res.* **39**, 302.

Versteeg, D. H. G. (1973). *Brain Res.* **49**, 483.
Vogel, S. A., Janowsky, D. S. and Davis, J. M. (1970). *Res. Commun. Chem. Pathol. and Pharmacol.* **1**, 451.
Vogt, M. (1954). *J. Physiol.* **123**, 451.
Vogt, M. (1969). *Brit. J. Pharmacol. Chemother.* **37**, 325.
Vogt, M. (1973). *Brit. Med. Bull.* **29**, 168.
Voogt, J. L. and Meites, J. (1971). *Endocrinology*, **88**, 286.
Walker, C. A. and Friedman, A. H. (1969). *Fed. Proc.* **28**, 444, No. 1050.
Weiner, R. I. (1973). *Recent Progr. Brain Res.* **39**, 165.
Weiner, N. and Rabadjija, M. (1968). *J. Pharmacol. Exp. Ther.* **164**, 103.
Weiner, R. I., Kragt, C. L. and Ganong, W. F. (1969). Proc. of 51st Meeting of Soc. Endocrin. No. 101.
Weiner, R. I., Blake, C. A., Rubinstein, L. and Sawyer, C. H. (1971). *Science*, **171**, 411.
Weiner, R. I., Shryne, J. E., Gorski, R. A. and Sawyer, C. H. (1972a). *Endocrinology*, **90**, 867.
Weiner, R. I., Gorski, R. A. and Sawyer, C. H. (1972b). *In* "Brain-Endocrine Interaction. Median Eminence Structure and Function". International Symposium Munich, 1971, p. 236. Karger, Basel.
Weissman, A. (1973). *In* "Serotonin and Behavior" (Eds J. Barchas and E. Usdin), p. 235. Academic Press, New York and London.
Werrbach, J. H., Gale, C. H., Goodner, C. J. and Conway, M. J. (1970). *Endocrinology*, **86**, 77.
Westman, A. and Jacobsohn, D. (1938). *Acta Pathol. Microbiol. Scand.* **15**, 445.
Whalen, R. E. and Luttge, W. G. (1970). *Science*, **169**, 1000.
Wheaton, J. E., Martin, S. K., Swanson, L. L. and Stormshak, F. (1972). *J. Animal Sci.* **35**, 801.
Wilson, C. (1974). Unpublished results.
Wilson, C. and McDonald, P. G. (1973). *Acta Endocrinol. Suppl.* **177**, 138.
Wilson, C. and McDonald, P. G. (1974). *J. Endocrinol.* **60**, 253.
Wilson, C., Endersby, C. and McDonald, P. G. (1974a). *J. Endocrinol.* **61**, xxv.
Wilson, C., Horth, C. E., Endersby, C. A. and McDonald, P. G. (1974b). *J. Endocrinol.* **60**, 293.
Wurtman, R. J., Axelrod, J. and Kelly, D. (1968). *In* "The Pineal Gland". Academic Press, New York and London.
Ying, S.-Y. and Greep, R. O. (1973). *Endocrinology*, **92**, 333.
Zarate, A., Canales, E. S., Jacobs, L. S., Maneiro, P. J., Soria, J. and Daughaday, W. H. (1973). *Fert. Steril.* **24**, 340.
Zemplan, E. P., Ward, I. L., Crowley, W. R. and Margules, D. L. (1973). *Science*, **179**, 1010.
Zigmond, M. J. and Wurtman, R. J. (1970). *J. Pharmacol. Exp. Ther.* **172**, 416.
Zigmond, M. J., Chon, C. and Wurtman, R. J. (1969). Proc. 51st meeting of Soc. Endocrin. No. 105.
Zitrin, A., Beach, F. A., Barchas, J. D. and Dement, W. C. (1970). *Science*, **170**, 868.
Zolovick, A. J. (1972). *J. Endocrinol.* **52**, 201.
Zolovick, A. J. and Labhsetwar, A. P. (1973). *Nature*, **245**, 158.
Zolovick, A. J., Pearse, R., Boehike, K. W. and Elefteriou, B. E. (1966). *Science*, **154**, 649.
Zschaeck, L. L. and Wurtman, R. J. (1973). *Neuroendocrinology*, **11**, 144.

Gastric Antisecretory and Antiulcer Agents

PAUL BASS, PhD

School of Pharmacy, University of Wisconsin, 425 North Charter Street, Madison, Wisconsin 53706 USA

1   Introduction

A conference on digestive diseases held in 1967 summarized the serious-
ness and incidence of illnesses affecting the gastrointestinal tract (National
Liaison Committee, 1967). Digestive diseases include disorders of the
esophagus, stomach, intestines, biliary passages, liver and pancreas. The
causes are numerous: infection, cancer, alcoholism, genetic defects and
reactions to life stress. In the United States, one-half of the population
has digestive complaints. Digestive diseases are the leading cause for
hospitalization and for inability to work because of illnesses.

In this organ system, peptic ulcers are the most common structural
disorders of the human gastrointestinal tract. They are circumscribed
defects through the epithelium of the organ, that is, through the muscularis mucosa. In contrast, erosions go down to but not through the
muscularis mucosa. The distinction is important because the latter
lesion tends to be superficial and temporary while the ulcer can be
permanent. An ulcer is localized and named according to the area of insult.
Thus peptic ulcers in the upper small bowel are referred to as duodenal
ulcers. Those in the stomach between the cardia and gastroduodenal
junction are called gastric ulcers. Peptic ulcers can also occur in the
esophagus.

Peptic ulcers affect approximately ten million Americans. They are
most common in men between the age of twenty and sixty. Among the

broad category of peptic ulcer diseases, duodenal ulcers are the most common. The etiology of peptic ulcers is unknown. Inheritance, emotion and environment appear to play major roles. Their formation requires the gastric secretion of acid and pepsin which are normally controlled by neurohormonal interactions. In some patients, e.g. those with duodenal ulcer, excessive acid and pepsin may be produced. These secretions are normally controlled by neurohormonal interactions. Patients with gastric ulcers do not necessarily produce excessive quantities of acid. Fragmentary evidence suggests that these people have a reduced capacity to resist the erosive action of gastric juice. A review on the etiology of gastric ulcer is available (Rhodes, 1972).

The physiological mechanisms affecting acid and pepsin secretion are under extensive investigation. The classical three phases of gastric secretion—cephalic, gastric and intestinal—are mutually interdependent and may work simultaneously. The cephalic or nervous phase is presumably more important in man than in animals since man has the ability to worry and possess anxiety about the future. The central phase is mediated both hormonally as well as directly through nervous channels. Animal models have been developed that respond to stress by developing ulcers. The production and properties of experimentally induced gastric lesions in animals have been reviewed (Brodie, 1968; Ader, 1971). The rat model has been extensively studied. The widely publicized "executive" monkey, confined to a chair and presented with making decisions developed ulcers. This is in contrast to a passive partner who showed no gastrointestinal lesion. Though this latter work has not been duplicated, it leads to interesting speculation. In any event, stress ulcers are common occurrences. They may be associated with CNS lesions (called Cushing's ulcer), ulcers associated with extensive body burns (called Curling's ulcer), and acute situations like myocardial infarction, a broken limb, or an operation remote from the abdomen. Thus "stress" can play a role in gastrointestinal lesions (Brady et al., 1958; Porter et al., 1958; Brady, 1964).

The gastric phase is initiated by several factors. The hormone gastrin, one of the most potent stimulants of acid known, is chemically released by the presence of secretagogues (from food) in the stomach. Gastrin can be released by mechanical distention of the lower third of the stomach (the antrum). The gastric phase has a built-in governor. Release of acid can reduce gastrin release. When the antrum and duodenum reach a pH of approximately 2, the output of gastrin is reduced. A rise of antral pH causes a release of gastrin. This delicate control of gastrin release does raise questions on the value of antacids in "turning off" the acid production in the stomach. The importance of histamine and gastrin in the gastric phase is much debated. The enzyme histidine decarboxylase is responsible for the formation of histamine in the mucosa. The enzyme levels increase whenever histamine stores are released. In rats, decreased histamine formation by either pyridoxine deficiency or histidine decarboxylase inhibition reduces the response to gastrin. Thus the complex hormonal–neuronal control of the gastric phase awaits further elucidation.

The intestinal phase of secretion is probably the least studied and least understood. Teleologically, the intestinal phase of gastric secretion should be mainly inhibitory and autoregulatory. This phase should protect the duodenum against the onrush of acid. In general, acid in the duodenum does inhibit gastric secretion. Again this is a complex mechanism that can be exerting its influence either through the vagus or through hormonal control. These factors can involve secretin, serotonin or some other enterogastrone. The pancreatic and biliary secretions may play a role in "neutralizing" duodenal contents. Nicotine administered to dogs can inhibit secretin-stimulated fluids and bicarbonate. The drug does not alter gastric acid secretion, gastric mucosal blood flow or the mucosal barrier to hydrogen or sodium ion diffusion (Konturek et al., 1971). Could this decrease in duodenal alkaline secretion lead to higher incidence of duodenal ulcers in people that smoke (Monson, 1970)? The role of duodenal alkalization in ulcer formation has not received extensive study.

The gastrointestinal tract consists of smooth muscle that demonstrates a remarkable degree of coordinated function. The stomach-duodenal area has an extensive interaction that controls the emptying properties of the stomach. Stomach emptying has been reviewed (Hunt and Knox, 1968). The integrative parameters of the muscle of the two organs have been studied by Weisbrodt et al. (1969) and McCoy and Bass (1963). These two organs function in a manner that favors passage of material in an aboral direction. However, in patients with gastric ulcers, bile is found in the stomach (Rhodes et al., 1969; Rhodes, 1972). Gastrin II and pentagastrin delay stomach emptying in man (Hunt and Ramsbottom, 1967) and in dog (Dozois and Kelly, 1971) respectively. The hormone also favors regurgitation of bile into the stomach of dog (Isaza et al., 1971). Whether a similar mechanism functions in the gastric ulcer patient awaits confirmation. The motor parameters of the antral duodenal area in a gastric ulcer patient have not been studied.

Bile in the stomach can cause transmucosal hydrogen ion flux which leads to damage of the mucosal barrier (Davenport, 1968). Whether motor abnormality and bile reflux are primary or secondary causes of gastric ulcers is unknown. Again, the motor properties of the antral-duodenal area in the diseased state are minimally understood.

The unknown etiology of peptic ulcer diseases and the fragmentary knowledge of the control of acid and pepsin production do not readily lend themselves to a rational approach to the development of therapeutic agents. Indeed, the search for effective agents for treatment of diseases related to gastric secretion has been long and controversial. Even the two established therapeutic classes, antacids and anticholinergics, are useful only for the relief of acute pain. They have not been shown to alter the progress or the frequency of exacerbation of the peptic disease (Piper and Heap, 1972). Agents affecting gastric secretion have been reviewed. The earlier literature is summarized in a review article (Code, 1951). More recent reviews are available (Brodie, 1970; Butler et al., 1970; Pfeiffer, 1971). The newer experimental agents proposed for treatment of peptic ulcer are reviewed periodically in the Annual Reports in Medicinal Chemistry (Hess, 1969; Evers and Ridley, 1971). Recent discussions of the clinical aspects of treatment of duodenal ulcers (Langman, 1968a; Kettering, 1971; Piper and Heap, 1972) or gastric ulcers (Cameron, 1971) are also available.

2 Experimental methods of evaluating antiulcer drugs

The experimental animal models used in pharmacological studies of potential antiulcer drugs usually involve several preparations in several species. The rat and dog remain the two most popular animals for this work. Some antisecretory drug studies have been done on the cat, pig and monkey. We have not had enough experience to know which animal model best characterizes the clinical conditions of gastric or duodenal ulcers; or indeed, whether the drugs that cause a decrease in secretory volume or acid concentration in animals will be beneficial in ulcer therapy in man. Thus, most drugs are evaluated in several models and several species of animals. The list below contains examples of experimental models employed in pharmacological studies of potential antiulcer agents. These are frequently modified by individual investigators. Reviews of methods of studying gastric secretion or experimental ulcers are available (Emås et al., 1967; Rudick et al., 1967; Pfeiffer, 1971).

2.1 PYLORIC LIGATED RAT (SHAY RAT)

This preparation is frequently used for the initial evaluation of antisecretory properties of drugs (Shay et al., 1945; Ishii, 1969). There is no indication that this model is capable of characterizing a drug that would have clinical usefulness. The rat stomach secretes gastric juice continuously at a constant rate. If a 2–6-hour ligation period is used, the effects of a test compound on the volume of gastric juice, acid and pepsin concentration and output can be measured. Ligation periods of 16–20 hours result in the development of lesions in the forestomach. This latter test has been used to evaluate a compound for its ability to reduce the incidence and severity of these lesions. Dose–response curves can be obtained with this animal preparation.

2.2 ACUTE OR CHRONIC GASTRIC FISTULA ANIMALS

Almost all experimental animal species and even man have been studied by gastric fistula. Dr Beaumont's classical study on Alexis St Martin was done through a gastric fistula created by a gunshot accident (Beaumont, 1833, republished, 1959). Currently, various models are used mainly to measure the antisecretory action of a test compound on gastric secretion induced by pharmacological doses of secretagogues, e.g. histamine, gastrin or insulin (Ghosh and Schild, 1958; Lai, 1964; Lee and Thompson, 1969). An elegant technique, which permits perfusion of the stomach through two cannulae in a chronic unanesthetized rat, should permit sensitive assay of antisecretory drugs (Borella and Herr, 1971). This method also permits the cephalic phase (visual and olfactory stimulation of food) to be studied in the rat. The gastric secretion parameters have also been characterized in the chronic fistula ferret (Pfeiffer and Peters, 1969; Basso et al., 1971). This species is a basal secretor, sensitive to histamine (like man, but unlike the rat) and possesses a gastric and intestinal morphology similar to man but unlike the rodent.

These preparations have several advantages: (i) the alimentary canal is minimally altered; (ii) all nerve innervations are intact; (iii) easy to construct and maintain; and (iv) can be used in studies in which stomach acid can be drained or permitted to enter the duodenum. The model does not permit study of secretion during a meal since this would plug the cannula. For this reason, Pavlov developed the pouch preparation that bears his name.

2.3 CHRONIC INNERVATED AND DENERVATED GASTRIC POUCH ANIMALS

Gastric pouch preparations permit the collection of gastric juice that is uncontaminated by saliva, duodenal reflux or food. Food may be added to the list of secretagogues administered to the animal (Markowitz et al., 1959; Rudick et al., 1967; Emås et al., 1967). These models have also been adapted to study the action of test compounds on endogenous secretagogues. The response following secretagogue alone is compared to that following secretagogue with test compound.

2.4   INDUCED ULCER PREPARATIONS

Gastric lesions of the glandular tissue of rodents may be induced by stress (Lambling *et al.*, 1953; Hanson and Brodie, 1960; Takagi and Okabe, 1968), chemicals (Bonfils *et al.*, 1954; Moreno and Brodie, 1962; Umeda *et al.*, 1971) like cortisone, phenylbutazone, polymyxin B, reserpine and cinchophen, excision (Mori *et al.*, 1964), heat injury (Skoryna *et al.*, 1958; Torgerson, 1961) or mechanical agitation (Hase and Scarborough, 1971). The latter type of mechanical rotation of either rats or guinea-pigs can be used in which the speed of rotation correlates with the time of onset, incidence, and severity of the lesions. Thus, the amount of stress can be controlled by regulating the rotating time and speed. The guinea-pig is the animal of choice for histamine-induced gastric and duodenal lesions (Marazzi-Uberti and Turba, 1961; Anderson and Soman, 1965a).

While the emphasis of the methods in the above models is in inducing or preventing lesions and ulcers, some studies have been conducted on enhancing healing rate of induced lesions (Skoryna *et al.*, 1958). The animal model in which acetic acid is injected into the gastric submucosa of rats leads to lesions which persist for at least 150 days (Takagi *et al.*, 1970). The technique has been extended to cats where the spontaneous healing rate was faster than in the rat (35 *vs* > 200 days respectively) (Okabe *et al.*, 1971a). The chronicity, severity and location of the experimental acetic acid ulcer model in the rat may make it useful as a model of the human disease.

It should be noted that only a few methods have been developed for inducing duodenal ulcers. Several models have been developed in the rat (Berg *et al.*, 1949; Seronde, 1963; Robert *et al.*, 1970). A chronic type of duodenal ulcer (lasting approximately 60 days) has been developed in the rat by placing acetic acid (100 per cent, 0·07 ml) onto the duodenum for 30 seconds (Okabe *et al.*, 1971b). A surgical procedure on the gastrointestinal tract of the dog can be performed that diverts the stomach effluent to the jejunum (Mann and Williamson, 1923). Under such conditions, a peptic ulcer comparable pathologically to that found in man develops in the intestinal mucosa, just adjacent to the gastric mucosa.

2.5   MISCELLANEOUS SECRETORY PREPARATIONS

The isolated stomach has not received extensive utilization for the initial studies of chemicals. The isolated gastric mucosa of the frog has been used for a few chemical studies (LeFevre *et al.*, 1964). This biological tissue may be used to characterize drugs that exert direct effects on hydrogen ion or pepsin-secreting cells. The isolated mouse stomach will remain viable for short periods of time. It has been used in biochemical studies (Davenport and Chavré, 1950) but not extended to extensive pharmacological tests. The action of drugs has not been assessed in isolated gastric parietal cells which are obtainable as a viable preparation (Croft and Ingelfinger, 1969; Blum *et al.*, 1971).

The central nervous system exerts an influence on gastric secretion (Brooks, 1967). Animal models that permit specific studies on centrally acting drugs have not been exploited in secretion studies. The biochemical approach to evaluate a secretory control has also not been extensively explored. The search for histidine decarboxylase inhibitors is a step in this direction. The search for chemicals that specifically antagonize the action of gastrin would also be of interest.

The role of secretion in the duodenum in preventing lesions has not been clarified. Further research in this area would be important. Studies indicate that nicotine may sensitize the duodenum to damage (Jacobson *et al.*, 1971; Robert *et al.*, 1971). The animal model for studying the alkalization of the proximal small bowel would be rewarding. Drugs could be forthcoming that enhance the alkalization of the upper small bowel.

2.6   MEASUREMENT OF PEPSIN ACTIVITY

Gastric secretions possess the property of proteolytic activity because of the pepsin content. This type of activity has been postulated to be a contributing factor to producing the peptic lesion. The gastric cells producing the pepsin can synthesize, store and secrete proteins. This property is different from the cells which produce the electrolytes. Because of its different function, the hormone–nervous interaction of the pepsin-producing cell may be controlled differently from that of the electrolyte-producing cell. A comprehensive review of pepsin secretion is available (Hirschowitz, 1967).

The peptic activity of gastric secretions and the *in situ* inactivation of proteolysis have been used by investigators for determining the antipepsin action of a test compound (Hunt, 1948; Klotz and Duvall, 1957; Piper, 1960; Bitch, 1966). Following administration of a test compound, the gastric secretions are collected and their peptic activity compared with that of secretions collected after treatment with placebo. In the *in vitro* studies, the test compound is added directly to the solution of commercial crystallized pepsin of known activity. The peptic activity of the mixture is compared to that of the pepsin solution alone (Bonfils *et al.*, 1960). Some investigators add the test compound to aliquots of gastric secretion rather than to dilutions of crystallized pepsin. By varying the amount of pepsin, or substrate, the investigator can determine if the compound is competing with pepsin for the substrate or is inactivating the pepsin itself.

2.7 ANTICHOLINERGIC TESTS

The potential nonanticholinergic antiulcer drug should be assessed for anticholinergic activity since it is desirable to develop a chemical devoid of this latter blocking action. Several tests are practical. The author has used the action of acetylcholine on blood pressure of the anesthetized dog; or the methacholine-induced chromodacryorrhea in rats (Bass *et al.*, 1967). The lack of blockade of the cholinergic action is the desired property of the potential antiulcer drug.

3 Nonanticholinergic antisecretory agents

It should be emphasized that the gastrointestinal tract is a multifunctional organ that is vital to the homeostasis of the organism. Secretion, absorption and contractile activity are integral parts of digestion and assimilation of the digested substances. This integrative function is performed under the influence of an extensive interaction between the neurogenic and hormonal systems. The interplay is accomplished by the tract producing and containing a host of various substances, some of which are biogenic amines (e.g. histamine, serotonin, and catecholamines); lipid soluble acids (e.g. Darmstoff and prostaglandins); and polypeptides (e.g. substance P, secretin, gastrin, and cholecystokinin-pancreozymin (CCK-PZ)). The gastrointestinal tract also contains many substances that are in need of purification and physiological verification. Some of these are villikinin and the gastrones, e.g. urogastrone, gastrogastrone, sialogastrone, and enterogastrone. Many of these substances are currently under study for their interaction with the neurogenic elements of the gastrointestinal tract.

It is legitimate to ask: What do we mean by inhibition of secretion? Most of the studies on the models described above indicate that inhibition occurs when the rate of secretion to some stimulus is decreased by an agent. It should be realized that inhibition can range from severe, irreversible mucosal damage to reversible decrease of response to a rebound increase in secretion either during or after cessation of the inhibitory effect. It is undesirable to elicit nonspecific actions like interfering with blood supply or with normal metabolic function. The desired action would be to block a physiological or biochemical secretagogue action. The desired action of a drug could be on nerve terminals which may directly control secretions or indirectly to release intestinal hormones that alter secretion. The drugs could also interact with specific receptors on the cell surface, or cause changes in the permeability of cell membranes. Drugs may also alter the induction of certain enzymes related to secretion. The direct action on cell metabolism and protein synthesis has been reported for the secretagogues caerulein and pentagastrin on the histidine decarboxylase enzyme (Melchiorri and Sopranzi, 1971). The blockade of the enzyme induction with cyclohexamide stopped the secretory action of the stimulants. However, the induction of histidine decarboxylase is not the exclusive process of secretagogues since increased activity levels may also be obtained with known antisecretory agents, e.g. SC-15396, CCK-PZ (Caren *et al.*, 1969). A possible explanation for the apparent paradoxical action of SC-15396 (**2**, see page 217) is given by Håkanson and Liedberg (1971). They postulated that the drug inhibits gastrin release which is the normal stimulus to increase histidine decarboxylase levels. We do not know whether drugs affecting secretion are altering nervous control, competitive or noncompetitive interactions at receptors, changing cell permeability, altering enzyme levels or a combination of actions. Drug mechanisms should be sought at a cellular and enzyme level to explain specific sites of action.

A potentially useful clinical agent could be one which effectively reduces the volume and acidity of gastric secretion through mechanisms other than the blockade of the cholinergic nervous system. To date, there has been no unequivocal clinical verification to support this hypothesis. Several chemicals, devoid of anticholinergic activity, have been characterized in animal models. Similarly, drugs may either inactivate pepsin in the stomach or alter its secretion. For either hydrogen ion or pepsin, multiple sites and mechanisms are theoretically possible.

3.1   2,2′-BIPYRIDINE, CI-588

A series of phenoxypyridines and arylpyridines were evaluated for their antisecretory action in the pyloric ligated rat (Butler *et al.*, 1971). Among the phenoxypyridines, compounds with substitutions in the 2′ position of 4-phenoxypyridine retained high activity ($ED_{50} < 10$ mg kg^{-1}). Substitutions in the 3′ and 4′ positions severely depress activity. The most active compounds with their ED_{50} in mg kg^{-1} were, 4-phenoxypyridine, 5; 3-phenoxypyridine, 4·5; 2-phenylpyridine *N*-oxide, 2·3; 2-(2-thienyl)pyridine, 4·2; 3-phenylpyridine, 2·0, and 2,2′-bipyridine, 2·4. The detailed pharmacology of the latter compound (**1**) is described below.

2,2′-Bipyridine, CI-588

(1)

CI-588 was evaluated for its antisecretory action in rats and dogs (Bass et al., 1966b). CI-588 decreased the secretory volume and hydrogen ion and pepsin output in the 4-h pylorus ligated rat preparation. A dose of 2·5 mg kg^{-1} s.c. reduced secretion by 50 per cent (ED$_{50}$). The substantially equal effect following intraduodenal administration indicated good absorption of the drug. In gastric-pouch dogs, CI-588 reduced food-stimulated secretions and hydrogen ion output, but had no effect on insulin- or histamine-stimulated secretions. It reduced the severity of stress-induced gastric lesions in guinea-pigs, but had a minimal effect against polymyxin B-induced gastric lesions in rats. The chemical possessed no demonstrable anticholinergic, ganglionic blocking or central nervous system activity.

CI-588's mechanism of action may involve the sympathetic or serotonergic systems (Bass et al., 1966b; Bapna et al., 1970). Both of these systems have been implicated in modulating gastric secretion. Reserpine antagonism of CI-588's antisecretory activity in rats was partially reversed by DL-3-(3,4-dihydroxyphenyl)alanine (DL-dopa) and by 5-hydroxytryptophan. Epinephrine and norepinephrine effects on dog blood pressure were partially antagonized by high doses (> 32 mg kg^{-1} i.v.) of CI-588 (Bass et al., 1966b). At doses (~ 100 mg kg^{-1}) far greater than needed to demonstrate antisecretory activity, CI-588 can decrease brain and heart norepinephrine levels and epinephrine concentration in the adrenals of rats. This is selective since dopamine and serotonin brain levels were not altered (Bapna et al., 1970). This action is presumably due to inhibition of dopamine β-hydroxylase (Goldstein et al., 1964; Green, 1964; Bapna et al., 1970). Since a dose–response curve was not studied, this type of enzyme inhibition may not be important to the antisecretory action of the drug.

Another possible action of CI-588 may be due to its chelating properties (Moss and Mellon, 1942). The chemical has been used as a quantitative indicator for some metals, e.g. iron. When a large number of other chelators were checked for antisecretory activity, only chelators which were structurally similar to 2,2′-bipyridine were active (Bass et al., 1967). In general, gastric antisecretory activity is not a common property of a chelator.

In preliminary clinical studies, a single dose as high as 1 g of CI-588 was well tolerated by man. The chemical has not been assessed in man for its antisecretory properties.

3.2 3-METHYLAMINO-2,1-BENZISOTHIAZOLE, CI-624

Several benzisothiazole derivatives (Table 1) were synthesized and evaluated for their antisecretory properties in the rat (Meyer *et al.*, 1965;

TABLE 1

Gastric antisecretory structure–activity relationship of some 3-amino-2,1-benzisothiazoles[a]

R_1	R_2	R_3	ED_{50} (mg kg^{-1} s.c.)
H	H	CH_3	1·8[b]
H	H	C_2H_5	3·0
H	H	$(CH_3)_2CH$	3·6
H	CH_3	CH_3	4·8
5–Cl	CH_3	CH_3	2·8
6–Cl	CH_3	CH_3	3·1
6–CH_3O	H	C_2H_5	4·2
H	H	H	58·0
H	H	$(CH_3)_2CHCH_2$	32·0
6–CH_3	H	C_2H_5	15·0

[a] Modified from Meyer *et al.* (1965).
[b] CI-624.

Bass *et al.*, 1966a). Detailed pharmacology was performed on CI-624. This chemical reduced pyloric ligated rat secretions by 50 per cent at 1·8 mg kg^{-1} s.c. and reduced food-, insulin-, and histamine-stimulated secretions in gastric-pouch dogs. It protected rats against stress-induced gastric lesions. CI-624 had no demonstrable anticholinergic or ganglionic blocking activity. CI-624 and congeners did possess antinociceptive action in the mouse and antibradykinin activity in the guinea-pig. Clinical assessment of the chemical has not been reported.

3.3 THIOACETAMIDES

Several research groups have independently reported a series of thio-acetamide derivatives, (2), (3), and (4), which possess gastric antisecretory actions (Lee *et al.*, 1972; Malen *et al.*, 1971; and Borsy *et al.*, 1970). There is some overlap in that all three groups reveal that 2-pyridyl-thioacetamide (4) is very active in reducing gastric secretions in rats.

2-Phenyl-2-(2-pyridyl)-
thioacetamide
(SC-15396)

(2)

2-Pyrazinyl-2-
ethylthioacetamide
(S-1897)

(3)

2-Pyridyl-
thioacetamide
(CMN-131)

(4)

The perfused rat preparation described by Ghosh and Schild (1958) was used by the Searle group to evaluate one of these series of thio-acetamides for their effectiveness in gastrin-induced secretions (Lee *et al.*, 1972). The structure–activity relationships of the active derivatives are listed in Table 2. 2-Pyridylthioacetamide and 3-methyl-2-(2-pyridyl)thiobutyramide were the most potent inhibitors. The chemical, 2-phenyl-2-(2-pyridyl)-thioacetamide (SC-15396) (2), also very active, was selected for more detailed pharmacology (see p. 220). Several of the series of chemicals were also studied on the gastric secretion in the 5-hour pyloric ligated rat (Table 2). The antisecretory tests were performed by giving the drug orally after pyloric ligation. This is a poor way of assessing drugs that may act systemically since they cannot empty into the duodenum. Their action may be due to local mucosal damage or a surface activity since gastric absorption would be expected to be minimal for this series of chemicals. These chemicals were all active in reducing acid concentrations but did not markedly influence gastric juice volume or proteolytic activity. It is difficult to interpret this test because of the intragastric dosage procedure. This series of drugs demonstrates antiulcer activity by protecting against lesions in the 19-hour pyloric-ligated rat, Δ'-cortisone-induced lesions in the rat and histamine-induced duodenal ulcers in the guinea-pig. SC-15396 can also prevent indomethacin-induced gastric lesions (Lee *et al.*, 1971).

The Servier Laboratories group have extended the series of chemicals that are capable of reducing secretion (Malen *et al.*, 1971; Pascaud *et al.*, 1971). If we take SC-15396 (Table 2) as a standard, this group has

TABLE 2

Gastric antisecretory structure–activity relationship of some thioacetamides $R_1R_2CHCSNH_2$

R_1	R_2	ED_{50}[a] (mg kg^{-1} i.d.)	ED_{50}[a] (mg kg^{-1} i.g.)	Antigastrin[b] (mg)
Cl—⟨phenyl⟩—	⟨2-pyridyl⟩		43	2
⟨phenyl⟩— (SC-15396)	⟨2-pyridyl⟩	5·4	11	2
CH_3—⟨phenyl⟩—	⟨2-pyridyl⟩			2
H	⟨2-pyridyl⟩		2·0	1
H	⟨2-quinolyl⟩		4·0	2
$(CH_3)_2CH$	⟨phenyl⟩		7·0	1
⟨phenyl⟩—CH_2	H			2
H (CMN 131 pyridine derivative)	⟨2-pyridyl⟩	1·4		
CH_3	⟨2-pyridyl⟩	2·3		

TABLE 2—*contd.*

R_1	R_2	ED$_{50}$[a] (mg kg^{-1} i.d.)	(mg kg^{-1} i.g.)	Antigastrin[b] (mg)
C_2H_5		5·1		
$CH_3(CH_2)_2$		4·1		
$(CH_3)_2CH$		1·9		
$CH_3(CH_2)_3$		2·6		
$CH_3(CH_2)_5$		3·7		
$CH_2{=}CH{-}CH_2$		3·3		
C_2H_5 (S 1897 Pyrazinyl, ethyl derivative)		4·3		
C_6H_5		4·3		

TABLE 2—*cont.*

R_1	R_2	ED_{50}^{a} (mg kg^{-1} i.d.) (mg kg^{-1} i.g.)	Antigastrin[b] (mg)
4-Cl—C$_6$H$_4$	(pyridazine ring)	1·5	
HN=C—CH$_3$ (with bond)	H	4·6	

[a] Dose of chemical administered intraduodenally (i.d.) that reduced the acid output by 50 per cent in the pyloric ligated rat; or the dose of chemical administered intragastrically (i.g.) that reduced acid concentration by 50 per cent in the pyloric ligated rat.

[b] Antagonism of pentagastrin stimulated secretion in the perfused stomach of an acute rat preparation. Dose in mg indicates level at which significant antisecretory activity was obtained. Data modified from Malen *et al.* (1971); Lee and Phillips (1972).

shown that most of their derivatives, whenad ministered intraduodenally, are more potent than SC-15396 (Table 2) in reducing acid output of the rat stomach.

From both studies, the structure–activity relationship indicates that activity is lost if: (i) oxygen replaces the S; (ii) when two N-C rings are substituted for R_1 and R_2; (iii) when no N is in either R_1 or R_2; (iv) by lengthening the distance between the non-amide N and the thioacetamide group; or (v) by steric hindrance on the alpha-carbon (Table 2).

The 2-pyridyl-2-thioacetamide, CMN-131, (4), has been studied in more detail (Dr X. B. Pascaud, personal communications; Pascaud and Laubie, 1971; Pascaud and Blouin, 1972). The chemical at 2·5, 5, or 10 mg kg^{-1} i.v. or orally can decrease for more than 4 h the acid concentration and output of histamine- (160 μg kg^{-1} h^{-1}) or pentagastrin- (6·4 μg kg^{-1} h^{-1}) induced secretions in dogs prepared with Pavlov pouches. This derivative also inhibited histamine- and pentagastrin-induced secretions in the acute, perfused rat preparation. It also prevents stress-induced lesions in rats. The chemical does not induce vomiting in dogs, is devoid of anticholinergic activity and does not block norepinephrine, epinephrine, histamine or serotonin effects on the dogs' blood pressure.

The most extensive studies have been performed on 2-phenyl-2-(2-pyridyl)thioacetamide (SC-15396) (2). Unfortunately rats receiving the drug (200 mg kg^{-1} per day for 1 year) developed (15/20 incidents) mammary adenocarcinomas (Y. H. Lee, personal communication). This precludes any further clinical studies with this most promising agent.

One must await to see if one of the other derivatives will survive pharmacological, toxicological and clinical evaluations.

The chemical SC-15396 was initially thought to be a specific gastrin-antagonist. It reduced gastrin-stimulated gastric secretions in the anesthetized acute rat preparation of Ghosh and Shild (Cook and Bianchi, 1967). In gastric fistula and gastric pouch dogs, SC-15396 was effective orally at 10 mg kg^{-1} against gastrin tetrapeptide-stimulated secretions but was not effective at doses as high as 50 mg kg^{-1} against food or histamine-stimulated secretions. Similar specificity was claimed, and the term "anti-gastrin" applied to SC-15396 when it was confirmed (10 mg per animal) to antagonize secretion in both Pavlov (innervated) and Heidenhain (denervated) pouch dogs, stimulated by gastrin II or pentagastrin but could not antagonize (at 20 mg per animal) histamine- or methacholine-stimulated secretions (Bedi et al., 1967a).

The specificity of SC-15396 was quickly refuted by several groups (Connell et al., 1967; Connell et al., 1968; Tiongco et al., 1968), and also by the original observers (Bedi et al., 1967b; and Gillespie et al., 1968). At higher doses (e.g. 200 mg per animal orally or parenterally), SC-15396 was capable of reducing histamine-, insulin-, or 2-deoxy-D-glucose-stimulated gastric secretion in dogs prepared with gastric fistula, Pavlov or Heidenhain pouches. The chemical can also antagonize food-induced secretions (Bedi et al., 1967a; Gillespie et al., 1968), and endo-genously released gastrin by antral irrigation with acetylcholine (Tiongco et al., 1968; Isaza et al., 1970). Though formal dose–response curves were not obtained, SC-15396 appears to antagonize the three secreta-gogues differentially: gastrin > insulin > histamine $\cong$ food. An unex-pected and unexplained species difference became evident when 20 mg i.v. of SC-15396 given to anesthetized cats failed to inhibit the acid or pepsin response which was stimulated by either gastrin tetrapeptide or by vagal excitation (Sewing et al., 1968).

A careful study in chronic fistula rats revealed that 25 mg kg^{-1} SC-15396 could significantly antagonize pentagastrin-, insulin-, or histamine-induced volume and acid concentration of stomach secretions (Lee and Thompson, 1968). This inhibition occurred when SC-15396 was given before or after the various secretagogues. In other studies on the acute perfused rat preparation of Ghosh and Shield, SC-15396 could antagonize pentagastrin-induced (Varró and Náfrádi, 1970) or gastrin-, bethanechol-, or histamine-induced secretions; and in acute perfused guinea-pig preparations it could antagonize gastrin- and hista-mine-induced secretions (Albinus and Sewing, 1969). SC-15396 can also decrease gastrin- or histamine-provoked pepsin secretion in the rat (Kahlson et al., 1968). The gastric antisecretory action, at least against gastrin-induced secretions, seems specific since SC-15396 does not antagonize gastrin-stimulated motor activity of the canine antrum (Isenberg and Grossman, 1969) or minimally depresses gastrin-stimulated canine pancreatic secretions (Stening and Grossman, 1968).

The mechanism of action of SC-15396 has not been explained. The gastrin-enhanced rate of histamine formation in the gastric mucosa of the rat and the increased urinary excretion of free histamine were not antagonized by SC-15396 (Kahlson *et al.*, 1968). These authors concluded that SC-15396 reduced the sensitivity of the parietal and peptic cells to secretory stimulation but did not have any direct action on the gastrin molecule *per se*. Another mechanism of action may be the antagonism between the SC-15396 molecule and phenylalanine amide, the C terminal of the gastrin molecule. SC-15396 may block the receptor for —$CONH_2$ groups of phenylalanine amide (Albinus and Sewing, 1969). A preliminary observation suggested that isoproterenol ($2\,\mathrm{mg\,kg^{-1}}$) can prevent the inhibitory effect of SC-15396 on gastrin-induced secretions in dogs, cats, or rats. Thus suggesting that SC-15396 inhibits gastric secretion through stimulation of β-adrenergic receptors (Amer, 1969). Further studies are needed to either confirm or expand on the mechanism(s) of this most interesting antisecretory series of drugs.

3.4   NONANTICHOLINERGIC QUATERNARY NITROGEN COMPOUNDS

This series (e.g. (5)) contains a quaternary nitrogen but does not possess the classical anticholinergic properties characteristic of these structures though it does have gastric antisecretory activity (Antonsen, 1968).

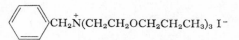

Benzyl-tri-(2-propoxyethyl)ammonium iodide,
(U 247–51)
(5)

This series was discovered accidentally when Antonsen, of Alfred Benzon Ltd, attempted to saturate gastrointestinal mucus with "inactive" quaternary compounds. The rationale was that if the binding sites were saturated, one should see a more uniform absorption of the active quaternary drugs. Some of the "inactive" drugs possessed gastric antisecretory activity. The two quaternary nonanticholinergic compounds, benzyl-tri-(2-propoxyethyl)ammonium iodide (U 247–51) and benzyl-tri-(beta butoxyethyl)ammonium bromide (U 247-73) could decrease acid secretion and stress-induced ulcers in rats when administered either intraperitoneally at 1·3 mg or orally. This latter route was effective when the chemical was given at > 10 mg kg^{-1} three hours before ligation. The corresponding tertiary chemicals were 10–16 times less potent (Antonsen, 1967).

This series of drugs was not evaluated in dogs for their antisecretory activity against various secretagogues because they cause vomiting at relatively low doses. U 247-51 does have antiinflammatory activity in rats, antagonizes reserpine-induced ptosis in mice, histamine-induced bronchial spasms in guinea-pigs, and polymyxin B-induced gastric lesions in rats. These effects were attributed in part to the weak sympathomimetic activity of U 247-51. The chemical did not antagonize acetylcholine, histamine, barium chloride or serotonin action on isolated ileal tissue.

The chemical, though devoid of anticholinergic activity, potentiated the mydriatic action of standard anticholinergic drugs. For example, mydriasis induced by Metropin (Strasenburgh Laboratories, Rochester, New York) was enhanced when given before or simultaneously with U 247-51. The toxicity of U 247-51 given i.v. in mice was enhanced by pretreatment with metropin. In contrast, physostigmine or pilocarpine reduced its toxicity. This quaternary compound apparently has a selective effect on the cholinergic system of the stomach. Toxicity trials in rats with these agents indicated that the compounds were well tolerated. Antisecretory trials have not been reported in humans.

3.5 XYLAMIDE (CR-242)

This agent (6) chemically is N''-benzoyl-N',N'-dipropyl-DL-isoglutamine and is on the European market under the trade name Milid® (Rotta

N''-Benzoyl-N',N'-dipropyl-DL-isoglutamine,
Xylamide, CR-242, Milid®

(6)

Research Laboratories, Milan, Italy). It is not very effective as an antisecretory agent in pyloric ligated rats since it requires 637 mg kg^{-1} s.c. to obtain an ED$_{50}$ value (Rovati et al., 1967a). In dogs, however, xylamide inhibited histamine-, gastrin-, and insulin-stimulated gastric secretions. The repeated daily administration of 35 mg kg^{-1} i.v. for 7 days resulted in strong gastric secretory inhibition. Secretions returned to normal when xylamide treatments were halted (Danhof, 1967; 1969). Xylamide also protected against pyloric ligation-, polymyxin B-, phenylbutazone-, and glucose-induced gastric lesions in rats (Rovati *et al.*, 1967b). It had no demonstrable anticholinergic, adrenolytic, antihistaminic or central nervous system activity.

Clinically, patients receiving corticoids have elevated uropepsinogen levels which were returned to normal levels by xylamide (Gobbi, 1967). Decreased gastric acid secretions were obtained in man with 600 to 800 mg daily in two doses (Giordano and Comi, 1967). In other clinical studies, oral and parenteral doses up to 8·0 g daily for 3 weeks was supposed to improve the condition of duodenal ulcer patients (Vallejo *et al.*, 1969a), suppress histamine secretion in patients with duodenal ulcers (Vallejo *et al.*, 1969b; Bianchi and Saccabusi, 1969), and "normalize" the secretion of duodenal ulcer patients (Borellini and Milvio, 1969; Rovati, 1969). No significant side effects were reported in any of these clinical trials. A critical double blind study is required with xylamide before the drug is worthy of being considered for ulcer therapy. The structure–activity relationships (Rovati *et al.*, 1969) that have been described for this series of drugs requires such high doses to be active in the rat that, if extrapolation from this study is possible, it would be predicted that a clinical dose could not be reached that was therapeutically effective.

4 Gastric antihistaminics

The establishment of histamine (**7**) as a specific physiological secretagogue has not been settled (Ivy and Bachrach, 1966; Code, 1965; Waton, 1971). *N*-Methylhistamine or *N*-dimethylhistamine, are two histamine metabolites that are more potent than histamine as secretagogues. One of these may be more intimately involved with the physiological mechanism of secretion (Lin *et al.*, 1962; Code *et al.*, 1971). In contrast to the above two derivatives, metabolites of the imidazole ring possess minimal

Histamine-preferred H$_2$ receptor tautomer

(**7**)

or no effect on acid secretion of the dog (Ivy and Liepins, 1958). Presumably, a chemical that would block gastric actions of histamine or its active metabolites would clarify the action of these substances and prove useful as a therapeutic agent.

Some of the early attempts to block histamine-induced secretions were on a variety of histamine analogues—pyrazole, triazole, tetrazole heterocyclic nitrogen compounds and β-aminoethyl derivatives. These studies were by two groups of workers who used the Heidenhain (denervated) or Pavlov (innervated) pouch dogs as secretion models (Grossman et al., 1952; Lin et al., 1962). Several of these chemicals acted as secretagogues. One or two analogues, for example 4-(β-aminoethyl)-2,1,3-triazole · 2HCl, of this series did decrease gastric secretion. These latter results are preliminary in nature and have not been confirmed. More recently, 5-methylhistamine was characterized as a potent (equal to, or greater than histamine) long-acting secretagogue in the cat. This histamine derivative is not known to occur naturally (Impicciatore and Grossman, 1973). Thus analogues of histamine may possess agonist or antagonist actions depending on their relative affinities for histamine receptors.

Physicochemical studies of histamine revealed that the molecule can exhibit tautomerism (Kier, 1968), i.e. react in isomeric structures which differ from each other in the position of a hydrogen atom and a double bond. One of the preferred conformations may be suitable for intramolecular metal binding (Margolis et al., 1971). The theoretical considerations (Kier, 1970; 1971) and the physical properties of the tautomer ratio of histamine and several derivatives (Ganellin, 1973a; 1973b; 1973c; Ganellin and Pepper, 1973) have been reviewed. These considerations imply that histamine (7) or one of its close analogues must assume a particular conformation to function at the secretory cell receptor.

Alternatively, there may be two distinct mechanisms by which histamine is made available to the mammalian organism. One is the release of bound histamine; the second is the production by new synthesis, catalyzed by an adaptive enzyme, histidine decarboxylase (Schayer, 1961). The dynamics of two histamine productions and the presence of at least two histamine-receptor interactions leads to four systems that may respond differently to various blocking agents.

4.1 H$_2$ RECEPTORS

The evidence that various histamine analogues differ in their ability to lower blood pressure, stimulate smooth muscle and alter gastric secretions would suggest that several types of histamine receptors exist in the body. For example, N-methylhistamine and N-dimethylhistamine are more potent than histamine in stimulating gastric secretion but are less potent than histamine in lowering blood pressure or stimulating smooth muscle contractility. The characteristics of histamine receptors on the smooth muscle of the guinea-pig ileum, which are blocked by conventional antihistaminic drugs, were compared to histamine receptors in rat uterus and rat gastric secretory cells (Ash and Schild, 1966). Specific structural requirements were needed for histamine analogues to stimulate the guinea-pig ileum. These histamine receptors were designated H_1. The histamine receptors of the rat uterus and stomach acid cells, which responded differentially to the same series of analogues, were designated H_2. These latter actions cannot be antagonized by conventional antihistaminics.

The postulation that two histamine receptors could exist prompted a group at Smith, Kline and French Laboratories to search for a specific gastric antihistaminic (Black et al., 1972). Over 700 compounds were synthesized and tested for their ability to inhibit histamine-stimulated gastric secretion in anesthetized rats. This would represent an H_2 receptor antagonist. Other types of gastric secretion inhibition in this series were eliminated by failure of compounds to block the H_2 receptors in other organs, e.g. rat uterus. On this basis, burimamide (8), N-methyl-N'-{4-[4(5)-imidazolyl]butyl}thiourea, was selected for further pharmacological studies.

$$HC{=\!=\!=}C-(CH_2)_4NHCNHCH_3$$

$$:N{\diagdown}{}{\diagup}NH \qquad \overset{\parallel}{S}$$

$$\underset{H}{C}$$

N-Methyl-N'-{4-[4(5)-imidazolyl]butyl}thiourea
Burimamide
(8)

Burimamide is a competitive inhibitor of histamine-stimulated gastric secretion in the rat ($ED_{50} = 6.1 \times 10^{-6}$ mol kg^{-1}). It is specific since the chemical did not block insulin- or electrical vagal stimulated-induced secretions. The specificity of blockade is further supported by the evidence that similar doses could competitively antagonize histamine on the H_2 receptor of the isolated guinea-pig atria and the rat uterus. No significant interaction occurred with histamine H_1 receptors (guinea-pig ileum), catecholamine β-receptors, or muscarinic receptors. The chemical can antagonize pentagastrin-induced secretion in the rat, histamine- and pentagastrin-induced secretion in the cat. Burimamide was active in studies on dogs with Heidenhain pouches against histamine- (ED_{50} 1.9×10^{-5} mol kg^{-1}), pentagastrin-, and food-induced secretions. It did not block carbachol-stimulated secretions in the dog. In a preliminary clinical study, burimamide given as an i.v. infusion to 2 volunteers significantly reduced the acid output.

A more detailed clinical trial has been completed on six subjects (Wyllie *et al.*, 1972). Histamine- or pentagastrin-induced gastric secretions were decreased an average of 57 per cent by intravenous infusion of approximately 90 minutes' duration (total dose of 5·6–9·8 mg kg^{-1}) of burimamide. There was mainly a decrease in acid output though acidity was also lowered. There was an excellent correlation between burimamide plasma levels and decreased acid output. Thus an exciting new chemical entity to specifically antagonize H_2 receptor-induced secretions has been introduced.

$$CH_3C\!\!=\!\!=\!\!CCH_2\!\!-\!\!S\!\!-\!\!(CH_2)_2NHCNHCH_3$$

N-Methyl-*N*'-[2-(5-methylimidazol-4-yl)methylthio]ethylthiourea
Metiamide

(9)

Burimamide is orally ineffective in experimental animals. A chemical analogue, metiamide (9), has been developed that possesses histamine H_2 receptor blockade, low animal toxicity and good oral bioavailability (Black *et al.*, 1973; Wyllie *et al.*, 1973). This chemical at doses of 2·5 to 10 mg kg^{-1} orally could cause a 31 to 80 per cent inhibition of hist-amine-induced secretions in Heidenhain pouch dogs. Metiamide was equally effective orally against pentagastrin-induced secretions in the dog. In another species, the rat, metiamide was orally effective in re-ducing both basal and histamine-induced secretions. Metiamide was also effective intravenously against histamine- or pentagastrin-induced secretions in the dog. The drug did not inhibit carbachol-stimulated secretions in the rat or dog. In man, metiamide at 2·5 mg min^{-1} i.v. for 90 minutes could reduce maximal histamine- and pentagastrin-induced secretions 74 per cent in three and 87 per cent in four people, respec-tively. Its oral effectiveness was shown in four subjects given 200 mg via a nasogastric tube. Pentagastrin was infused intravenously. One hour later, metiamide was administered, and gastric aspiration continued 30 minutes later. Acid output was suppressed by 60 per cent. Metiamide has been administered to 32 volunteers with no adverse side effects. We await a thorough clinical evaluation of metiamide. Will it prove useful in treating duodenal ulcer patients?

Other pharmacological studies have been performed on the two H_2 receptor antagonists. Burimamide does not decrease mucosal blood flow in the dog (Curwain et al., 1973a) but may do so in the anesthetized cat (Albinus and Sewing, 1973a; Albinus and Sewing, 1973b). This latter action may be due to an adrenal catecholamine releasing effect of burimamide.

A direct receptor interaction was further demonstrated in the isolated rat stomach, where the blood supply was not a factor (Assem et al., 1973). Burimamide could antagonize histamine-induced secretion in this isolated tissue. Preliminary studies on the effect of burimamide on histamine distribution in the mouse suggest that the drug occupies histamine binding sites and does not possess any histamine catabolism inhibitory properties (Schayer, 1973). It has been postulated that cAMP may be involved as a second messenger in the histamine-induced acid secretion (see section 9.2). At least in minced gastric tissue of guinea-pigs, a dose dependent histamine-stimulated production of cAMP could be competitively inhibited by burimamide (Karppanen and Westermann, 1973).

The H_2 receptors are also present in the uterus, atrium, lungs, and even the mast cells. They may also influence peripheral vasoconstriction. The blockade of H_2 receptors in these other organs or cells could possibly limit a potential gastrointestinal clinical candidate for H_2 receptor blockade. Burimamide can prevent the depressor effect of histamine on the pulmonary vascular bed of guinea-pig (Türker, 1973; Goadby and Phillips, 1973). It can also potentiate vasoconstriction in the pulmonary vasculature of calves (Eyre and Wells, 1973). Burimamide can also inhibit the uptake of histamine in the guinea-pig atrium and mouse neoplastic mast cells (Fantozzi et al., 1973). Are the blockade of H_2 receptors in the lungs and cardiovascular system potential sites for "side effects" for the H_2 antagonist gastric antisecretory agents? Extensive clinical studies should indicate whether pulmonary or cardiac side effects will limit the use of these agents for ulcer therapy.

4.2 H_1 RECEPTORS

In contrast to the above rational design of a drug, the studies with H_1 receptor antihistaminics on gastric secretion were controversial and mainly equivocal. They are summarized in this section to demonstrate the massive effort that can be expended in the wrong direction. The initial enthusiasm (Loew et al., 1945; 1946; McGavack et al., 1946) that the antihistaminic diphenhydramine would be useful in lowering gastric secretions and treating ulcer diseases was not substantiated. This inability of antihistaminics to block histamine secretion was demonstrated in man (Moersch and Rivers, 1946; Gilg, 1948; Doscherholmen, 1949; Ashford and Heller, 1949; Reitter, 1952; Ferrando and Lozzio, 1957; and others), dog (Loew and Chickering, 1941; Burchell and Varco, 1942; Linde, 1950; Ragins et al., 1958), cat (Emmelin and Frost, 1947; Wood, 1948; Dutta and Tamhane, 1953; Howat and Schofield, 1954), and mouse (Davenport and Chavré, 1950). In fact, the antihistaminics, promethazine, methapyrilene, diphenhydramine, and tripelennamine can actually increase the secretory response to histamine in cats, rats, or dogs (Lin et al., 1962). This observation confirmed what was first shown for the original Fourneau histamine antagonists, thymoxyethyl-diethylamine (929F) and N-phenyl-N-ethyl-N'-diethylethylenediamine (1571F), that they do not alter or may even increase gastric secretory responses to histamine in Heidenhain pouches in dogs (Burchell and Varco, 1942; Hallenbeck, 1943; Loew and Chickering, 1941). Paradoxically, these two agents were effective in antagonizing food-induced secretions (Hallenbeck, 1943). The slight increase in secretion after these various antihistaminics may be due to the blockade of peripheral histamine receptors and consequently a higher circulating level of histamine. These agents may also act as secretagogues by blocking histamine methyltransferase (Barth et al., 1973). This differential blocking property of drugs on histamine acting on smooth muscle function or gastric secretion is further evidence that the histamine receptors in these biological responses are different or at least differentially accessible to blocking agents.

The effect of established antihistaminic drugs on experimental ulcers is variable. Part of the variability may be due to lesions being caused by different mechanisms. For example, simply dosing guinea-pigs with histamine by two different regimens can give different types of lesions. A single intraperitoneal injection leads to acute gastric lesions within six hours (Eagleton and Watt, 1965), while repeated half-hourly intramuscular administration of histamine causes duodenal ulceration within four hours (Eagleton and Watt, 1967). A list of studies in which antihistaminics can protect against a variety of ulcerogenic agents and situations is presented in Table 3. The two antihistaminics, chlorothen and mepyramine, can protect against histamine-induced lesions in the guinea-pig (Van Meter and Oleson, 1949; Watt and Eagleton, 1964). The protective action of the antihistaminics, promethazine, cyproheptadine, tripelennamine, AHR-224-B and brompheniramine have also been reported (Alphin and Ward, 1969). It appears paradoxical that brompheniramine, which could protect against histamine-induced

TABLE 3

Protective effects of antihistamines on various experimental ulcers[a]

Ulcerogenic treatment	Species	Antihistamine used	Protection[b]	References
Histamine	guinea-pig	promethazine	−	Halpern and Martin (1946)
			−	Zaidi and Singh (1958)
			+	Alphin and Ward (1969)
		diphenhydramine	−	Crane et al. (1947)
		brompheniramine	+	Alphin and Ward (1969)
		AHR-224-B	+	
		tripelennamine	+	
		cyproheptadine	+	
		chlorothen	+	Van Meter and Oleson (1949)
		mepyramine	+	Watt and Eagleton (1964)
	rat	antisdine	−	Deutsch and Thaler (1951)
	dog	diphenhydramine	−	Friesen et al. (1946)
Polymyxin	rat	chlorpheniramine	+	Moreno and Brodie (1962)
		pyrilamine	+	
		cyproheptadine	+	
		promethazine	+	Franco-Browder et al. (1959)
		chlorpheniramine	+	
		dexbrompheniramine	+	
		phenindane	+	
		chlorpromazine	−	
Restraint	rat	diphenhydramine	−	Thayer et al. (1965)
	guinea-pig	brompheniramine	−	Alphin and Ward (1969)
Pyloric ligation	rat	brompheniramine	−	Alphin and Ward (1969)
Reserpine	rat	thenalidine	±	Nikodijevic and Vanov (1960)
		brompheniramine	−	Alphin and Ward (1969)
Serotonin	rat	thenalidine	+	Nikodijevic and Vanov (1960)

[a] Table modified from Schwartz (1971).
[b] + Protection; − no protection in various studies.

lesions in the guinea-pig at doses less than 1 mg kg^{-1} s.c. did not reduce histamine-induced secretions, or restrained stress-induced lesions in the guinea-pig or reserpine-induced lesions in the rat. The gastric lesions produced by polymyxin B in the rat, presumably due to histamine release, can be prevented by cyproheptadine, chlorpromazine, chlorpheniramine, and pyrilamine (Moreno and Brodie, 1962), promethazine, chlorpheniramine, dexbrompheniramine, and phenindane (Franco-Browder et al., 1959). This latter group saw no protection with chlorpromazine or lysergic acid diethylamide. In contrast, diphenhydramine did not prevent histamine induction of ulcers in dogs (Friesen et al., 1946) or guinea-pigs (Crane et al., 1947; Alphin and Ward, 1969). The ability of certain antihistaminics to reduce either direct or indirect histamine-induced ulcers in guinea-pigs and rats without a concomitant decrease in gastric acidity suggests that other factors are important.

These antihistaminic drugs may be exerting some nonspecific effects, e.g. altering blood flow or exerting blood pressure alterations. Promethazine, as well as mepyramine and chlorpromazine, when applied directly to gastric mucosa may be antisecretory because they cause nonspecific damage (Blair and Forrest, 1960; MacDougall *et al.*, 1964; Kay and Forrest, 1956). The complexity of action is exemplified by pyrilamine and promethazine when given i.v. to dogs. These drugs exert an inhibitory action on gastric secretions induced by endogenous release of gastrin from the antrum, no effect on insulin- or histamine-induced secretions and a non-specific inhibitory effect when applied topically (Ragins *et al.*, 1958).

Promethazine may possess a unique action in preventing the release of endogenous gastrin from the antrum (Dombro and Ragins, 1967). The drug can block secretion induced by locally perfusing the antrum of a dog with an acetylcholine solution but not prevent exogenous-induced secretions by i.v. administered gastrin pentapeptide. In contrast, atropine blocks both of the above types of induced secretions. This unique drug action has not been extended to other chemicals. Promethazine can also inhibit basal and histamine-induced secretion in man (Konturek and Radecki, 1963). Thus with one or two exceptions we are left to conclude that most of the antihistaminics have no effect on secretion and a variable, controversial effect on altering the response to ulcerogenic drugs.

The dichotomy between secretory and ulcerogenic response to H_1 receptor antagonists raises important questions about the ulcer animal model. How typical is it of the clinical counterpart? Do animal ulcer models have any value in predicting the usefulness of a clinical candidate?

4.3 DYNAMICS OF HISTAMINE PRODUCTION

Gastric secretion may be decreased by altering the production or catabolism of histamine or one of its analogues. Studies have been designed to decrease histamine-induced gastric secretions by decreasing the conversion of L-histidine to histamine by blocking the enzymatic action of histidine decarboxylase. The properties of the enzyme and the chemistry of the various inhibitors have been thoroughly described (Schayer, 1966; Pletscher *et al.*, 1966). The formation of histamine from histidine by bacterial decarboxylase was first recognized in 1910 (Dale and Laidlow, 1910). More than one decarboxylase enzyme exists in tissues. One is a nonspecific aromatic aminoacid decarboxylase while the other is a specific histidine decarboxylase (Weissbach *et al.*, 1961; Aures *et al.*, 1969). The latter, an adaptive enzyme, can be lowered in concentration by prolonged fasting or raised by feeding or by the administration of gastrin, reserpine or caerulein (Kahlson *et al.*, 1964a; 1967; Rosengren and Svensson, 1969; Schwartz *et al.*, 1969; Melchiorri and Sopranzi, 1971). The gastrin effect on secretion in the rat may exert its physiological function by stimulating gastric body histidine decarboxylase (Håkanson and Liedberg, 1972; Bersimbaev *et al.*, 1971). Variable amounts of histidine decarboxylase activities were found in the gastric mucosa of a variety of species. The following three species showed some activity—rat, mouse, and hamster—but no detectable activity was present in the mucosa of monkey, pig, dog, cat, rabbit, or guinea-pig (Aures *et al.*, 1969). The latter study confirmed the species differences already reported where only trace amounts of the enzyme histidine decarboxylase were present in the mucosa of several of the above species and man (Kahlson *et al.*, 1964). The species differences in the distribution of histidine decarboxylase prevent sweeping generalizations on the role of gastric histamine and histidine decarboxylase in affecting parietal cell secretions. Possibly in the rat, histamine acts directly on the parietal cell while other secretagogues act indirectly via the histidine decarboxylase system. This theory explains why drugs may be antisecretory by inhibiting gastrin or cholinergic mechanisms but do not block histamine-induced secretions (Levine, 1965a).

The enzyme histidine decarboxylase has been inhibited in several ways. An extensive series of chemicals have been evaluated *in vitro* for their effects on inhibiting the specific histidine decarboxylase activity from the glandular portion of the stomach of the rat (Mole and Shepherd, 1972; 1973). A series of benzyloxyamines can also inhibit specific histidine decarboxylase (Hamor *et al.*, 1970; Huszti *et al.*, 1973). Thiazol-4-ylmethoxyamine can inhibit histidine decarboxylase and cause a depletion of histamine from rat brain (Menon *et al.*, 1971). *In vivo* antisecretory studies are not available on the above series of chemicals.

Rats placed on diets deficient in pyridoxine, a co-enzyme necessary for aminoacid decarboxylase, caused an 80 per cent decrease in urinary histamine. The administration of semicarbazide, a weak histidine decarboxylase inhibitor, inconsistently decreased urinary histamine. The combination of pyridoxine deficiencies and administration of semicarbazide promptly dropped the histamine levels in the urine. Two other histidine decarboxylase inhibitors, α-methyl histidine and α-methyl-dopa (α-methyl-3,4-dihydroxyphenylalanine) were tested in rats. The former lowered while the latter had no effect on histamine levels in the urine (Kahlson *et al.*, 1963). Two compounds, a hydrazine analogue of histidine D-2-hydrazino-3[4(5)-imidazole]propionic acid, HH, or MK-785 and 4-bromo-3-hydroxybenzyloxamine (NSD-1055, brocresine) were found to be potent inhibitors of specific histidine decarboxylase *in vitro* (obtained from homogenates of whole fetal rats) and effectively decreased histamine levels in the stomach tissues and urine of the rat (Levine *et al.*, 1965). In rats with both the esophagus and gastroduodenal junction ligated, pretreatment with either HH (200 mg kg^{-1} i.p.) or NSD-1055 (150 mg kg^{-1} i.p.) decreased basal acid secretion, or secretion stimulated by reserpine, insulin, gastrin or bethanechol. The inhibitory responses were not due to nonspecific tissue damage, since animals pretreated with NSD-1055 or HH could still demonstrate secretory response to histamine (Levine, 1965b). Partial confirmation of Levine's results were obtained in a study on rats when histamine formation was blocked by either pyridoxine deficiency or by NSD-1055. Both basal and gastrin responses in the pyloric ligated rat were inhibited. In contrast these workers could not demonstrate an inhibition of insulin- or bethanechol-induced secretions (Thayer and Martin, 1967). The picture is more confusing since NSD-1055 and other decarboxylase inhibitors had minimal or no effects on secretion of the pyloric ligated rat (Bass and Patterson, 1967). Another study in which NSD-1055 was given orally, intraperitoneally or intravenously to gastric perfused rats stimulated by tetragastrin, histamine or bethanechol resulted in minimal or no inhibitory effects (Becker and Sewing, 1971). Similar negative effects were obtained when gastrin or histamine was administered to dogs with innervated or denervated pouches that had been dosed acutely (160 mg kg^{-1} p.o. in individual doses), or chronically (rising doses to the point of side effects) with NSD-1055 (Fletcher *et al.*, 1969). Paradoxically the enzyme can also be increased by the antisecretory agents SC-15396 (Kobayashi and Maudsley, 1968; Kahlson *et al.*, 1968), burimamide and metiamide (Maudsley *et al.*, 1973), and after repeated injections of prostaglandin E$_1$ (Håkanson *et al.*, 1973). NSD-1055, in addition to inhibiting the synthesis of histamine, can inhibit the histamine catabolic enzyme diamine oxidase in rats (Binder and Sewing, 1973). This action would tend to "antagonize" the chemical's inhibitory secretory effects. Part of the controversial antisecretory effects of NSD-1055 may also be due to its rapid metabolism (Ellenbogen *et al.*, 1973). The specificity of histidine decarboxylase inhibitors has been studied and discussed in greater detail (Johnston and Kahlson, 1967). The entire topic of histidine decarboxylase properties and its physiological role has been reviewed (Kahlson and Rosengren, 1968). Thus a promising, rational approach to inhibiting acid secretion by inhibiting an enzyme cannot be confirmed. In addition, the different biological levels of histidine decarboxylase activities between rodents and other species reflect that a more potent or more specific enzyme inhibitor may be very effective in rodents but not active in man.

The physiological actions of histamine could be altered by influencing its catabolic process. Histamine catabolism has been reviewed (Schayer, 1959). Enzymes responsible for oxidative deamination (diamine oxidase, histaminase) or methylation by imidazole N-methyltransferase are the main pathways involved in inactivating histamine. No chemicals are known that can enhance the rate of catabolism. Chlorpromazine and bromolysergic acid diethylamide can decrease the rate of catabolism of histamine in the rat and hence enhance its secretory response (Amure and Ginsburg, 1964). This route of potentiating histamine action does not appear important since chlorpromazine when not followed by exogenous histamine is a potent antisecretory agent in man (Haverbach *et al.*, 1955; Sun and Shay, 1959a), dog (Sun and Shay, 1959b), and rat (Tiede *et al.*, 1963; Konturek and Radecki, 1963; Bass and Patterson, 1967). The inhibitory response of secretion may reflect the alpha-adrenergic blocking properties of chlorpromazine. In any event, the balance of pharmacological properties present in chlorpromazine leads to predominantly antisecretory rather than secretory responses. The antimalarial drug, amodiaquine, also characterized as a histamine methyltransferase inhibitor, can potentiate pentagastrin-induced secretions in the dog (Troidl *et al.*, 1973). Indeed, both H_1 and H_2 receptor antagonists can inhibit histamine methyltransferase (Taylor, 1973; Barth *et al.*, 1973). These actions are presumed to act by inhibiting imidazole N-methyltransferase, the enzyme that catalyzes the transfer of the methyl group of S-adenosylmethionine to the nitrogen of the 1 position of the imidazole ring to yield 1-methylhistamine (Brown *et al.*, 1959a). The physiological significance of agents possessing this enzyme inhibitor action as well as antisecretory activity is not known.

5 Catecholamines and sympatholytics

The role of the sympathetic nervous system and catecholamines in affecting gastric secretion has not been subjected to the same degree of scrutiny as that of the parasympathetic nervous system or the histaminergic system. The sympathetic nervous system through its mediator, though controversial, predominantly produces gastric antisecretory effects (Code, 1951). The antisecretory action has been postulated to be due to vasoconstriction (Forrest and Code, 1954).

5.1   ANTISECRETORY PROPERTIES OF VASOACTIVE DRUGS

Several experiments refute the statement that gastric secretion is intimately related to vascular flow. In the dog, three known vasodilators, histamine, gastrin and bradykinin, act as secretory agents at much lower concentrations than can cause a decrease in vascular resistance (Jacobson, 1964). Isoproterenol, a potent vasodilator, as well as epinephrine, and norepinephrine both predominantly vasoconstrictors, are antisecretory in dogs against food-, bethanechol-, and histamine-induced secretions (Pradhan and Wingate, 1962). The isoproterenol effect was confirmed against food-induced secretion in dogs and was highly potent (0·20–2·0 µg kg⁻¹ min⁻¹) in inhibiting pentagastrin-induced secretions in both conscious and unconscious dogs (Curwain and Holton, 1972). This isoproterenol inhibition of gastric secretion was not blocked by propranolol. Mucosal blood flow measurements indicated that the isoproterenol antisecretory effect was not due to a decrease in mucosal blood flow. Salbutamol and terbutaline, two other β-receptor agonists, also reduced pentagastrin-induced secretions in the dog. The action of both of these agents was blocked by propranolol. Again, the antisecretory action is not secondary to a fall in mucosal blood flow (Curwain et al., 1972).

In the rat, the three catecholamines, isoproterenol, epinephrine and norepinephrine, and vasopressin reduced while angiotensin and L-dopa had no effect on secretion in the pyloric ligated rat (Bass and Patterson, 1967). The antisecretory action of isoproterenol has been confirmed in the chronic fistula rat. No consistent correlation was observed between vascular responses and gastric secretion in the acute fistula rat when four vasopressors (clonidine, vasopressin, angiotensin, norepinephrine) or five vasodepressors (methacholine, isoproterenol, phenoxybenzamine, sodium nitrite, diazoxide) were administered (Brodie and Hooke, 1971). A similar lack of relationship between blood pressure and gastric secretion was obtained for isoproterenol and phenylephrine in the chronic fistula rat (Misher et al., 1969). The action of phenylephrine is controversial since it exerts a biphasic effect in the chronic fistula rat, initially stimulating and then inhibiting gastric secretion (Misher et al., 1969). It is relatively inactive in the pyloric ligated rat, requiring 230 mg kg⁻¹ s.c. to reduce secretion by 50 per cent (Bass and Patterson, 1967). Yet phenylephrine is active at lower doses (10–50 mg kg⁻¹ i.p.) in producing gastric ulcers in the rat (Djahanguiri et al., 1969a) and mouse (Lynch et al., 1964). The latter group could not consistently demonstrate the ulcerogenic effect of phenylephrine at doses as high as 300 mg to rats. General hemodynamic pharmacological mechanisms cannot be totally implicated in the action of catecholamines and other vasoactive substances on secretion.

Drugs possessing adrenergic and/or vasoactive properties have been studied for their effect on induced gastric bleeding. Certain types of stress conditions inflicted on rats can cause bleeding without the accompaniment of lesions (Brodie and Valitski, 1963). Chlorpromazine, trifluoperazine as well as certain anticholinergics and ganglionic blocking agents can effectively prevent the bleeding. In a series of vasodilators studied, methacholine did not prevent the hemorrhage while histamine, isoproterenol, phenoxybenzamine, sodium nitrite and diazoxide effectively prevented the bleeding. In the group of vasoconstrictors tested, epinephrine and clonidine decreased hemorrhage while norepinephrine, angiotensin and vasopressin did not alter the hemorrhage (Brodie and Hooke, 1971). Both epinephrine and clonidine possess an inherent vasodilator component in their actions. Thus there does not appear to be a consistent effect among vasoconstriction, vasodilation, gastric secretion and bleeding tendencies.

5.2   EFFECTS OF ALPHA- AND BETA-ADRENERGIC RECEPTOR BLOCKING AGENTS ON SECRETION

It may appear paradoxical that the agonists, norepinephrine, epinephrine and isoproterenol, and their antagonists, alpha- and beta-receptor blocking agents, should both possess antisecretory properties. However, the following all caused a decrease in acid secretion in the rat: phenoxybenzamine (Brodie and Hooke, 1971; Jow et al., 1960; Bass and Patterson, 1967), SY-28, hydralazine, ergotamine, phentolamine, piperoxan, tolazoline, dibenamine, and yohimbine (Bass and Patterson, 1967; Okabe et al., 1970). Phenoxybenzamine and dichloroisoproterenol were antisecretory in the dog against basal, food-, bethanechol-, and histamine-induced secretions. In contrast, two blockers, phentolamine and tolazoline, acted as secretagogues in the dog (Jacobson, 1961; Pradhan and Wingate, 1966). Phentolamine could not prevent ulcers induced by stress, reserpine or after 17 hours of pyloric ligation in the rat (Boissier et al., 1970). These blocking agents can alter catecholamine effects by preventing norepinephrine uptake, blocking receptors or interfering with storage. The administration of alpha-receptor blocking agents, regardless of mechanisms, prolongs the biological half-life of catecholamines in blood and urine (Benfey et al., 1959a; 1959b; Millar et al., 1959). This leads to the hypothesis that the antisecretory effect produced by various chemicals may be due to the prolonged biologic half-life of the catecholamines (Bass and Patterson, 1967).

The beta-receptor blocking agents, dichloroisoproterenol, propranolol, pronethalol, MJ 1999 and alprenolol, when administered to a rat possess antisecretory activity comparable to the weaker α-adrenergic blocking agent (Jow et al., 1960; Bass and Patterson, 1967; Okabe et al., 1970; Danhof and Geumei, 1972). In man, 10 mg i.v. of propranolol could reduce basal secretory volume (Geumei *et al.*, 1969) and histamine-induced secretions (Geumei *et al.*, 1972a). In another clinical study, propranolol at a lower dose (~ 7 mg i.v.) exerted no effect against basal or pentagastrin-induced secretions. In fact, slight stimulatory results were obtained (Konturek and Oleksy, 1969). Similar potentiation of pentagastrin-induced secretion by propranolol has been seen in the dog (Curwain *et al.*, 1973a). Propranolol at 25 mg kg^{-1} p.o. had no effect on secretions on the chronic fistula rat (Misher *et al.*, 1969). In another species, the pigeon, nylidrin, a beta-receptor agonist, increased gastric secretions which could be blocked by propranolol. In the same species, propranolol could also block histamine-induced secretions (Geumei *et al.*, 1972b). As a group, the beta-receptor blocking agents are not as potent as several of the alpha-receptor blocking drugs in decreasing gastric secretions.

5.3 DRUGS THAT BLOCK NOREPINEPHRINE UPTAKE MECHANISMS

A major route of inactivating either endogenous or exogenous norepinephrine is by neuronal uptake of this agonist into sympathetic nerve terminals. Drugs which inhibit this inactivation process can potentiate the actions of norepinephrine. Chemicals that interfere with norepinephrine uptake (Lippmann, 1968a), but do not cause alterations in the endogenous tissue levels of catecholamine have been extensively studied for antisecretory actions (Lippmann, 1968b; 1969a; 1970a; 1970b; 1970c; 1971a). Several series of chemicals have been shown to block the uptake of norepinephrine in rat or mouse heart. The ability of a chemical series to block uptake correlates with gastric antisecretory properties of the series. We do not know whether these chemicals increase the biological half-life of the catecholamines. We also do not know what these chemicals do to either catecholamines or the sympathetic nervous system in the stomach. The degree of inherent anticholinergic activity has not been satisfactorily assessed in these series of chemicals. In spite of these criticisms, chemicals with this imipramine-like action could prove useful clinically for gastrointestinal secretory problems.

The first of the series studied was aralkylamine derivatives (Lippmann, 1968a; 1968b). The three chemicals that were active against reserpine-induced secretions in the rat were: AY 14,948 (**10**), AY 18,627 (**11**), and AY 20,214 (**12**). The AY 18,627 was the most potent (ED_{50} in rats, ~ 10 mg kg^{-1} s.c.) demonstrating an activity similar to that of imipramine.

Another series, the cycloheptadiene (AY 8794) (**13**), was found to be the most active ($ED_{50} \sim 5$ mg kg^{-1} i.p.) in decreasing the secretion in the pyloric ligated rat (Lippmann, 1969a). This series expands the studies on

Cl—⟨benzene⟩CH₂—C(CH₃)(CH₃)—NH—CH₂—C(=O)—CH₃

4-Chloro-α,α-dimethylphenethylaminopropan-2-one
AY 14,948
(10)

⟨benzene⟩—CH₂—C(CH₃)(CH₃)—NH—CH₂—C(=O)—C

α,α-Dimethylphenethylaminopropan-2-(
AY 18,672
(11)

Cl—⟨benzene⟩—CH₂—C(CH₃)(CH₃)—NH—CH₂—CH(OH)—CH₃

4-Chloro-α,α-dimethylphenethylaminopropan-2-ol
AY 20,214
(12)

tricyclic compounds, which includes imipramine, desmethylimipramine and chlorpromazine, that can block norepinephrine uptake and also act as antisecretory agents. The following structural elements in the tricyclic series are of importance for antisecretory activity: two benzene rings, or one benzene and one hexane ring, a seven-membered central ring which may be carbocyclic or heterocyclic (nitrogen in the five position), and a linear, three-carbon aliphatic side chain attached to the seven-membered ring by a single or double bond.

5-(3′-Dimethylaminopropyl)dibenzo[a, d][1,4]cycloheptadiene
AY 8794
(13)

Another antidepressant that blocked norepinephrine uptake, 2-(p-chlorophenyl-2′-pyridyl-hydroxymethyl)imidazoline, (Sch-12650), was approximately twice as potent as imipramine in decreasing basal- and pentagastrin-stimulated secretion in the rat (Lippmann, 1970a).

A bicyclic drug, Lu3-010 (14), is one of a series that can block norepinephrine uptake and is antisecretory (Lippmann, 1970b; 1971a). In the rat, its ED_{50} was approximately $1\cdot3$ mg kg^{-1} i.p. or p.o. against basal secretions. This is four times as potent as imipramine. Lu3-010 is also active in the rat in decreasing pentagastrin-, histamine-, or reserpine-induced secretions and reserpine-induced ulcers. Lu3-010 (ED_{50}

3,3-Dimethyl-1-(3-methylaminopropyl)-1-phenylphthalan;
Lu3-010
(14)

$6\cdot3$ mg kg^{-1}) could also protect against stress-induced ulcers in rats, though imipramine was three times as potent. It also protected against lesions in the 17-hour pyloric ligated rat. The prior dosing of a rat with α-methyltyrosine, an inhibitor of norepinephrine synthesis, could prevent the antisecretory action of Lu3-010 but did not alter the antisecretory actions of imipramine or atropine. The administration of dopa after dosing with α-methyltyrosine, which would bypass the blocked synthesis step, could reverse the blockade of antisecretory activity of Lu3-010 caused by α-methyltyrosine. This pharmacological evidence suggests that newly synthesized norepinephrine is important for the actions of Lu3-010.

A final series of chemicals possessing antisecretory and norepinephrine uptake blocking properties was described (Lippmann, 1970c), of which AY 9928 **(15)**, is one of the more active. It decreased basal secretion in

trans-1,4-Di(naphth-1-ylmethylaminomethyl)cyclohexane
AY 9928
(15)

the rat (ED_{50} 5 mg kg^{-1} i.p.) though requiring four times more drug for an ED_{50} in the guinea-pig. AY 9928 also reduced histamine-, reserpine-, and pentagastrin-stimulated secretion in the rat. The potency of the *cis* and *trans* isomers of some members of this series differed, but this was not so for AY 9928.

Thus several series of chemicals can exert an antisecretory response and appear capable of altering norepinephrine uptake. The action of these chemicals has not been extensively assessed for their α-receptor blocking activity or ability to block various cholinergic pathways. The most obvious mechanism of action of the antisecretory property of the thymoleptic drugs is by their anticholinergic blocking activity. This is certainly characteristic of the tricyclic compounds. The inadequate reference (Petersen *et al.*, 1966) to some incidental anticholinergic studies done on the above series does not exclude the possibility that an anticholinergic component may be present in the molecule. One also awaits studies with these chemicals on secretions in dog and ultimately studies in man.

In addition to the above series of chemicals, other drugs can block norepinephrine uptake; for example, cocaine, chlorpromazine, haloperidol and imipramine. Other tricyclic neuroleptics have been shown to depress secretion in the pyloric ligated rat (Yamaguchi *et al.*, 1973). However, these agents are not specific for altering just a single phase of catecholamine bioactivity. Chlorpromazine is antisecretory in the rat (Shay *et al.*, 1958; Konturek and Radecki, 1963; Amure and Ginsburg, 1964; Bass and Patterson, 1967; Pendleton *et al.*, 1970), dog (Sun and Shay, 1959b), and man (Haverback *et al.*, 1955; Sun and Shay, 1959a) and has potent alpha-receptor blocking properties (Huidobro, 1954). Imipramine and desmethylimipramine, which also have been reported as antisecretory in rats (Bonfils *et al.*, 1962a; Lippmann, 1969a; Pendleton *et al.*, 1970), possess anticholinergic properties (Domenjoz and Theobald, 1959), or may even act as antisecretory agents through a central mechanism (Pendleton *et al.*, 1970). Both imipramine and desamethylimipramine have minimal effects in man against basal secretion and no effect against insulin-induced secretion (Baume and Powell, 1966).

Several drugs that release catecholamines have minimal or no effect on secretion (Bass and Patterson, 1967). For example, DMPP releases catecholamines from tissues (Lindmar and Muscholl, 1961), guanethidine and CI515[1] are known to release heart norepinephrine (Cass and Spriggs, 1961) but do not alter secretions in the rat. Drugs classified as indirect or mixed sympathomimetics, e.g. (+)-amphetamine, tyramine or ephedrine also exerted minimal antisecretory actions. Since tissue catecholamines consist of two or more pools with different turnover rates, the

[1] 3-phenoxypropyl)-guanidine hemisulfate.

various releasers may not affect the depot that is critical to antisecretory activity; or the catecholamines released, may be transient and not demonstrate any antisecretory action.

5.4 CATECHOLAMINE METABOLISM

Drugs acting on the enzymes that affect the catecholamines have variable effects on secretion. The monoamine oxidase inhibitors pheniprazine and pargyline had weak antisecretory actions while iproniazid had no effects at doses tested (Bass and Patterson, 1967). Pheniprazine did not prevent insulin-induced gastric lesions or reduce insulin-stimulated gastric secretion in the rat (Kim and Shore, 1963). Modaline has been reported as antisecretory (Rider et al., 1965). The equivocal results agree with other studies (Bonfils et al., 1962b). Drugs affecting dopamine β-hydroxylase or catechol O-methyltransferase, e.g. tetraethylthiuram and tropolone, exert no antisecretory actions. The variable response to drugs affecting decarboxylase enzymes has been discussed in section 4.3. Since inhibition of most of these enzymes decreases the synthesis of catecholamines, little reduction in gastric secretion would be expected. For example, α-methyltyrosine in the rat can inhibit tyrosine hydroxylase, which is the enzyme that is the limiting step in the biosynthesis of catecholamines. This does not reduce secretions in the rat (Lippmann, 1971a). The mucosa of the rat contains both dopa decarboxylase and histidine decarboxylase (Schayer, 1956; Håkanson, 1965). Inhibition of both enzymes could lead to equivocal results since inhibition of histidine decarboxylase produces a gastric antisecretory effect while inhibition of dopa decarboxylase gives a gastric secretory response. More specific drugs are needed to evaluate the role of catecholamine enzyme inhibitors on gastric secretion.

5.5 ADRENERGIC DRUG EFFECTS ON EXPERIMENTAL ULCERS

Equivocal results are also obtained in evaluating drug effects on experimental ulcers. This complexity may be due to the ability of chemicals to produce ulcers by different mechanisms. They may possess vasodepressor actions like histamine which causes extreme dilatation, stasis and pooling. They may exert a vasopressor action like vasopressin which leads to vascular contractions and anoxia. These two vascular extremes can be antagonized and the incidence of lesions reduced. Posterior pituitary hormones, which are ulcerogenic, can prevent histamine-induced lesions in the dog (Kowalewski et al., 1958) or in the guinea-pig (Kowalewski, 1967). Thus adrenergic drugs may either aggravate or prevent lesions depending on the conditions of the experiment (Gaetani and

Debeus, 1972) and the lesion inducing agent (Bhargava *et al.*, 1973). Also, few studies exist in the literature which evaluate a dose–response relationship of drugs affecting gastric lesions. Consequently, conflicting reports are present in the literature.

Acute stress of rats can increase the turnover rate of norepinephrine in the gastric mucosa (Djahanguiri *et al.*, 1973). The author speculated that this may be related to the development of restraint-induced ulcers. The adrenergic drugs bretylium (20 mg kg^{-1}), phenoxybenzamine (20 mg kg^{-1}), phentolamine (15 mg kg^{-1}), and α-methyldopa (40 mg kg^{-1}) could reduce the incidence of lesions. Unfortunately, these drugs were not evaluated for their effects on norepinephrine turnover characteristics in the mucosa. At low doses of 1 mg kg^{-1} s.c. and 1·5 mg kg^{-1} i.p. neither phenoxybenzamine nor propranolol prevented stress-induced ulcers in the rat (Rosoff and Goldman, 1968). Phenoxybenzamine at 1 mg kg^{-1} i.p. could prevent while chlorpromazine (10 mg kg^{-1} i.p.) had no effect on polymyxin B-induced lesions in the rat (Franco-Browder *et al.*, 1959). In a separate study, the following drugs expressed as ED$_{50}$ dose, mg kg^{-1} i.p., in the rat were effective in reducing poly-myxin B-induced lesions: cyproheptadine 0·5; phenoxybenzamine 9·0; chlorpromazine 12·0 (Moreno and Brodie, 1962). In another study, phenoxybenzamine at 20 mg kg^{-1} (route not given), could not prevent stress-, reserpine-, or 17-hour pyloric ligated-induced ulcers in the rat (Boissier *et al.*, 1970). In contrast, phenoxybenzamine at 5 mg 100 g^{-1} rat i.m. protected against the pyloric ligated- and reserpine-induced lesions but not the stress-induced lesions (Gáti *et al.*, 1971). Other studies have shown chlorpromazine to be effective in preventing lesions in the pyloric ligated rat (Tiede *et al.*, 1963). α-Methyldopa at 3 mg doses could prevent restrained- and swimming-induced ulcers (Djahanguiri *et al.*, 1967). Imipramine at 5 mg kg^{-1} i.m. could reduce stress-induced ulcers (Bonfils *et al.*, 1962a), while the monoamine oxidase inhibitor isocar-boxazid gave a "U-shaped" curve in that 10 mg kg^{-1} s.c. reduced reserpine- and stress-induced lesions while 20 mg kg^{-1} s.c. was ineffec-tive (Doteuchi, 1968). Pheniprazine at 5 mg kg^{-1} i.p. prevented reser-pine-induced lesions in the rat (Kim and Shore, 1963). Species specificity is evident, since phentolamine (2 mg kg^{-1}) can prevent aspirin- or stress-induced ulcers in rats (Djahanguiri *et al.*, 1968a; Djahanguiri, 1969a), but not histamine- or promethazine-produced lesions in guinea-pigs (Djahanguiri *et al.*, 1968b; Djahanguiri, 1969b). Neither MJ 1999 (10 mg kg^{-1}) or isoproteranol (1 mg kg^{-1}) were active against several of the above types of lesions. In contrast, propranolol at 20 mg and 50 mg kg^{-1} s.c. could reduce the ulcers produced in the pyloric ligated rat (Takagi *et al.*, 1969). Though at 5 mg kg^{-1} i.p. propranolol could not protect against pyloric ligated-, restraint-, or reserpine-induced lesions (Gáti *et al.*, 1971). In a comparative study, imipramine and desmethyl-imipramine are more potent than amitriptyline and desmethylamitriptyline in preventing the combined effects of reserpine and stress-induced gastric lesions in the rat (Garattini *et al.*, 1962).

Clonidine (ST 155) is a useful hypotensive agent in man. It is believed to exert its pharmacological effect by acting centrally to depress the sympathetic vasoconstrictor tone (Hoefke and Kobinger, 1966; Van-Zwieten, 1973; Sherman *et al.*, 1968). It initially causes an increase (Brodie and Hooke, 1971) followed by a decrease in blood pressure (Rand and Wilson, 1968). The drug could not prevent the increase in acidity in the rat produced by either vagus nerve stimulation or after the injection of methacholine. On another system, ST 155, at 100 μg kg^{-1} s.c., significantly reduced the volume and acidity in a 6-hour pyloric ligated rat and could prevent reserpine-induced lesions (Hoefke and Kobinger, 1966). This potency was confirmed for ST 155. At doses of 1 mg kg^{-1} or less, it could prevent stress-, reserpine-, or 17-hour pyloric ligated-induced ulcers in the rat but had no effect on histamine-induced ulcers in the guinea-pig (Boissier *et al.*, 1970). The control of ulceration by a central mechanism will have to be further explored.

A detailed study on the rat has been reported on the conditions that lead to gastric lesions by epinephrine (Sethbhakdi *et al.*, 1970a; Sethbhakdi *et al.*, 1970b). The presence of acid in the stomach was an important factor since the lesions could be prevented by the prior oral administration of sodium bicarbonate or by vagotomy. The administration of acid to animals with vagotomies returned the ulcerogenic action of epinephrine. Phenoxybenzamine (20 mg kg^{-1} i.m.) prevented the epinephrine-induced lesions, but a low dose of propranolol (0·4 mg kg^{-1} i.m.) had no preventive effects. In addition both adrenalectomy and hypophysectomy could prevent the epinephrine-induced lesions.

5.6   ADRENERGIC DRUG EFFECTS ON PEPSIN SECRETION

A study on the effects of various sympathomimetic agents on pepsin secretion in the dog revealed that the chief cells responded differentially (isoproterenol > epinephrine > norepinephrine) in increasing the secretion of pepsin. This response could be blocked by dichloroisoproterenol but not by phenoxybenzamine. α-Methyldopa also exerted an inhibitory response to pepsin secretion. Thus the cells producing pepsin appear to be controlled by a β-adrenergic receptor sensitive system (Anichkov and Grechiskin, 1969).

Chemicals affecting the sympathetic nervous system may mimic the nerve transmitter, cause or inhibit release, or prevent uptake of the nerve mediators. These drugs may exert some indirect action by their complex influence on the vascular supply of the stomach. The multiple actions of drugs on this nervous system has been the subject of several reviews (Acheson, 1966; Schümann and Kroneberg, 1970). The literature implies that the catecholamines, and in turn the sympathetic nervous system, play an important role in regulating gastric secretion. The dominant evidence indicates that the acid secreting cells are predominantly under alpha-receptor influence with minimal beta-receptor response while the pepsin-secreting cells are mainly sensitive to beta-receptor stimulation.

6 Gastrin inhibitors

The release of the secretory hormone gastrin from antral mucosa can be influenced by vagal, cholinergic mechanisms (Uvnäs, 1942; Pe Thein and Schofield, 1962), is pH sensitive (Woodward et al., 1954; Pe Thein and Schofield, 1962; Rheault et al., 1965a) and can be blocked by local anesthetics (Zeljony and Savich, 1911). A minority, controversial point of view exists in which it is claimed that the suppression of gastrin release is accompanied by the elaboration of an inhibitory antral hormone that decreases gastric secretion (Harrison et al., 1956; Longhi et al., 1957; Thompson et al., 1964). The role of the antrum in regulating gastric secretions has been the subject of several reviews (Woodward and Dragstedt, 1960; Thomson and Peskin, 1961).

6.1 LOCAL ANESTHETIC EFFECTS ON GASTRIN RELEASE

Early studies demonstrated that cocaine applied to the antral mucosa of dogs reduced acid secretory response to either mechanical or chemical stimulation (Zeljony and Savich, 1911; Uvnäs, 1942). It has been confirmed that either a 2 per cent cocaine or a 5 per cent procaine solution has a similar effect (Lim et al., 1925; Gregory and Ivy, 1941). It has been postulated that the antrum can secrete gastrin in response to a local neuronal reflex that is both excitatory, responding to distention and high pH, and inhibitory, responding to low pH (Redford and Schofield, 1965). These workers utilized a dog prepared with both antral and denervated gastric pouches. The irrigation of the antral pouch with meat extract or 1·0 per cent acetylcholine at pH 5·5–6·0 was assumed to release gastrin as evidenced by an increase in secretion from the denervated gastric pouch. The excitatory phase of gastrin release stimulated by meat extracts could very effectively be blocked by 5 per cent cocaine, 3 per cent lignocaine,

1 per cent lignocaine benzyl chloride or 2 per cent amethocaine. Amethocaine, a quaternary ammonium anesthetic, which is presumably ionized at the antral pH, could also prevent vagal gastrin release when it is stimulated by feeding (Redford et al., 1962; Schofield et al., 1967). The ability of ionized local anesthetics to effectively block neurogenic secretory processes is contrary to the current pH partition coefficient hypothesis. These agents may be acting by some other pharmacological action. Alternately, sufficient drug may be in the unionized state to permit some diffusion of the drug into the nerve elements of the antrum.

The local anesthetics, with the exception of 3 per cent procaine, could not block acetylcholine-stimulated secretion or prevent the marked inhibitory response of acidifying (pH 1·2) the antral pouch after initiating secretions with acetylcholine. These negative results may be due to the ionization of either the tertiary and certainly the quaternary nitrogen local anesthetics when the pouch is acid in character. The inability to inhibit acetylcholine-induced secretions when the pouch is neutral is not clear. Another unexplained pharmacological result is the ability of systemic hexamethonium bromide (1 mg kg^{-1}) to abolish the response to secretagogue stimulation but not reduce the local action of acetylcholine. Possibly the acetylcholine has diffusion characteristics that permit the direct effect on the cells containing the gastrin or may influence the synapse that is not permeable to the local anesthetics or blocked by hexamethonium. The antral mucosa is more permeable than the mucosa in the body of the stomach to the hydrogen ions (Dyck et al., 1969). This differential permeability property may play a role in allowing certain chemicals to penetrate to the effector organ, though the gastrin-containing cells are part of the surface mucosal epithelial cells of the antral pyloric glands (McGuigan, 1968a). Alternately, acetylcholine or acid media releases an endogenous inhibitory mediator that can act by bypassing the pathways blocked by these local anesthetics or hexamethonium. Another study indicated that 2 per cent procaine placed in an antral pouch was effective in reducing acetylcholine-induced secretions in two out of three dogs. In contrast, the local anesthetic oxethazaine in combination with aluminum hydroxide had no effect on acetylcholine-induced secretions (Rheault et al., 1965b). Also, the injection of 1 per cent dibucaine into the lumen of the stomach of the rat after pyloric ligation had no antisecretory effect (Ishii, 1969). Thus, the experimental data is not conclusive that local anesthetics can block acetylcholine-induced secretions though they seem effective in blocking mechanical and other chemical-induced secretions.

A series of local anesthetics that would effectively block gastrin release was prepared at Wyeth Laboratories (Seifter et al., 1962). One of these, oxethazaine (16), is a weak base and relatively nonprotonated in acid solution. At gastric pH, the efficiency of oxethazaine was higher than that of the other local anesthetics tested (Rheault, *et al.*, 1965b). Most local anesthetics are protonated at low pH and therefore are not active in an

2,2′-[2-Hydroxyethylimino]bis-[N-(α,α-dimethylphenethyl)-N-methylacetamide]
Oxethazaine

(16)

acid stomach. Partition studies at ∼ pH 1 indicated that oxethazaine could be expected to penetrate the nerve sheaths and thereby effect anesthesia. In both the pyloric-ligated rat and the acute gastric-fistula rat, the intragastric administration of oxethazaine increased the pH and lowered the volume of histamine-stimulated secretions (Malis, 1966).

The clinical studies with oxethazaine do not lead to definitive conclusions for the objective usefulness of the agent. In most cases the clinical trials are confounded since they are performed with oxethazaine in combination with aluminum hydroxide gel. Claims of usefulness have been made for the combination against pain from gastritis, duodenal ulcer, and hiatus hernia peptic esophagitis (Deutsch and Christian, 1959; Jankelson and Jankelson, 1959; Hollander, 1960; Somogyi *et al.*, 1965). In a double-blind study, patients hospitalized with recurrent peptic ulcers were relieved of symptoms in 85 per cent of the cases (47/56) when treated with oxethazaine–aluminum hydroxide mixture in comparison to a 53 per cent relief (34/64 patients) when treated with antacid alone (Bower and Myerson, 1964). In two cross-over studies on people with duodenal ulcers, there was no difference in the relief of symptoms from the antacid–local anesthetic combination in comparison to when antacid alone was utilized (Balmforth *et al.*, 1964; Grabham, 1964). These essentially negative results may be due to the presence of the antacid which may be enhancing stomach emptying and not permitting sufficient time for oxethazaine to be in contact with the antrum. Clearly, a definitive clinical trial is needed in which oxethazaine alone is tested for its effects on various clinical conditions of hypersecretion of the stomach.

6.2 GASTRIN ANTAGONISTS

The isolation, purification and identification of the two heptadecapeptide gastrin molecules from the antrum of several species including man is an important factor in attempting to develop a specific antigastrin chemical. This topic was reviewed in a symposium (Levine, 1968). The observation that all of the biological activities of the seventeen-member polypeptide, gastrin, can be duplicated by the carboxyl-terminal tetrapeptide amide of gastrin (Try-Met-Asp-Phe-NH_2) has permitted the chemist to alter this portion of the molecule in an attempt to develop a gastrin antagonist (reviewed by Morley, 1968; Gregory, 1970). Over 500 analogues were synthesized! The approach was to retain three of the aminoacids and to replace the fourth with a different one. The permutation of this approach is massive. A poor correlation was obtained between the *in vitro* evaluation of these analogues in preventing gastrin-stimulated contractions of the *in vitro* guinea-pig stomach and the *in vivo* studies on histamine- or gastrin-induced secretions in the anesthetized rat or cat or the unanesthetized dog. *In vivo*, the agents were either weak inhibitors or stimulators of gastric secretion. It is intriguing to speculate about the role of the N-terminal tridecapeptide. It is inactive by itself. Does it promote the effective transport of the active tetrapeptide end to the secretory receptor? Does it act as a protector to the tetrapeptide from N-terminal degradation? It is known that on a molar basis, the tetrapeptide is approximately one-twentieth as active as the parent molecule. The challenging question is: Can a chemical be synthesized that will occupy the receptor site of gastrin and inhibit the physiological functions of gastrin?

A unique action has been reported for the phenothiazine antihistaminic, promethazine (**17**) (Dombro and Ragins, 1967). Dogs were prepared with

10-[2-Dimethylamino)propyl]phenothiazine
Promethazine

(**17**)

both a denervated antral and body pouch. Secretions, stimulated by antral perfusions of either a meat homogenate or acetylcholine, could be markedly inhibited by the i.v. administration of 1 mg kg^{-1} promethazine. This dose of promethazine had no effect on the secretory response to i.v. pentagastrin, that is, exogenous gastrin. In contrast, atropine blocks both exogenously administered or endogenously released gastrin. Therefore, promethazine is characterized as inhibiting the release of gastrin from its cells of origin. Once released, and circulating, promethazine does not block the secretory effects of gastrin. Promethazine at 50 mg orally can also inhibit basal and histamine-induced secretions in man (Konturek and Radecki, 1963). Is this "antigastrin release" common to the phenothiazines or unique to promethazine? The definitive studies to clarify this intriguing mechanism of action have not been performed.

Bombesin, a tetradecapeptide in the skin of certain European frogs, has secretory activity in the dog and rat (Bertaccini *et al.*, 1973). The aminoacid sequence is different from the other secretagogues, caerulein and gastrin. This is not likely to act on the same receptor site. Bombesin can increase the plasma level of gastrin. It is postulated to act as a gastrin-releasing factor. If so, promethazine should block the secretory effect of bombesin. This experiment, when done, will help confirm the action of bombesin and promethazine on secretion.

6.3   GASTRIN ANTIBODIES

It is possible to develop gastric antibodies to rat gastric antigens by injecting rat gastric mucosa or gastric secretion into rabbits (Kawashima and Takagi, 1972). These antisera cause an inhibition of gastric acid and pepsin (Kawashima, 1972). This is a broad approach to developing an antisecretory agent. A more specific approach would be to antagonize gastrin by the development of antibodies to the hormone (Jaffe *et al.*, 1968; McGuigan, 1968b; McGuigan, 1968c). Antibodies were obtained by immunizing rabbits or guinea-pigs with the C-terminal tetrapeptide or gastrin I molecule covalently coupled to bovine gamma-globulin. These antibodies were effective in reducing secretions in rats. The effect of the gastrin antibodies has not been reported in chronic studies in animals or man. The ability to produce the fluorescent pharmacologically active derivative of the tetrapeptide should aid in determining the site of binding of gastrin (Sachatello *et al.*, 1971; Sachatello and Tritsch, 1971).

Several possibilities appear on the horizon for preventing gastrin action. The aborted pharmacological study with antisecretory agents, like SC-15396, or the preliminary studies of an endogenous inhibitor like promethazine await further development. The further elucidation of the mechanism of action of local anesthetics could yield a fruitful clinical candidate. A specific gastrin polypeptide antagonist is still a possibility. Finally, immunization against one's own hormones could be a major breakthrough in the control of gastric secretion.

7 Pepsin inactivation

Pepsin is a generic term for protease substances produced in the stomach and consisting of several enzymes and possibly isoenzymes which, on secretion, have different substrate specificity and pH optima. The physiological properties of pepsinogen and pepsin have been reviewed (Turner et al., 1967; Sun, 1967a; Turner, 1968). The chemical characterization of pepsinogen has also been elucidated (Marciniszyn and Kassell, 1971). The role of these proteolytic enzymes in causing gastric or intestinal lesions has not been elucidated. One theory suggests that the back diffusion of hydrogen ions into an abnormally permeable gastric mucosa creates a critical pH environment for sulfated glycosaminoglycan to activate the pepsinogen. This creates a proteolytic situation within the mucosa (Anderson, 1969). The physiological control of pepsin secretion has been reported (Schofield, 1957; Menguy and Thompson, 1967).

Drugs which decrease the volume and acidity of gastric secretions also usually decrease pepsin secretion. To date, no one has reported a specific pepsin secretory inhibitor. The secreted pepsin activity can be inhibited in the gastric lumen by raising the pH of the gastric contents. Pepsin can also be inactivated by compounds which combine with either pepsin itself or the protein substrate. Currently, the lumen of the stomach is the arena for most substances to decrease pepsin activity.

7.1 PEPSIN INHIBITION BY SEVERAL CHEMICALS

Studies in vitro have shown that many compounds can inhibit pepsin activity. Antacids can inactivate pepsin by altering the pH of the digestive media (Shoch and Fogelson, 1942; Persson and Bunke, 1962; Kuruvilla, 1971). Some antacids have been shown to complex with or adsorb pepsin (Bateson, 1954; Piper and Fenton, 1961a; Bergman et al., 1962). In general, antacids can protect the pyloric ligated rat preparation against ulceration and reduce the acidity and pepsin output (Shay et al., 1947a). In a noncontrolled clinical trial, bismuth aluminate was beneficial in reducing the presence of the lesions and relieving the symptoms in 80 per cent of patients with either gastric or duodenal ulcers without decreasing the acid or pepsin secretions (Flavell Matts and Swan, 1965). The relief of symptoms by antacids may be due to pepsin inactivation, acid neutralization or some other mechanism that has not been clarified.

An impressive number of heterogenous chemicals have been shown to exert antipepsin activity in both *in vitro* and *in vivo* tests. The detergents, sodium lauryl sulfate, sodium heptadecyl sulphate, sodium *m*-xylene sulfonate and sodium 1,2-ethylenedisulfonate dihydrate all inhibit protein digestion by pepsin *in vitro* (Ravin *et al.*, 1962). Sodium lauryl sulfate could inhibit pepsin digestion without alteration in pH (Shoch and Fogelson, 1942). Sodium dodecyl sulfate (2 per cent solution) when applied topically to the mucosa of the dog's stomach could inhibit histamine-induced acid concentration and output, pepsin output and stimulate mucus production. The agent effectively protected the pyloric ligated rat against lesions and reduced the pepsin concentration and output towards zero while stimulating mucus production (Shay *et al.*, 1947b).

In a clinical trial on three people with duodenal ulcers, sodium lauryl sulfate at doses as high as 780 mg hourly did not lower the peptic activity of the gastric juice (Kirsner and Wolff, 1943). The clinical assessment of the surfactants did not correlate with either *in vitro* pepsin inhibition results or animal data.

Several types of macromolecules can inhibit pepsin activity. An acidic polymer, produced by condensation of formaldehyde and hydroquinone sulfonic acid, can prevent pepsin action *in vitro* (Heymann *et al.*, 1959). The majority of these antipepsin substances have a high percentage of divalent anions as part of their chemical structures. In an *in vitro* test, the following sulfated polysaccharides had antipepsin activities, listed in decreasing order of activity: heparin, degraded carrageenin, fucoidan, and chondroitin sulfate. Chemicals with no antipepsin activity were sodium sulfate and nonsulfated polysaccharides, hyaluronic acid, agar, starch and tragacanth (Bonfils *et al.*, 1960; Anderson, 1961). This observation was extended to a larger series of macromolecules (Ravin *et al.*, 1962) where the *in vitro* antipeptic activity of these substances closely parallels their sulfate content (Table 4). Even sulfated disaccharides like sucrose, lactose and maltose can exert an *in vitro* antipepsin effect (Namekata *et al.*, 1967). Compounds can be rendered inactive by removing the SO_4 portion. When the sulfate content of degraded carrageenin is decreased by acid hydrolysis, the antipepsin activity is also decreased. Thus, the greater the sulfate content the greater the antipepsin activity.

Dextran sulfate, a sulfated polymer of 40 000 molecular weight, effectively inhibits pepsin digestion *in vitro* and when placed in the stomach of pyloric ligated rat can protect from ulceration and death (Namekata, 1962a; Barnes *et al.*, 1967). The *in vitro* inhibition of pepsin

TABLE 4

Relationship between sulfate content and antipeptic activity for
several naturally occurring and synthetic polymers[a]

Polymer	Antipeptic activity %	Sulfate %
Polyvinyl sulfonate	310	59·0
Sulfated polyvinyl alcohol	247	42·5
Sulfated rice starch	230	45·3
Amylose sulfate	182	38·0
Lambda-carrageenan	150	32·2
Kappa-carrageenan	110	24·0
Heparin	103	27·0
Carrageenan, C-16	114	27·1
Sodium alginate	13	0
Carboxymethylcellulose	0	0
Polyvinyl alcohol	15	0
Pectin N.F.	12·5	2·07
Sea Kem, type 8	73	23·0
Alginic acid sulfate	40	15·8
Carrageenan, standard	100	29·0

[a] Adapted from Ravin et al. (1962).

has been confirmed for dextran sulfate and dextran phosfate (Anderson et al., 1968). This study further confirmed that the ester sulfate content of the molecule paralleled the antipepsin activity.

In another study, dextran (anionic component not given) was effective ($ED_{50} = 8·5$ mg per 100 g rat) in reducing the acid, pepsin output and ulceration in the pyloric ligated rat when given intravenously but had not gastric effects via the subcutaneous, intraduodenal or intragastric route. It could also inhibit histamine- and compound 48/80-induced secretions in the dog but could not block betazole- or gastrin-induced secretions. These actions were speculated to be due to a histamine binding property of dextran (Rudick et al., 1968; Rudick et al., 1969). Dextran has also prevented gastric ulceration caused by hemorrhagic shock or by gastric bleeding (Atik et al., 1965; Goodale et al., 1964; and Harjola and Sivula, 1966). A preliminary clinical study suggests that dextran may be useful as an antiulcer drug (Lösel, 1964).

A series of oxidized starch sulfates could inhibit pepsin activity in vitro. The activity in this series was also directly related to the degree of sulfation of the macromolecule, though the amount of polymerization was also a factor (Namekata, 1962a). The in vitro activity parallels the *in vivo* actions in protecting the pyloric ligated rat against ulcers when given orally but not by the subcutaneous route. This protection was presumably due to the loss of peptic activity in the gastric juice. These agents were ineffective against stress-induced lesions in the rat (Namekata, 1962b). The mechanism of protection was thought to be due to the formation of a complex between the sulfated molecule and pepsin (Namekata, 1962c).

Lignin sulfates, obtained as a by-product of wood processing, is another substance that can inactivate pepsin. The chemical administered either p.o. or i.p. could protect the pyloric ligated rat against ulcers (Fletcher *et al.*, 1957). This agent was also active as an anticoagulant. The purified polymer (approximate molecular weight 5000) preparation of calcium lignosulfate (4-hydroxy-3-methoxy y-phenylpropane)$_n$ which is abbreviated LS$_5$ could protect rats from gastric ulcers (approximate oral ED$_{50}$ = 20 mg kg^{-1}) through inhibition of pepsin proteolysis and possessed minimal blood anticoagulant properties (Vocac and Alphin, 1968). The substance can also inhibit the digestion of egg albumin within the dog stomach (Alphin *et al.*, 1972). It did not decrease secretory volume or acidity. A series of twenty polymers of lignosulfates was studied and the majority demonstrated similar activities to LS$_5$ (Vocac and Alphin, 1969). Since this antipepsin activity does not parallel the sulfate content of this series of chemicals, the protective action must be due to some other chemical property.

Two relatively small molecules, bisdiazoketone 1, 1-bis-(diazoacetyl)-2-phenylethane and 1-diazoacetyl-2-phenylthane, were developed as chemical means of inactivating pepsin *in vitro*. These act stoichiometrically with pepsin in a 1:1 ratio (Husain *et al.*, 1971). Whether such an approach could yield a useful drug has not been explored.

7.2 CARRAGEENIN

Extensive studies have been reported on carrageenin, a naturally occurring sulfated polysaccharide, which is obtained from seaweed. The biological actions and possible toxicity of this polymer have been reviewed (Watt and Anderson, 1961; Editorial, 1962). For formulation reasons, carrageenin is degraded to decrease viscosity and gel formation. This procedure decreases the molecular weight from 100 000–700 000 to approximately 20 000 (Anderson, 1961). It is a branched polymer of galactose, containing approximately 1 mol of sulfate per mol of sugar (Houck *et al.*, 1960). Based on *in vitro* studies, the fraction with highest sulfate content is associated with the greatest antipeptic activity (Bonfils *et al.*, 1961; Ravin *et al.*, 1962; Figueroa and Klotz, 1963; Hawkins and Leonard, 1962; also see Table 4).

Degraded carrageenin, administered orally, protected against histamine-induced ulcers in guinea-pigs and dogs and against pyloric ligated and delta[1]-cortisol-induced gastric ulcers in rats (Anderson and Watt, 1959; Houck *et al.*, 1960). In comparison to heparin it possesses relatively weak anticoagulant activity (Hawkins and Leonard, 1962). The macromolecule on chronic administration can cause a 50 per cent reduction of volume and acidity of histamine-stimulated gastric juice in the guinea-pig (Anderson *et al.*, 1962). It prevents parietal cell hyperplasia caused by repeated injections of histamine to guinea-pigs (Anderson and Soman, 1965b). Carrageenin can also protect dogs against ulceration induced by the chronic endogenous release of gastrin without reducing the gastric acidity (Ellis and Nicoloff, 1969). Feeding carrageenin in doses of 20 g per day could not protect dogs against cinchophen-induced ulcers (Figueroa and Klotz, 1963). Nor could the drug protect guinea-pigs against aspirin-induced ulcers (Anderson, 1965).

The degraded carrageenin preparation Ebimar (Evans Medical Laboratories, Liverpool, England) is used clinically in Europe. Degraded carrageenin was administered at doses of 0·5–5 g orally to 60 people (10 normal, the rest with various gastric and other diseases). There was a marked decrease of peptic activity and acidity of gastric juice (Bonfils *et al.*, 1959). Several other uncontrolled trials suggest beneficial effects from degraded carrageenin (Lambling *et al.*, 1961; Esposito and Nicolini, 1961; Garcia, 1960; Bonfils *et al.*, 1965; Berthet, 1961). One study did compare degraded carrageenin and aluminum hydroxide in two separate series, consisting of a total of 35 and 53 patients respectively (Evans *et al.*, 1965). The two series were double-blind trials but clinical assessment and supervision were poorly controlled. Both drugs gave equally effective symptomatic relief but neither influenced the natural history of the disease. An objective double-blind clinical test has not been performed.

A postulated mechanism of action for the sulfated polysaccharides is complexation with the protein substrate thus protecting it from digestion by pepsin (Piper and Fenton, 1961b; Anderson, 1961; Martin *et al.*, 1968). It does not inhibit the effects of the enzyme pepsin. Thus, the ratio of protein substrate to sulfated polysaccharide determines the inhibition. The relative affinity of degraded carrageenin for a series of proteins is: hemoglobin, plasma protein, gastric-mucoprotein and pepsin, the latter three actions being very slight (Anderson, 1961). The affinity for the substrate was the same whether purified pepsin, gastricsin or whole gastric juice was used as the proteolytic enzyme (Anderson *et al.*, 1968), indicating that the nonenzymatic components of gastric juice have minimal effect on carrageenin-substrate interaction. This agent may reduce ulcers by several mechanisms. It may complex with the protein in the ulcer floor and protect it from further attack. Alternatively, it may complex with mucus, increasing its viscosity and preventing pepsin action. The disadvantage of such a mechanism is that the drug must first overcome the substrate competition from the protein in food. As for any chemical that works locally, the emptying rate of the stomach is a factor in maintaining an effective level of sulfated polysaccharide in the stomach.

The mechanism of action of the various pepsin inhibitors differs. Several of the sulfated polysaccharides complex with the protein substrate. The sulfated oxidized starch forms a complex with pepsin (Namekata, 1962c). The surfactants do not precipitate the substrate protein (Ravin et al., 1962). Degraded carrageenin, in addition to complexing with substrate, possesses an indirect effect on gastric secretion and lesion induction. This activity is present though degraded carrageenin is minimally absorbed from the gastrointestinal tract (Anderson and Soman, 1966b). When administered into the small bowel or subcutaneously, it can protect the animal against a gastric or duodenal insult (Anderson and Soman, 1966a; Eagleton et al., 1969). For example, carrageenin can prevent histamine-induced gastric ulcers when administered intraduodenally to pyloric ligated guinea-pigs (Anderson and Soman, 1963). This latter action may be due to carrageenin possessing a histaminase or diamine oxidase liberating effect since carrageenin can antagonize the actions of the histaminase inhibitor, aminoguanidine. The net effect is that the antiulcer effect of carrageenin is abolished by aminoguanidine (Anderson and Soman, 1966b). A single injection of 400 mg kg^{-1} s.c. of the drug can inhibit gastric secretions for more than 24 hours (Eagleton et al., 1968). This prolonged action may be due to a "depot" effect of carrageenin and the slow release of this drug from a relatively insoluble subcutaneous injection. The subcutaneous route of administration of carrageenin to the guinea-pig reduced histamine-induced gastric ulceration and protected against duodenal-induced ulceration (Eagleton et al., 1969). Paradoxically, it could not prevent subcutaneously administered betazole-induced secretions (Watt et al., 1966). This type of protection against histamine-induced lesions was not attributed to the local antipepsin action. Thus, part of the antiulcer effect may be due to binding with histamine or releasing diamine oxidase. This action may be in addition to complex formation with the substrate.

Is it possible to prevent the pepsin activity by reducing its synthesis? Gossypol, a yellow, polycyclic phenol obtained from cottonseed, can bind pepsinogen in vitro, and prevent the conversion of pepsinogen to pepsin (Wong *et al.*, 1972; Finlay *et al.*, 1973). This may be another approach to reduce the amount of pepsin present in the stomach.

7.3 SULFATED AMYLOPECTIN (SN-263, DEPEPSIN®)

A rational approach to develop a synthetic sulfated polysaccharide was undertaken by the people in Searle's Research Laboratories (Cook *et al.*, 1963). A series of polysaccharides differing in size, shape, nature of constituent sugars and configuration of glucosidic linkage were sulfated and assessed for various biological activities. Several of the larger macromolecules were active in inhibiting pepsin digestion *in vitro* and in reducing ulcers in the pyloric ligated rat. This action, though not a perfect correlation, seemed to vary directly with sulfate content and molecular size of the molecule. Detailed pharmacological and clinical studies were done on SN-263 or Depepsin®, one of the synthetic inhibitors. This substance is a sodium salt of sulfated potato amylopectin which has 1·6 sulfate groups per glucose molecule which contains 15–16·5 per cent sulfur and has a molecular weight of 2×10^7 to 8×10^7. SN-263 could protect the rat against pyloric ligation-induced-ulcers without affecting gastric juice or titratable acidity. The proteolytic activity of the gastric juice decreased with increasing dosage of SN-263. The drug was also effective against cortisone-induced gastric ulcers in rats, histamine-induced duodenal ulcers in guinea-pigs, but not against reserpine-, or indomethacin-induced ulcers in the rat. SN-263, given every 4 hours for 60 days (dose not given) could protect dogs against ulceration produced by the endogenous release of gastrin (Ellis and Nicoloff, 1969). The agent does prolong blood clotting time, being half as active as heparin (Bianchi and Cook, 1964; Cook and Drill, 1967; Lee *et al.*, 1971). SN-263 appears effective in preventing experimental lesions.

A symposium on gastric pepsin and mucus contained several reports on SN-263 (Sun, 1967a). It was confirmed that SN-263 could inhibit pepsin *in vitro* (Klotz, 1967; Texter *et al.*, 1967). In man, SN-263 could also inhibit pepsin activity stimulated by a test meal (Klotz, 1967). In noncontrolled clinical studies, SN-263 in a dose of 500 mg 6 times daily apparently could relieve the symptoms of patients with peptic ulcers (Cayer and Ruffin, 1967; Sun, 1967b). The agent in doses of 100–800 mg could significantly decrease gastric peptic activity. The effect of the higher dose lasted for approximately 75 minutes. The gastric acidity was not altered. The antipepsin activity of SN-263 could be enhanced by concurrent administration of an anticholinergic agent. Presumably the latter delayed stomach emptying and prolonged the direct contact of SN-263 with the gastric contents.

Several carefully controlled double-blind clinical trials have given conflicting results (Zimmon *et al.*, 1969; Sun and Ryan, 1970; Cocking, 1972). Zimmon demonstrated an enhanced healing rate of gastric lesions in 10 inpatients receiving SN-263 for five weeks. No other medication was used. In man, SN-263 has an affinity to bind in the gastric ulcer crater (Zimmon and Mazzola, 1973). This demonstrates an important substrate-binding action for SN-263. The mucosal surface coating may also prolong the duration of action of this antipepsin drug. In Sun's study, the recurrence of symptoms in 75 chronic duodenal ulcer patients receiving various drugs for 1 year were: 75 per cent in the placebo, 39 per cent in the propanthelene-treated group (15 mg, 4 times daily), 16 per cent in the SN-263 (250 mg every 2 hours during waking periods) treated group and 12 per cent in the group receiving both SN-263 and propanthelene. A recurrence was defined as the reappearance of ulcer-like symptoms for more than 3 days. Cocking's results indicate that SN-263 (500 mg at 3-hour intervals) and propanthelene (15 mg 3 times daily and 30 mg at night), either alone or in combination, were no more effective than placebo in controlling the symptoms of 65 chronic duodenal ulcer patients for a period of 48 weeks. Two editorials commenting on the latter two trials (Littman and Chalmers, 1970; Littman, 1972) emphasize the minor differences between these two studies. It is possible on a statistical basis to periodically obtain either a false negative or a false positive result. The problem of conducting objective clinical trials is clearly exemplified. The solution to the problem is not readily available. Does SN-263 have a greater differential effect against gastric than duodenal peptic ulcers? We shall have to await further objective studies, e.g. the use of the fiberscope to assess duodenal healing, before final clinical assessment can be made on SN-263 or any other antiulcer drug.

7.4 PEPSTATINS

An antibiotic, isovaleryl-L-valyl-L-valyl-4-amino-3-hydroxy-6-methyl-heptanoyl-L-alanyl-4-amino-3-hydroxy-6-methylheptanoic acid, called pepstatin A, was the first to be isolated from culture filtrates of streptomycetes and purified (Umezawa *et al.*, 1970; Morishima *et al.*, 1970). It is a polypeptide that is effective in *in vitro* inhibition of pepsin digestion of albumin. It could protect against lesions in the 22-hour pyloric ligated rat. Apparent effects were evident at doses as low as 0.5 mg kg^{-1} orally. This dose also decreased the pepsin activity of the gastric juice. Neither the volume nor pH were affected by pepstatin A. Pepstatin A binds tightly to pepsin in an equimolar ratio (Kunimoto *et al.*, 1972). In titrating pepsin with pepstatin A, the binding ratio is 1 mg pepstatin A to 65 mg of pepsin. Considering that the molecular weight of pepstatin A and pepsin are 686 and 35 000 respectively, there must be a $1:1$ molecule combination. Pepstatin A also inhibits the *in vitro* and *in vivo* effects of renin (Miller *et al.*, 1972) and can lower blood pressure in rats (Lazar *et al.*, 1972). It can also inhibit cathepsin D, obtained as a pig brain proteinase (Marks *et al.*, 1973). A comparison of the inhibitory action (Table 5) has been reported for pepstatin A and several analogues against pepsin,

$$
\begin{array}{c}
\text{CH}_3 \qquad\qquad\qquad\qquad \text{CH}_3 \\
\text{CH}_3 \quad \text{CH}_3 \quad \text{CHCH}_3 \qquad\qquad \text{CHCH}_3 \\
\text{CHCH}_3 \quad \text{CHCH}_3 \quad \text{CH}_2\,\text{OH} \qquad \text{CH}_3 \quad \text{CH}_2\,\text{R}_2 \\
\text{R}_1\text{NHCHCONHCHCONHCH}-\text{CHCH}_2\text{CONHCHCONHCH}-\text{CHCH}_2\text{R}_3
\end{array}
$$

	R_1	R_2	R_3
Pepstatin A	isovaleryl	H⟨OH	—COOH
Pepstatin B	caproyl	H⟨OH	—COOH
Pepstatin C	isocaproyl	H⟨OH	—COOH
Pepstatin D	heptanoyl	H⟨OH	—COOH
Pepstatin E	isoheptanoyl	H⟨OH	—COOH
Pepstatin F	anteisoheptanoyl	H⟨OH	—COOH
Pepstatin G	capryl	H⟨OH	—COOH
Pepstatin H	isocapryl	H⟨OH	—COOH
Pepstanone A	isovaleryl	=O	—H

TABLE 5

Biological inhibitory activities of pepstatins

Structural variations of pepstatins

	ID_{50} (μg ml^{-1})		
	Pepsin	Renin	Cathepsin D
Pepstatin A	0·01	4·5	0·011
Pepstatin B	0·01	3·0	0·0003
Pepstatin F	0·01	1·8	0·002
Pepstatin G	0·01	1·2	0·003
Pepstanone A	0·013	25	not examined

Adapted from Aoyagi *et al.* (1972).

cathepsin D and renin (Aoyagi *et al.*, 1972). Further trials on this potent pepsin inhibitor should help elucidate the role of pepsin in ulcer diseases.

7.5 ENDOGENOUS PEPSIN INHIBITORS

The gastric mucus has been postulated to contain an antipepsin factor which prevents the autodigestion of gastric mucosa (see Babkin, 1950, for review of early concepts). The early workers had demonstrated that various mucus components, e.g. chondroitin sulfuric acid, or mucoitin sulfuric acid, inhibited the peptic activity of canine gastric juice. In a completely uncontrolled study, 12 patients with gastric ulcers were given a crude preparation of "gastric mucin" and observed some relief of symptoms (Fogelson, 1931). More recently, several biological substances, heparin, chondroitin sulfate and sodium polyhydromanuronic acid (a purified heparin), were shown to inhibit pepsin *in vitro* and to protect against ulceration (Anderson *et al.*, 1968; Barnes *et al.*, 1967; Piper and Fenton, 1961b; Houck *et al.*, 1960; Placer *et al.*, 1958; Bonfils *et al.*, 1960; Levey and Sheinfeld, 1954). These antipepsin agents can be depleted by ulcerogenic procedures like restraint or the administration of cinchophen (Häkkinen *et al.*, 1966; and Häkkinen and Hartiala, 1966). Hyaluronic acid, which contains no sulfate groups, and sodium sulfate are inactive *in vitro* (Levey and Sheinfeld, 1954). The anionic moiety may be important for this macromolecule to exert antipepsin activity.

In a pyloric ligated rat, the intragastric administration of a gastric mucus preparation from hog stomach protected the animal against ulcers. The ester sulfate moieties of mucus were essential for this protective action because blocking them with protamines eliminated the protective action of the mucus. The mucus protective action could be increased by chemically increasing the sulfate content of the material (Placer *et al.*, 1958). Sulfated glycosaminoglycans are normal constituents of gastric cells which may be the physiological substance by which intracellular pepsinogen disruption is normally prevented. At low concentrations, this substance may enhance pepsinogen release (Anderson, 1969). Both a natural, named GLP, and a sulfated glycopeptide, named GLPS, obtained by sulfuration of GLP (14 per cent sulfur molecular weight 81 000) were derived from pig duodenum. GLPS when given orally could protect rats against pyloric ligation-hydrocortisone-, or restraint-induced ulcers (Bertellini *et al.*, 1971; Prino, 1971). It was also active i.v. or i.p. in preventing pyloric ligated-induced ulcers and in reducing acid and pepsin secretion. GLPS at 1 mg kg^{-1} i.v. could also antagonize dibutyryl cAMP-, histamine-, pentagastrin-, bethanechol-, but not theophylline-induced secretions in the perfused rat stomach preparation (Niada and Prino, 1973).

It is surprising that GLPS is effective by the parenteral route since it is essentially not absorbed from the gastrointestinal tract of rat, dog, or man (Chasseaud *et al.*, 1972). GLPS, given orally, could protect guinea-pigs against histamine-induced gastric or duodenal lesions (Prino *et al.*, 1972a). Lesions of the stomach were less severe in animals dosed with 100 mg kg^{-1}. A higher dose (245 mg kg^{-1}) was needed to decrease the small bowel lesions though complete protection was not obtainable at even higher doses of GLPS. Pepsin was inhibited at doses less than 100 mg kg^{-1}. In a clinical study, GLPS at 50 mg orally inhibited the peptic activity of human gastric juice within 15 minutes (Prino *et al.*, 1972b). The agent also has the ability to reversibly bind to gastric and intestinal mucosa for several hours (Chasseaud *et al.*, 1972). A sulfated galactopyranose, called DB 1550, has also been implicated in preventing or reducing the incidence of animal and clinical ulcers (Tournut and Boisson, 1973). These biological substance derivatives may prove useful in ulcer therapy. Current literature does not lead to a firm conclusion at this time.

Heparin can exert antipepsin actions *in vitro* (Levey and Sheinfeld, 1954; Houck *et al.*, 1960). Heparin i.v. given to a series of dogs can inhibit a broad spectrum of secretogogue actions. It could markedly suppress the secretion induced by food, insulin, methacholine, histamine, gastrin, and local antral stimulation with acetylcholine (Lerner and Thompson, 1963; Thompson *et al.*, 1966a). Heparin also decreased insulin- or histamine-stimulated acid output in normal and duodenal ulcer patients (Thompson *et al.*, 1966b).

An *in vitro* pepsin inhibitor may also be present in the pituitary (Hilliard and West, 1957; Carsten and Pierce, 1957). The polypeptide fragments produced when pepsingogen is split in acid media may also inhibit pepsin (Anderson and Harthill, 1973). Further studies are needed on the biological properties of these biological substances.

8 Enhanced healing rate of mucosal lesions

It is difficult to objectively assess drugs in either man or animals that apparently enhance the healing of gastrointestinal lesions. Several agents reputed to possess enhanced healing properties were first introduced clinically, and then characterized for their pharmacological properties. Many of the factors controlling mucosal healing are still to be identified and verified. The current specific animal models, e.g. stress ulcers, histamine-induced, drug-induced, or burn lesions are highly variable and much more time consuming to assess than simple antisecretory tests.

Possibly the acetic acid-induced lesion rat model (Takagi *et al.*, 1970) may prove useful in assessing drugs that increase tissue granulation. Thus more objective criteria in both man and animals are needed to evaluate healing of a mucosal lesion. In general such a drug should find an important place in therapy. Presumably it would be devoid of autonomic action and possess local regenerative properties. This would minimize systemic toxicity. Below are several candidates for this type of agent.

8.1   GERANYL FARNESYLACETATE (GEFARNATE)

This drug was discovered in 1958 at the research laboratories of the Istituto De Angeli, Milano, Italy. Professor E. Adami was a principle investigator in this discovery, and an Italian and English review by him is available from the Institute. The basis of the discovery was an attempt to isolate and identify an alleged antiulcer factor present in fresh vegetables, particularly white-headed cabbages (Cheney, 1940; 1950). This approach was unsuccessful but did lead to the investigation of a series of terpine derivatives (Adami *et al.*, 1962). This series, evaluated for their protective action against histamine-induced lesions in guinea-pigs, led to the selection of gefarnate as the active member of the series (**18**). Gefarnate, a water-insoluble, fat-soluble substance, consists of three isoprene units (farnesol) linked to two isoprene units (geraniol) through an acetate grouping.

Geranyl farnesylacetate (gefarnate)

(**18**)

Gefarnate has no demonstrable antisecretory action in pyloric ligated rats and is virtually devoid of anticholinergic, ganglionic blocking or antihistaminic properties (Adami *et al.*, 1964). Its gastric action is mainly demonstrated by enhanced healing or prevention of a variety of experimental gastric ulcers in three animal species (Table 6). The table

TABLE 6

Gefarnate effect on various types of experimental ulcer

Type of ulcer	Animal species	Kind of test	Dose (mg kg^{-1}) and route of administration		Result	Reference
Histamine-induced	guinea-pig	curative	1·25	s.c.	active	Adami et al. (1964)
			1·25	oral	active	
Restraint	rat	preventive	50	s.c.	active	
Reserpine-induced	adrenalec-tonized rat	preventive	20	i.p.	active	
			50	i.p.	active	
Fasting	rat	preventive	20	i.p.	active	Adami et al. (1966)
Pyloric, ligated	rat	preventive	10	s.c.	active	
			10	oral	inactive	
Pyloric, ligated	rat	preventive	100	i.p.	active	
Reserpine-induced	rat	preventive	100	i.p.	active	
Fasting	rat	preventive	100	i.p.	active	Ichiki and Isoda (1973)
Mann–Williamson	dog	curative	50	s.c.	active	
	dog	curative	100	oral	active	Marullo and Cuzzocrea (1964)
Pyloric, ligated	rat	preventive	120	i.m.	active	Mori et al. (1964)
Induced by excision of a portion of gastric mucosa	rat	curative	100	s.c.	active (histologic and histochemical evaluation)	
Indomethacin-induced	rat	curative	200	oral	active (spectrofluorimetric evaluation of Schiff positive gastric mucins)	Mori et al. (1969)
Prednisolone-induced	rat	preventive	20	oral	active	Murari (1964)
Phenylbutazone-induced	rat	preventive	20	oral	active	
Stress ulcer-induced	rat	preventive	200	oral	inactive	Takagi and Okabe (1968)
By immersion in cold water	rat	curative	100	oral	active	
			100	s.c.	active	

contains the references and the variety of tests in which gefarnate has altered lesion formation.

The most convincing experimental evidence for the antiulcer action of gefarnate was obtained in the Mann–Williamson dog ulcer preparation, which is considered to be a good model of duodenal ulcers in man (Ichiki and Isoda, 1973). The ulcer in an untreated preparation has no tendency toward spontaneous healing, is progressive and ultimately perforates, causing morbidity and death of the animal. Gefarnate was used in such a dog preparation by the s.c. route (50 mg kg^{-1}) daily in 6 animals, orally (100 mg kg^{-1}) daily in 7 animals and compared to 6 operated, untreated dogs. All treated animals survived a 30-day period, whereas 4 out of 6 untreated animals died within one to three weeks. Macroscopic ulcers were less frequent and enteritis was absent in the treated dogs. Histologically, the few ulcers in the treated animals showed signs of granulation and an absence of progressive degeneration and edema in the surrounding ulcer area. Thus the drug was effective by the oral and parenteral route of administration in reducing experimental ulcer in the dog.

The mode of action of gefarnate is speculative. It is not a simple local action, since it can alter an ulcerogenic situation via either oral or parenteral administration. It appears more regenerative than protective in animal models (Takagi and Okabe, 1968). Mucosal hexosamine levels are decreased in rats by stress and cortisone treatment. These tissue levels of hexosamine gradually return to normal eight days after the insult. Gefarnate enhances the return, normal levels of hexosamine being present in three days (Takagi and Yano, 1972). It has also been speculated to increase acid mucopolysaccharides of gastric mucosa in experimental ulcers in rats (Mori et al., 1969), to protect capillary vessels (Marullo and Cuzzocrea, 1964), and to possess an antihyaluronidase activity (Adami et al., 1964). It can increase the O_2 uptake of heart and liver tissue (rat), which is indicative of metabolic activation (Adami et al., 1964). The chemical can also prevent or reduce the rise of uropepsinogen levels in man or that induced in the rat by stress, pyloric ligation, reserpine, or fasting lesion-producing preparations (Adami et al., 1966; Pastor Franco, 1966).

Pharmacokinetic studies in the rat with ^{14}C-labelled drug indicate that either after oral or intramuscular route, it is rapidly absorbed and is slowly metabolized in a 24-hour period (Coppi et al., 1969). It is found mainly in the liver as well as in other organs including the digestive tract. Approximately 30 per cent of ^{14}C-drug is recovered in the urine and some in expired air as ^{14}CO$_2$. The drug is singularly devoid of other pharmacological activity. It lacks diuretic, antiinflammatory, analgesic, local anesthetic actions and does not modify blood pressure, respiration, or glucose blood levels. Gefarnate has a very low toxicity; its LD_{50} in mice could only be determined by the intravenous route and was $\sim 2 \cdot 8$ g kg^{-1} (Adami et al., 1964). The definitive mechanism of action of gefarnate awaits elucidation.

Clinically, an impressive number of case records have been accumulated by the Angeli Institute. Gefarnate has a widespread use in Italy and in other countries but is not available in the United States. I shall not attempt to review the clinical literature. An extensive list of tables is available from the Angeli Institute. To date, close to 3000 case records have been analyzed, of which 210 involve pediatric gastrointestinal problems. In the adult group, 1518 were suffering from various forms of peptic ulcers, 214 from gastritis, duodenitis and gastroduodenitis, forty from dyspepsia induced by corticosteroid treatment and 111 from colitis and rectocolitis. These clinical series include various standards like clinical (remission of symptomatology), radiographic, endoscopic evaluations and/or uropepsinogen level determinations. Gefarnate was used either intramuscularly (daily dose of 50 to 100 mg) or orally (daily dose 150 to 400 mg) from 10 to 210 days, depending on the test.

The drug appears highly effective in eliminating both the ulcer pain and reducing or "healing" the ulcer. For example, in the clinical studies of the various types of peptic ulcers (1283 patients) gefarnate was effective in 93 per cent of the patients. These were both gastric and duodenal lesions. The results of a double-blind radiological study by Newcomb et al. (1970) is an example of the type of results reported in the literature. This was carried out at various centers on 20 outpatients with gastric ulcers. Each group of 10 patients received either gefarnate (150 mg daily by oral route) or placebo. Treatment lasted 4 weeks. Radiological studies indicated that the ulcer niche in the gefarnate treated group was reduced by 72 per cent, as compared to only a 20 per cent reduction in the placebo group.

Other mucosal aberrations also appear to respond to the drug. Gastritis, colitis, rectocolitis and corticosteroid-induced mucosal changes appear responsive to therapy. In addition, pediatric studies indicate a positive response of conditions requiring a high regenerative and protective action on the digestive mucosa. The drug has been used after extensive antibiotic therapy and malabsorption syndromes. In the latter condition, gefarnate treatment allowed the return to a normal dietary regimen.

The drug appears as a new therapeutic agent in a complex field of peptic ulcers and other disorders of the digestive mucosa. Both the experimental and clinical data, plus the virtual absence of toxicity in man or animal ranks gefarnate as an agent of high therapeutic value. Studies indicate a reasonably effective agent in relieving gastrointestinal symptoms with a negligible amount of side effects. We await with interest to see whether gefarnate will replace current therapeutic ulcer regimens. This latter action would be the test that the drug is acceptable to both physician and patient.

8.2 LIQUORICE DERIVATIVES

Since ancient times, liquorice has been used as a flavour in candy and in a variety of medical concoctions. In modern medicine, it has found use as a demulcent and an expectorant. In 1946, a Dutch physician, Revers, noticed that some of his patients with peptic ulcers were greatly improved after taking a proprietary preparation containing liquorice. He started to utilize a liquorice preparation in his practice, but the treatment was abandoned (Doll *et al.*, 1962). The apparent benefit of the crude liquorice has led to the introduction of several preparations for experimental and clinical studies.

8.3 CARBENOXOLONE

Carbenoxolone sodium is an example of a substance that is synthesized from the glycoside, glycyrrhizic acid, a sweet substance which is one of a large number of substances present in liquorice root. Hydrolysis of the glycoside yields glycyrrhetinic acid. The active drug is the disodium salt of glycyrrhetinic acid hemisuccinate with the generic name of carbenoxolone (**19**). The drug is in two trade preparations, Biogastrone® and Duogastrone®. It was synthesized by Turner and Watton, at Biorex Laboratories, London, England (Brown *et al.*, 1959b). The action and clinical trials of carbenoxolone have been discussed at three symposia (Robson and Sullivan, 1968; Baron and Sullivan, 1970; Avery Jones and Sullivan, 1972). The detailed pharmacology has been documented by Sullivan and others in the above three symposia. A review is also available (Sircus, 1972).

The antiulcer activity of carbenoxolone in animals is difficult to demonstrate (Sullivan, 1972). Early studies of carbenoxolone on lesions induced by restraint or serotonin in rats showed no healing rate changes. The difficulty of assessing an animal model can be seen in the following experiments. Using cold, restraint-stressed rats, it was demonstrated that carbenoxolone had significant antiulcer activity following intraperitoneal administration in nonfasted but no protective action in either 24- or 48-hour fasted animals. The oral administration had no protection even in the nonfasted rat (Perkins and Vars, 1973). Several other positive

Disodium salt of glycyrrhetinic acid hemisuccinate
Carbenoxolone

(19)

models have been reported. Carbenoxolone can enhance the healing rate of electrocautery-induced gastric lesions in the rat (Sullivan, 1972). Pretreatment of rats with carbenoxolone for two weeks will give some protection against a low ulcerogenic dose of compound 48/80 (Dean, 1968). In another chronic dosing (for 1 week) experiment, carbenoxolone could give some protection to the guinea-pig against stress-induced lesions (Lipkin and Ludwig, 1968). In both of these latter experiments the authors attribute the protection to an enhanced mucus production. Prednisolone-induced ulcers in rats can also be prevented by carbenoxolone pretreatment (Hoffmeister and Hoffmeister, 1971). Thus careful handling of ulcerogenic drug doses and animal preparation can yield a model for testing this type of agent.

The difficulty in demonstrating the healing of gastric ulcers in the rat by oral carbenoxolone may be related to the different metabolism of the drug by rat (Iveson et al., 1966; Parke, 1967) and man (Parke et al., 1972a; 1972b). In patients with gastric ulcers, the isotope form of carbenoxolone appears as 70–80 per cent in the faeces, 0·2–1 per cent in urine and 12–20 per cent as expired radioactive CO_2. In contrast, in the rat, ^{14}C-carbenoxolone given orally is excreted as 60–75 per cent as $^{14}CO_2$, 12–35 per cent in faeces and 2 per cent in urine. Rats pretreated with orally administered antibiotics metabolize carbenoxolone similarly to man. These findings suggest that carbenoxolone given orally to rat is hydrolyzed into β-glycyrrhetic acid and succinate by the bacteria in the rat stomach. Thus in the rat, the drug is altered before it is absorbed. This also suggests that the parent compound and not its metabolite is the antiulcer agent.

Possibly, carbenoxolone exerts its action topically. However, it is difficult to attribute its action in the stomach to absorption across the gastric mucosa. In man, the drug is best absorbed when ingested on an empty stomach and gives progressively lower blood levels if taken after a light or heavy meal respectively (Parke et al., 1972b). This indicates that blood levels correlate best when carbenoxolone has access to the small intestine. Alternately, the food in the stomach prevents the absorption of the drug. In contrast to the above study, several other studies in man are interpreted to suggest that stomach absorption is relatively complete (Parke *et al.*, 1972a; Parke, 1972). Carbenoxolone is a weak acid and in its nonionized form is highly lipid soluble. It also gives higher blood levels when given to an individual with a normal (pH $\cong 2$) acid stomach than when preceded by the administration of an alkali (Downer *et al.*, 1970). These properties are interpreted to be indicative of stomach absorption.

In distribution studies, carbenoxolone possesses an extensive bile excretory rate in man and rat since 80 per cent of an oral dose can be collected in the bile (Parke *et al.*, 1963). One of the drug's outstanding features is its affinity for plasma proteins in rat, dog, monkey and man. Over 99·9 per cent of the drug in the blood is protein bound. The drug, if given parenterally to rats, is excreted across the gut wall and binds to various areas of the mucosa. Aldosterone administered at different concentrations subcutaneously to carbenoxolone-pretreated rats can displace the drug from nonspecific renal binding sites. The competitive nature of carbenoxolone and aldosterone is detailed in a study on the subcellular distribution of the two substances in various tissue fractions of the kidney (Humphrey *et al.*, 1972). This displacement results in potentiation of aldosterone by carbenoxolone which may account for the mineralocorticoid side effects seen in humans. The ability of carbenoxolone to potentiate aldosterone is in agreement with *in vitro* studies on the frog skin (Porter, 1970). Thus the avid binding properties of carbenoxolone may be the reason for its gastric healing properties as well as its edema-producing side effects.

Carbenoxolone does possess other pharmacological actions. At oral doses of 12·5 to 200 mg kg^{-1}, it can give a dose-dependent decrease in the peptic activity of gastric secretions from a 4-hour pyloric ligated rat preparation. Carbenoxolone also possesses *in vitro* antipeptic activity (Henman, 1970). The antipepsin activity has been confirmed in *in vitro* studies on human gastric juice. Also, carbenoxolone at 100 mg orally to man can reduce the peptic activity of gastric juice by a mean of 52 per cent. The effect lasted for 40–60 minutes (Berstad, 1972). This antipepsin activity in man could not be confirmed (Ivey and Gray, 1973b; Domschke *et al.*, 1972). In man, carbenoxolone increases the appearance of visible mucus in gastric aspirates. It does not change volume or pH (Hausmann and Tárnoky, 1966). At laparotomy, people previously treated with carbenoxolone have a gastric mucosa covered by extensive amounts of viscid adherent mucus (Goodier *et al.*, 1967). In an *in vitro* study, carbenoxolone inhibited gastric histidine decarboxylase from converting histidine to histamine. Since other antiinflammatory drugs exert the same action, this carbenoxolone effect does not appear to be unique (Skidmore and Whitehouse, 1966). In the rat, the drug has one-third the antiinflammatory properties of hydrocortisone. This action may be due to potentiating endogenous corticosteroids. It is paradoxical to see both antiinflammatory and antiulcer actions in the same molecule, since most antiinflammatory agents are ulcerogenic rather than protective. The drug also possesses marked antidiuretic and sodium-retaining activity. Carbenoxolone is devoid of autonomic nervous system activity. It does not alter the action of histamine, 5-hydroxytryptamine, nicotine or barium on isolated smooth muscle. It is also devoid of *in vivo* effects on motility (Finney and Tárnoky, 1960).

It has also been postulated that carbenoxolone may heal gastric ulcers by its ability to reduce the back diffusion of hydrogen ions. In the dog with a Heidenhain pouch, carbenoxolone in the pouch could reduce the back diffusion of hydrogen ions induced by an instillation of human bile (Cross and Rhodes, 1972). In human volunteers, carbenoxolone, orally as a single 100-mg dose or 300 mg in three divided doses, over a three-week sequence of dosing, did not alter the back diffusion of hydrogen ions caused by the intragastric instillation of taurocholic acid (Ivey and Gray, 1973a). A similar acute or chronic carbenoxolone regimen in patients with gastric ulcers also failed to alter the permeability to 160 mM HCl (Ivey and Gray, 1973b). The "trapped" drug in the dog's pouch may reach a higher concentration than is obtainable in the stomach of man. In any event, it is not practical to use higher doses in man since 100 mg three times daily is already associated with a high incidence of side effects.

Objective, impressive evidence is available that carbenoxolone is effective clinically for enhancing the healing rate of gastric ulcers in a group of outpatients (Doll et al., 1962). In a double-blind study, carbenoxolone as either the disodium salt or the acid or a placebo was given orally at 100 mg 3 times a day to 50 outpatients with gastric ulcers. The gastric lesions of the individuals were examined radiologically before the therapy and five weeks after continuous therapy. The drug was highly effective in comparison with the placebo in reducing the size or eliminating the gastric ulcers. There was no significant decrease in the incidence of pain between the two groups. In a separate study on 46 patients, the healing benefits and the unaltered effect on pain was confirmed within the same institution (Doll et al., 1965). In another group of 42 patients with duodenal ulcers, Doll et al. (1962) could not demonstrate that carbenoxolone had any significant effect on either the pain pattern or small bowel lesion history. The enhanced healing of gastric ulcers was confirmed in other clinical trials. Table 7 summarizes the results of

TABLE 7

Clinical trials of carbenoxolone in gastric ulcer

Investigator	Number studied	Outpatients or in hospital	Response
Doll *et al.* (1962)	50	ambulant	benefit
Doll *et al.* (1965)	46	ambulant	benefit
Horwich and Galloway (1965)	33	ambulant	benefit
Middleton *et al.* (1965)	31	in hospital	no benefit
Turpie and Thomson (1965)	12	in hospital	benefit
Scobie (1966)	23	in hospital	no benefit
Bank *et al.* (1967)	20	ambulant	benefit
de Marcos Perez (1967)	27	ambulant	benefit
Montgomery (1967)	70	ambulant	benefit
Doll *et al.* (1968a)	56	ambulant	benefit
Doyle *et al.* (1968)	27	in hospital	benefit
Cocking and MacCaig (1969)	36	ambulant	benefit
Geismar and Mosbech (1970)	8	ambulant	no benefit
MacCaig (1970)	53	ambulant	benefit
Ottenjahn and Rosch (1970)	36	ambulant	benefit
Kunz (1971)	9	in hospital	benefit
Lenz *et al.* (1971)	7	ambulant	benefit
Rosch and Ottenjahn (1971)	70	ambulant	benefit
Stadelmann *et al.* (1972)	41	ambulant	benefit
Von Schiemann (1972)	33	ambulant	benefit
Wilson (1972)	37	ambulant	no benefit
Geismar *et al.* (1973)	34	ambulant	no benefit
Langman *et al.* (1973)	33	ambulant	benefit
Wolf (1973)	24	in hospital	no benefit

several of these studies. The majority report that carbenoxolone had real benefit. Since bed rest alone is an effective way of treating gastric lesions, carbenoxolone is less effective in enhancing an ongoing healing effect. Thus the drug appears more effective in outpatient trials than for treating patients confined to a hospital.

Carbenoxolone produces serious side effects. In most clinical trials, approximately one-fifth of the patients treated with carbenoxolone demonstrate an aldosterone-like response. Patients develop reversible hypertension which may be associated with water retention and hypokalemia. Thus the drug must be used under good medical management. The following should be monitored in patients receiving carbenoxolone, serum potassium, bicarbonate and glutamic pyruvic transaminase (Hausmann and Tárnoky, 1966). To minimize side effects but retain ulcer healing, carbenoxolone was administered in combination with either spironolactone or a thiazide derivative to outpatients with gastric ulcers (Doll et al., 1968a). The spironolactone blocked both the side effects and the healing properties of carbenoxolone! In contrast, the thiazide diuretic did not interfere with the healing property of carbenoxolone. Unfortunately, it is not practical to treat patients with gastric ulcers with both carbenoxolone and thiazide diuretics.

Two mechanisms are possible for the aldosterone-like action. (i) Carbenoxolone may stimulate the adrenals to produce aldosterone, inhibit aldosterone metabolism or displace aldosterone from binding sites. These effects should lead to higher excretion of aldosterone. (ii) Carbenoxolone possesses intrinsic aldosterone-like action. In this instance, aldosterone secretion and excretion would be suppressed. A study indicates that carbenoxolone can cause a decrease in plasma aldosterone levels (Baron et al., 1969). Spironolactone, an aldosterone antagonist, can block carbenoxolone's therapeutic and side effects (Doll et al., 1968a). Aldosterone-like actions are still evident when carbenoxolone is administered to either adrenalectomized rats or dogs (Sullivan, 1972). Thus carbenoxolone apparently possesses intrinsic aldosterone-like actions.

Data on the relapse rate of gastric ulcers in patients after carbenoxolone treatment is still needed. In one study, patients who had healed gastric ulcers following carbenoxolone therapy had a relapse rate similar to other forms of therapy, e.g. bed rest (Montgomery et al., 1969). There was a 25 per cent recurrent ulceration within 12 months of healing. This was not prevented by a maintenance dose of 25 mg twice a day.

Summing up possible modes of action for carbenoxolone, it does have a direct binding affinity for gastric mucosa and enhances the secretion of gastric mucus. It can possibly inhibit pepsin. It is also excreted in high concentrations in the bile which may be of benefit in the ulcer patient. The drug can decrease the turnover rate of gastric cells in the mouse stomach. This increased life span could decrease the requirement for cell replacement. The unfortunate side effects of the drug suggest that an agent with similar healing actions without aldosterone-like properties is needed (Langman, 1968b).

A comparative trial between carbenoxolone and gefarnate was performed in the same institute (Langman et al., 1973). A total of 73 randomized patients with gastric ulcers received for 4 weeks either carbenoxolone 100 mg three times daily or gefarnate 50 mg four times daily. A succeeding group of patients received gefarnate at 100 and 200 mg four times daily. Both drugs significantly reduced the diameter of the gastric ulcer, though carbenoxolone was superior to even the higher doses of gefarnate. The ulcers healed an average of 80·6 and 51·7 per cent respectively as shown on radiological examination. The incidence of side effects was greater with carbenoxolone than with gefarnate.

People with gastric or duodenal ulcers respond differently to carbenoxolone. Doll *et al.* (1962) first reported that carbenoxolone sodium tablets were ineffective in treating duodenal ulcers. Since the drug may be absorbed or bound mainly in the stomach, its ineffectivness against duodenal ulcers may be that insufficient concentrations of original drug reach the small bowel. A "positioned-release" capsule was developed to deliver carbenoxolone into the duodenum (Galloway, 1968; Hunt, 1972). This medication consists of a mixture of 50 mg carbenoxolone combined with sugar and small amounts of tartaric acid and sodium bicarbonate. The production of gas swells the capsule and the hypertonic sugar concentration absorbs fluid. This expanded mass enters the antral area, is ruptured by the antral contractions and theoretically delivers the carbenoxolone to the duodenum. Studies with X-rays indicate that 80–90 per cent of the capsules do rupture in the antrum.

Several clinical trials with carbenoxolone in a "position-release" capsule were reported at the first carbenoxolone symposium (Robson and Sullivan, 1968). Since it is difficult to assess objectively the healing of duodenal ulcers, several of these preliminary trials are controversial, not properly controlled and lead to equivocal conclusions. Also, the evidence that the carbenoxolone is really "delivered" to the duodenum is weak. A series of controversial, equivocal results were again presented at the second symposium (Baron and Sullivan, 1970). Several of these studies on the use of carbenoxolone for duodenal ulcers have been reported in the conventional journals (Montgomery *et al.*, 1968; Amure, 1970; Cliff and Milton-Thompson, 1970). Problems of dosage, delivery systems and assessment of the small bowel lesion do not permit the conclusion that carbenoxolone is beneficial in treating duodenal ulcers.

8.4 LAUROYLGLYCYRRHETIC ACID (BX24)

The effect of a carbenoxolone analogue, BX24, on gastric ulcers in man was studied in outpatients for four weeks (Fraser *et al.*, 1972). Doses of BX24 at 300, 600, or 1200 mg were not clinically useful. The drug was also devoid of aldosterone-like properties. The pharmacology of the analogue is not available in the literature. In the same report, BX24 combined with zinc sulfate tended to heal gastric ulcers better than either substance alone. This combination will require confirmation before it is accepted therapy.

8.5 DEGLYCYRRHIZINATED LIQUORICE

A commercial preparation with the trade name Caved-S®, consists of several antacids, frangula bark, and powdered liquorice which has had the glycyrrhetinic acid, the aglycone of glycyrrhizic acid removed. Favorable results were reported in a subjective study on 30 patients with duodenal ulcers (Gassman and Forster, 1963). This has led to several other studies which yielded conflicting results. In a double-blind study on 16 patients with gastric ulcers and 32 patients with duodenal ulcers, an effect was noted on the gastric lesions but not on the duodenal disease (Russell and Dickie, 1968). Favorable results have been claimed for healing duodenal ulcers (Tewari and Trembalowicz, 1968) and reducing the frequency of recurring ulcer symptoms (Tewari and Kirk Wilson, 1973). In several other double-blind studies, Caved-S has not enhanced the healing effect on either gastric or duodenal ulcers (Feldman and Gilat, 1971; Engqvist et al., 1973). Larger, properly controlled studies are needed to assess the effect of this liquorice extract–laxative–antacid mixture in treating either gastric or duodenal ulcer patients.

Trials with Caved-S are confounded because it is a mixture. An important double-blind study was performed on deglycyrrhizinated liquorice alone at 380 mg given to 16 patients and placebo given to 17 patients with gastric ulcers (Turpie et al., 1969). The patients were treated for four weeks. The liquorice extract was significantly more effective than the placebo in healing the gastric lesions. This was accomplished without evidence of aldesterone-like side effects.

In a multicenter trial, involving 7 hospitals, deglycyrrhizinated liquorice, at 760 mg, three times a day daily after meals for six weeks, was evaluated on 90 men with proven chronic duodenal ulcers (Multicenter trial, 1971). The group consisted of outpatients who were advised to take antacids as required. The results showed no advantage for the drug when compared to the placebo for effects on frequency and severity of pain, amount of alkali consumed, or the doctors' and patients' rating of clinical response. Two criticisms of the study are apparent. Could taking the medication after meals prevent the pharmacological action of the medication? Animal studies (see below) indicate that deglycyrrhizinated liquorice is active parenterally. Possibly the medication has to be absorbed before it is effective. Secondly, could the presence of antacids alter the absorption and hence the action of the drug? As concluded by the people in the multicenter trial: "Further clinical trials are needed if the usefulness of glycyrrhizinic-acid-reduced liquorice for the treatment of duodenal ulcer is to be established."

Deglycyrrhizinated liquorice was compared to carbenoxolone in a clinical trial on 37 ambulatory patients with gastric ulcers (Wilson, 1972). Medication was: carbenoxolone, 100 mg 3 times a day for 7 days, then 50 mg 3 times a day for 3 weeks after meals, deglycyrrhizinated liquorice 760 mg 3 times a day for 4 weeks. Only a nonsignificant trend on healing was reported although each drug reduced the size of the ulcer crater by an average of 89 and 74 per cent respectively. Apparently, liquorice extract may contain "a healing substance" that is beneficial for treating gastric but not duodenal ulcers.

In an experimental study, deglycyrrhizinated liquorice in graded doses of 25–200 mg, given intraperitoneally, prevented gastric lesions in a 24-hour pyloric ligated rat preparation. The extract also reduced the acid and volume of stomach secretion (Andersson et al., 1971). Effectiveness on both the lesion and secretion parameters was evident at the 50-mg dose. The antiulcer, antisecretory effects in rats for deglycyrrhizinated liquorice have been confirmed (Aarsen, 1973). This latter author suggests that the pyloric ligated rat preparation be used to bio-assay the liquorice extract. Deglycyrrhizinated liquorice at 200 mg kg^{-1} i.p. was also antisecretory in the chronic fistula rat. Paradoxically, it also increased plasma gastrin and gastric mucosa histidine decarboxylase (Håkanson et al., 1973). How liquorice extract affects secretion and gastrointestinal lesions is not clear. More experimental information on electrolyte diffusion, mucus production and antral-duodenal motility is needed for this fascinating new group of substances. Clearly carbenoxolone and deglycyrrhizinated liquorice exert a different spectrum of pharmacological responses.

8.6 F_M100

A fraction of liquorice, called F_M100, has been studied on experimental animals (Takagi and Ishii, 1967; Ishii, 1968; Takagi and Harada, 1969). It is antisecretory and protects against lesions in the pyloric ligated rat. Its ED_{50} dose, by the intraduodenal route, in the rat is 400 mg kg^{-1}. F_M100 can inhibit histamine-, methacholine-, but not gastrin-induced secretions in acute fistula rats. It also decreases histamine-induced secretions in the acute fistula anesthetized dog. Speculation that F_M100 exerts its action by inhibiting the release of gastrin from the antral mucosa is not supported by objective evidence (Ishii, 1970). Another crude plant extract, Platycodin, also is antisecretory and protective in the pyloric ligated rat (Kawashima et al., 1972). Both F_M100 and Platycodin can enhance the healing rate of acetic acid-induced lesions. Both agents require more extensive pharmacological evaluation to assess their worth for clinical trials.

8.7 ESTROGENS

Peptic ulcers are much less common in females of child-bearing age than in males of the same age group. This differential is lost in women that are postmenopausal (Clark, 1953; Winkelstein, 1940). Gastric events associated with the menstrual cycle are a rise in acid concentration and output during the first half and a fall in the second half of the cycle (McDonald, 1956). Women with chronic peptic ulcers become symptom free during pregnancy (Sandweiss *et al.*, 1939; Clark, 1953). A single clinical case report suggests that pregnancy decreases gastric acid and pepsin output in a woman with a duodenal ulcer (Spiro *et al.*, 1959). In the dog, pregnancy exerts equivocal effects on gastric secretions (McCarthy *et al.*, 1954; Clark 1957). Experimentally, pregnancy as well as lactation are effective in preventing prednisolone-induced lesions in the rat (Kelly and Robert, 1969), though acid secretions may be elevated (Lilja and Svensson, 1967). Polymyxin-B is less ulcerogenic in pregnant than in nonpregnant rats. Also, suckling rats offer protection to the mother rat against polymyxin-B-induced lesions (Kahlson *et al.*, 1964b). Diethylstilbestrol can reduce acid secretory responses to histamine in the cat, with the female more sensitive than the male cat (Ojha and Wood, 1950). There may be a species difference since 1·25 mg i.m. daily of conjugated equine estrogens (Premarin®) has no effect on either acid or pepsin secretion in the monkey (Kaufmann and Spiro, 1968). Chorionic gonadotrophins can decrease secretion in the rat (Ghosh, 1959) and dog (Culmer *et al.*, 1939a; 1939b). Ovariectomized rats treated with 17β-estradiol showed a diminished secretory response to carbachol, histamine or gastrin (Amure and Omole, 1970). Thus female hormones or pregnancy could offer protection against duodenal ulcers and possibly reduce acid secretion.

These observations, along with a few isolated clinical and experimental reports (Winkelstein, 1940), suggest that estrogens may have antiulcer activity. A properly designed trial in male patients with duodenal ulcers was performed (Truelove, 1960). Stilbesterol, 0·5 mg twice daily, was given for six months and found to significantly alter the short- and long-term course of the disease. Truelove reported a 79 per cent remission to the hormone versus only a 33 per cent placebo response. The two major side effects, reduction in sexual potency and gynacomastia, were reversible at the end of therapy. A small clinical trial confirmed that oral stilbesterol could control the symptoms of duodenal ulcers, but had no effect on basal, or histamine-induced secretions of acid or pepsin. An increase in mucus production was observed (Parbhoo and Johnston, 1966). Conjugated equine estrogens (Premarin®) at 1·25 mg twice daily orally for three months had no effect on basal or histamine-induced pepsin or acid secretory parameters in three gastric and five duodenal ulcer patients (Kaufmann and Spiro, 1968). A preliminary report indicated that 1 mg of estriol was not beneficial in treating duodenal ulcers in man (Connell *et al.*, 1966). Two double-blind clinical trials were conducted in which male patients with gastric ulcers received 0·5 mg stilbesterol or female patients with gastric ulcers received 0·5 mg estriol (Doll *et al.*, 1965; 1968b). Neither sex benefited from the therapy. At present, estrogens may be helpful in people with duodenal ulcers, but not useful for treating gastric ulcer patients. However, the use of female hormones is not practical. Possibly a steroid analogue with minimal feminizing activity would be a useful addition to ulcer therapy.

9 Prostaglandins

Prostaglandins are currently undergoing extensive investigation. This series of hydroxy fatty acids are highly potent biological substances that are distributed throughout all organ systems, including the gastric mucosa and secretions from the stomach (Table 8). Extensive reviews of the pro-

TABLE 8

Prostaglandins isolated from rat gastric mucosa and stomach perfusates

	PGE_1	PGE_2	$PGF_{1\alpha}$	$PGF_{2\alpha}$
Gastric mucosa	+[a]	+	+	−
Spontaneous release	+	+	+[a]	−
Gastrin i.v.	+[a]	+	+	−
Vagal stimulation	+[a]	+	+	trace
Theophylline-cyclic AMP	+[a]	−	+[a]	+

[a] Denotes the prostaglandin which predominates. Shaw and Ramwell (1968).

staglandins are available (Ramwell and Shaw, 1970; Bennett and Fleshler, 1970; Bergström *et al.*, 1968; Weeks, 1972; Waller, 1973; Wilson, 1972; 1973; Oesterling *et al.*, 1972).

Little is known about the physiological function of prostaglandins but theories abound that they are involved in some pathological processes affecting the gut. The prostaglandins consist of a 20-carbon molecule with a five-membered ring between C_8 and C_{12} (see Table 11). The prostaglandin E series (PGE) is characterized by a carbonyl group at C_9 and hydroxyl groups at C_{11} and C_{15}. The prostaglandin F series (PGF) contains hydroxyl groups at C_9, C_{11}, and C_{15}. The prostaglandin A series

(PGA) is the $\Delta^{10, 11}$ analogue derived from PGE. Slight chemical modifications contribute marked differences in the biological properties of the different types of prostaglandins. Secretion studies have been done with prostaglandins PGE_1, PGE_2, $PGF_{2\alpha}$ and to a lesser extent PGA_1 and $PGF_{1\alpha}$. The subscript characters denote different locations of double bonds and stereoisomerism (see also p. 84).

Two independent laboratories have shown that small amounts of prostaglandins are released from unstimulated rat stomach but severalfold more PGE_1 is released after vagal or transmural stimulation (Bennett et al., 1967). The second group found that PGE_2, $PGF_{1\alpha}$, and $PGF_{2\alpha}$ were present in the rat stomach perfusate after vagal stimulation (Coceani et al., 1967; 1968). This release of prostaglandins is not from preformed stores but is formed during the period of stimulation. Stimulation of periarterial sympathetic nerves could antagonize the release induced by vagal stimulation. PGE_2 has been extracted from the mucosa of the body and antrum of human stomach. Its concentration was approximately 400 $\mu g\ g^{-1}$ wet weight mucosa (Bennett et al., 1968). The PGE_2 was mainly at the luminal surface of the mucosa with much smaller amounts in the submucosa and muscles (Bennett et al., 1972; 1973a; 1973b). PGE_2-like substances are also present in human basal gastric secretions (2·4 $ng\ ml^{-1}$). This concentration in the secretions can be reduced by submaximal amounts of pentagastrin or histamine (0·3 and 40 $\mu g\ kg^{-1}$ h^{-1} i.v., respectively). Thus the prostaglandin levels within the stomach can be altered by hormonal and nerve influences.

The prostaglandins appear to be locally synthesized and degraded. The stomach of the rat has been shown to metabolize $PGF_{1\alpha}$ (Pace-Asciak et al., 1970) and synthesize PGE_2 and $PGF_{2\alpha}$ from arachidonic acid (Pace-Asciak and Wolf, 1970; Pace-Asciak, 1972). The synthesis is by a membrane-bound enzyme system referred to as prostaglandin synthetase. This enzyme system can be stimulated by norepinephrine, epinephrine, and dopamine to produce mainly the E-type of prostaglandin (Pace-Asciak, 1972). The adrenergic neurotransmitters may prolong prostaglandin anti-secretory activity by their effects on prostaglandin synthetase. The enzyme system can be inhibited by nonsteroid anti-inflammatory agents (Vane, 1971; Eckenfels and Vane, 1972). Clinically, 200 mg of indomethacin, administered rectally, reduces pentagastrin-induced secretions by 32 per cent (Bennett et al., 1973b). The ability of a prostaglandin synthesis inhibitor exerting an antisecretory effect argues against the prostaglandins being directly involved in the physiological control of secretions. The prostaglandin synthetase inhibitors (aspirin, indomethacin, phenylbutazone) produce vasoconstriction which leads to local ischemia, tissue necrosis, and bleeding. The nonsteroid antiinflammatory drugs may initiate the back diffusion of the hydrogen ion and its sequelae by decreasing the synthesis of the endogenous prostaglandins which are thought to be vasodilators (Main and Whittle, 1973a).

Several of the prostaglandins have been tested for their antisecretory properties in different species, administered by different routes and against either basal or stimulated secretions. Table 9 summarizes the re-

TABLE 9

Effects of prostaglandins on gastric secretion in animals

Species	Route of administration	Prostaglandins tested	Stimulus for acid secretion	Inhibition
Rat	s.c.	E_1	none	+
			pentagastrin	+
		synthetic PGs	none	+
			pentagastrin	+
	i.v.	E_1, E_2	pentagastrin	+
		A_1, A_2	histamine	+
	oral	E_2	pentagastrin	−
		synthetic PGs	none	+
	gastric perfusion	E_1, E_2	none	+
			pentagastrin	+
			histamine	+
			vagal stimulation	+
Dog	i.v.	E_1	food	+
			histamine	+
			2-deoxyglucose	+
			pentagastrin	+
			carbachol	+
			reserpine	+
		synthetic PGs	histamine	+
		E_2	food	+
			histamine	+
		A_1	histamine	−
			pentagastrin	+
			food	+
			2-deoxyglucose	+
		arachidonic acid	histamine	+
		$F_{2\alpha}$	histamine	−
	oral	E_2	histamine	−
		synthetic PGs	histamine	+
Cat	i.v.	E_2	pentagastrin	−
Ferret	s.c.	E_1	none	+
			pentagastrin	±
Frog	topical	E_1	histamine	+
			gastrin I	+

sults. In the initial studies of prostaglandins on the secretory function of dogs with either innervated (Pavlov) or denervated (Heidenhain) pouches, PGE_1 and PGE_2 at $1~\mu g~kg^{-1}~min^{-1}$ could give near total inhibition of either food- or histamine-induced volume, acid or pepsin output (Robert et al., 1967). The antisecretory action of PGE_1 against histamine-induced secretions in the dog has been confirmed (Wilson and Levine, 1972). PGE_1 was also effective in inhibiting 2-deoxyglucose-, pentagastrin-, carbachol-, or reserpine-induced secretions in dogs (Robert, 1968; Robert et al., 1968a). The detailed experiments for the potent action of PGE_1 against several secretagogues are well documented (Nezamis et al., 1971). The agent is not selective but has a broad spectrum of inhibitory actions against several secretagogues. The potency of PGE_1 to block secretion is: 2-deoxyglucose > pentagastrin > food = histamine. PGA_1 at $1~\mu g~kg^{-1}~min^{-1}$ did not affect histamine-induced but strongly inhibited food-induced secretion in the dog. Also $PGF_{2\alpha}$ did not block histamine-induced secretion. Thus all prostaglandins do not exert a similar action on the gastric secretions of the dog.

PGE_1 is also antisecretory in the pyloric ligated rat (Robert et al., 1968b). Volume, concentration and output of acid and output of pepsin could be reduced by 50 per cent with doses as low as $200-300~\mu g~kg^{-1}$ s.c. Similar effects have been obtained in chronic fistula rats (Håkanson et al., 1973). PGE_1 could also inhibit either histamine-, pentagastrin-, or vagal stimulated-induced secretions in the perfused rat stomach preparation (Shaw and Ramwell, 1968). The antisecretory action of exogenous PGE_1 is apparently direct on the parietal cell since doses as low as 10^{-7} M could markedly block either histamine or synthetic human gastrin I secretory response on isolated gastric mucosa of the bullfrog (Way and Durbin, 1969). Gastric lesions in the rat induced by 21-hour pyloric ligation, steroids, prednisolone (Robert, 1968) or serotonin (Ferguson et al., 1973) were reduced in number and severity by PGE_1.

Prostaglandin E_2 was found to be stable in an iso-osmotic, pH 7·4, Na_2HPO_4 buffer (Lee et al., 1973). In this vehicle, the PGE_2 was active i.v. but not orally, in decreasing pentagastrin-induced acidity in the rat. The buffered PGE_2, given orally, however, could reduce or prevent gastric lesions induced by pyloric ligation or reserpine in the rat, histamine-induced duodenal lesions in the guinea-pig or pentagastrin-induced duodenal lesions in the guinea-pig and cat. PGE_2 could not protect the rat against cortisone-induced lesions. These studies are further evidence that the prostaglandins possess a broad spectrum of antisecretory and antiulcer activity rather than specific antagonist activity. Possibly the natural prostaglandins could be formulated to be useful in treating ulcers in man.

Arachidonic acid, the endogenous metabolic precursor of PGD_2, can

TABLE 10

Effect of prostaglandins on gastric secretion in man

Route	Prostaglandin	Dose	Stimulants to acid secretion	Ratio of subjects with decreased volume and/or output	Unwanted effects
Oral	15(r)15 MePGE$_2$	100–200 µg	none	31:31	nil noted
		200	pentagastrin 6 µg kg^{-1} i.m.	8:8	nil noted
I.v. injection	15(s) MePGE$_2$	100–200 µg	none	0:5	nil noted
Oral		25–50 µg	pentagastrin 6 µg kg^{-1} i.m.	4:4	nausea, borborygmi
I.v. injection	16-di-MePGE$_2$	3·1 µg	none	0:5	nil noted
		6·3 µg	none	0:5	nil noted
		12·5 µg	none	4:5	nil noted
		25 µg	none	4:6	nil noted
		50 µg	none	10:10	nil noted
		25–50 µg	pentagastrin 6 µg kg^{-1} i.m.	9:11	nil noted
				9:11	nil noted

Route	Agent	Dose		Ratio	Effects
Oral		25 µg	none	0:5	bile contamination of aspirate
		50 µg	none	5:7	
		100 µg	none	3:5	
		200 µg	none	5:5	
		200 µg	pentagastrin 6 µg kg^{-1} i.m.	7:7	nil noted
Oral	PGE_1	10–40 µg kg^{-1}	pentagastrin 6 µg kg^{-1} s.c.	0:4	diarrhea
	PGE_2	2·5 mg	none	0:1	nil noted
		4·0 mg	none	0:3	
I.v. infusion	PGE_1	4 µg kg^{-1} per 30 min	none	8:8	cardiovascular desire to defecate
		7 µg kg^{-1} per 30 min	pentagastrin 2 µg kg^{-1} h^{-1} i.v.	7:8	
	PGA_1	0·5–0·6 µg kg^{-1} min^{-1}	none	1:1	
			histamine 0·015 mg kg^{-1} h^{-1} i.v.	9 ($p < 0·01$)	pulse rate occasional nausea
		1–1·25 µg kg^{-1} min^{-1}	none	0:2	
			histamine 0·015 mg kg^{-1} h^{-1} i.v.	9 (p-ns)	
	$PGF_{1\alpha}$	0·5 µg kg^{-1} min^{-1} for 20 min	pentagastrin 0·01 µg kg^{-1} min^{-1} i.v.	0:5	nil noted
Oral	PGA_1	10–50 mg	none	4:11	hypotension
	15-Epi-PGA_2	5–20 mg	none	1:6	nil noted
	PGA_2	5–20 mg	none	0:6	nil noted

also reduce histamine-induced secretions in the dog with a Heidenhain pouch (Bieck et al., 1971).

Several of the prostaglandins have been tested for antisecretory action in man. Results are summarized in Table 10. In three subjects, oral doses of 10–40 $\mu g\ kg^{-1}$ of PGE_1 had no effect on pentagastrin-induced gastric secretion (Horton et al., 1968). PGE_2 (2·5 and 4 mg) was also ineffective orally against basal secretions (Karim et al., 1973a). PGE_1 via an i.v. infusion (300 μg per 30 min) caused a 40 per cent decrease of basal gastric secretion (Classen et al., 1970). It could also reduce the volume, and acid output but not the hydrogen concentration of pentagastrin-induced secretions (Classen et al., 1971). In contrast to animal studies, i.v. infusions of PGA_1 could reduce the volume and acid output of histamine-induced secretions in man. Hydrogen ion concentration was not affected. A dose–response curve was not obtained since the antisecretory effects were less with the higher (0·6 versus 1·25 $\mu g\ kg^{-1}\ min^{-1}$) doses (Wilson et al., 1970; Wilson et al., 1971). Prostaglandins A_1, A_2 and 15-epi-A_2 were evaluated by the oral route on basal secretions in man (Bhana et al., 1973). PGA_1 (up to 20 mg) and 15-epi-A_2 (up to 20 mg) exerted equivocal results on secretions. In contrast, PGA_2 (up to 20 mg) could raise the pH of gastric juice, though the effects were relatively brief and not dose dependent. The need for the intravenous route, brevity or lack of oral action and the incidence of side effects, e.g. diarrhea and hypotension, prohibit the use of either PGE_1, PGE_2, PGA_1, or PGA_2 for controlling acid secretion in man.

9.1 SYNTHETIC PROSTAGLANDINS

Clinical experiences suggest that a prostaglandin analogue may be orally effective and clinically useful. An attempt to develop prostaglandin derivatives that are secretory inhibitors has been reported (Lippmann, 1969b; 1970d; 1971b). A series of analogues which were evaluated by the s.c. route on the pyloric ligated rat preparation are presented in Table 11. AY-20,524, a PGE_1 analogue, is one-tenth as potent as PGE_1. The synthetic PGF analogues AY-16,809, AY-21,669 and AY-21,670 were even weaker antisecretory agents. However, AY-22,093, a prostaglandin E_1 analogue which lacks the hydroxyl group at position C-11 and is saturated at position C_{13} was one-half as active as PGE_1. AY-22,093 could also prevent pentagastrin-induced secretions in the rat.

Several analogues were evaluated orally in the pyloric ligated rat (Lippmann, 1973; Lippmann and Seethaler, 1973). AY-22,093 up to 50 mg kg^{-1} was orally inactive. AY-22,469 administered orally, one hour before pyloric ligation, had an ED_{50} of 44 mg kg^{-1}. Oral dosing

TABLE 11

Prostaglandin analogues with gastric antisecretory activity in the rat

	A	B	C	D	Dose mg kg^{-1} s.c.	Per cent inhibition	
PGE$_1$	O	—CH=CH—	H OH	H OH	0·8	85[a]	65[a]
					0·4		48[a]
AY-20,524	O	—CH=CH—	H H	H OH [e]	8·0	72[a]	
					4·0	49[a]	
AY-22,093	O	—CH$_2$—CH$_2$—	H H	H OH	2·0	NS	
					1·6	77[a]	
					0·8	52[a]	41[b]
					0·4	NS	NS
AY-16,809	H, OH	—CH=CH—	H H	H OH	32	35[a]	43[a]
					16	NS	
AY-21,669	H, OH	—CH$_2$—CH$_2$—	H H	H OH	32		33[c]
AY-21,670	OH, H	—CH$_2$—CH$_2$—	H H	H OH	32	37[b]	
					16	NS	
AY-22,469	O	—CH$_2$—CH$_2$—	H H	CH$_3$ OH	oral ED$_{50}$ 3		
AY-22,443[d]	O	—CH$_2$—CH$_2$—	H H	CH$_3$ OH	6·3		

[a] P < 0·001. [b] <0·02. [c] <0·05. [d] methyl ester at carbon 1. [e] not resolved
From Lippman (1971b).

after ligation produced an ED$_{50}$ of 3 mg kg^{-1}. AY-22,443, when dosed orally after ligation had an ED$_{50}$ of 6·3 mg kg^{-1}. AY-22,469 was also evaluated orally in the rat against several experimental ulcer models. The chemical had a protective ED$_{50}$ of 1 mg kg^{-1} when administered after ligation in the 19-hour preparation, and a 30 mg kg^{-1} ED$_{50}$ against a cold-restraint rat preparation. It did not prevent (10–30 mg kg^{-1} p.o.) reserpine-induced gastric lesions.

Another PGE$_1$ derivative, SC-24665 (**20**), was found to be orally active against pyloric ligation-induced lesions in rats (ED_{50} 0·32 mg kg^{-1}), and histamine-induced duodenal lesions in guinea-pigs (ED_{50} 3·2 mg kg^{-1}). It could also protect against reserpine- or stress-induced lesions in rats and pentagastrin-induced lesions in guinea-pigs and cats (Lee and Bianchi, 1972). Clinical studies will be needed to evaluate these prostaglandin analogues.

(−)—11α,15α-Dihydroxy-5-oxoprostynoic acid
SC-24665
(20)

Another approach to developing an orally active prostaglandin derivative was reported by Robert and Magerlein (1973). The inability of PGE_2 to inhibit gastric secretions when given orally to man (Horton et al., 1968; Karim et al., 1973a) may be due to rapid enzyme degradation. The natural prostaglandins are readily broken down by dehydrogenation at carbon-15 by the enzyme prostaglandin 15-OH dehydrogenase. Prostaglandin analogues modified at carbon 15 and 16 to avoid being dehydrogenase substrate have been synthesized and several derivatives have received biological evaluation. These prostaglandin derivatives are: 15(S)-15-methyl-PGE_2 methyl ester (15(S)-MePGE_2) (21) and its isomer 15(R)-15-methyl PGE_2 methyl ester (15(R)-MePGE_2) (22), a third derivative is 16-dimethyl-PGE_2 methyl ester (16-diMePGE_2) (23). The structure may be compared to prostaglandin E_2 (24). The methyl substitution may protect the 15(S)-hydroxyl from metabolism by prostaglandin 15-hydroxy dehydrogenase.

The 15(S)-MePGE_2 and 16-diMePGE_2 were tested on dogs with denervated gastric pouches against histamine-induced secretions. Both derivatives, when given i.v., were respectively 30 and 50 times as potent and of longer duration of inhibition than the PGE_2 administered by the same route. The relative ED_{50} antisecretory potency of the three substances by the i.v. route is 10 μg kg^{-1} for PGE_2, 0·3 μg kg^{-1} for 15-MePGE_2 and 0·1 μg kg^{-1} for 16-diMePGE_2. When 16-diMePGE_2 was given orally in a 10 per cent ethanol solution, it was highly effective in reducing secretions; however, it caused a high degree of vomiting. Thus, these derivatives were evaluated for their antisecretory action by ad-

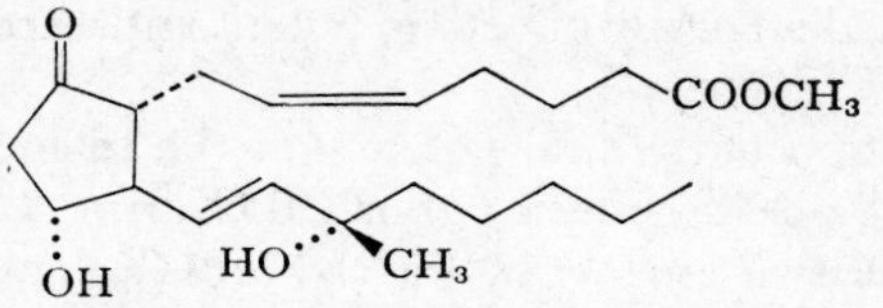

Prostaglandin-15(S)-15-methyl-E₂ methyl ester

(21)

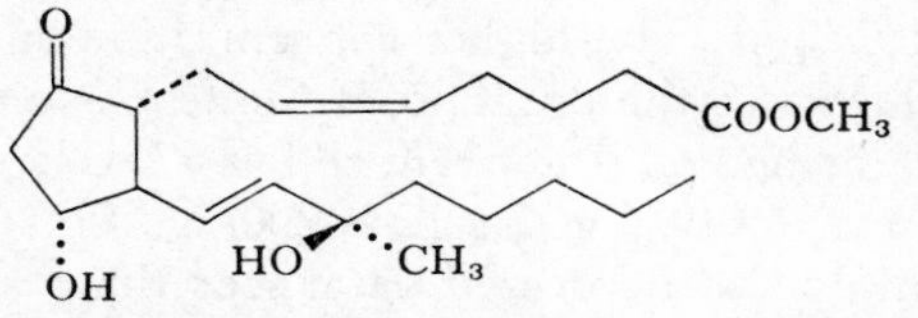

Prostaglandin-15(R)15-methyl-E₂ methyl ester

(22)

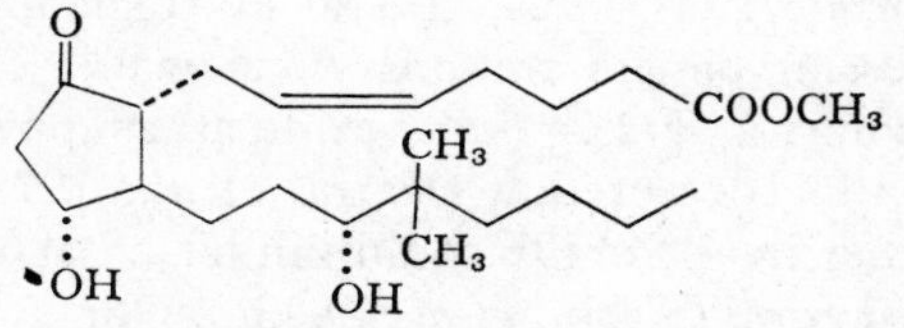

Prostaglandin-16-dimethyl-E₂ methyl ester

(23)

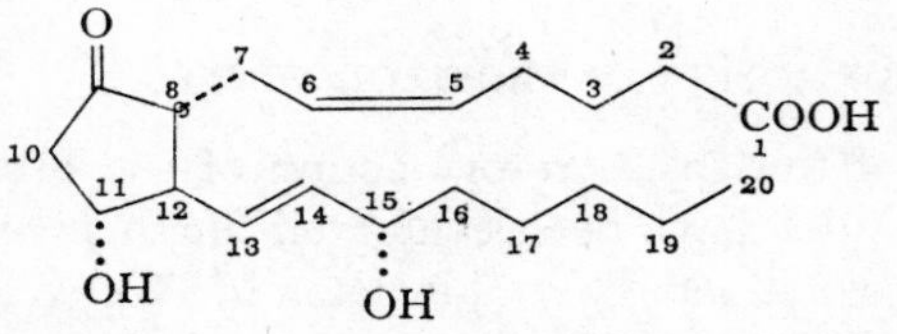

Prostaglandin E₂

(24)

ministering them into the jejunum. Both 15(S)MePGE₂ and 16-diMe-PGE₂, at 20 μg kg⁻¹ were effective in suppressing the volume and acid output of histamine-induced secretions. The 16-diMePGE₂ derivative was 2·8 times as potent, and did not produce vomiting in dogs. In contrast, PGE₂ was inactive by the jejunal route at doses of 400 μg kg⁻¹ or 10 mg per dog. Thus, methylation at either C-15 (monomethyl) or C-16 (dimethyl) produced an orally effective, potent antisecretory derivative of PGE_2.

Clinical verification of the oral potency of the 15-methyl analogues as antisecretory substances has been published (Karim *et al.*, 1973a; Karim *et al.*, 1973b). The two analogues $15(S)$-MePGE$_2$ and $15(R)$-MePGE$_2$ as well as PGE_2 were evaluated against basal secretion for their effects on volume, pH, acid output and concentration. While PGE_2 in doses as high as 4 mg had no effect, $15(R)$-MePGE$_2$ at doses of 100 (five tests), 150 (three tests) and 200 (seven tests) µg orally, effectively reduced acid concentration and output. The higher concentration suppressed acidity for three hours which was the duration of the test. No side effects were noted. The $15(R)$ analogue did not reduce basal levels of acid secretion when given i.v. in a dose range of 12·5–200 µg. Prostaglandin $15(R)$-MeE$_2$ at 100 µg orally also depressed basal secretions without excessive uterine stimulation in 16 pregnant patients at term (Amy *et al.*, 1973). Doses of $15(S)$-MePGE$_2$ at 25 (two tests) and 50 (two tests) µg orally were highly effective in decreasing acidity. One individual did complain of nausea and borborygmi. Thus, several prostaglandin analogues are effective in suppressing basal secretions. As shown in eight patients, the $15(R)$-MePGE$_2$ isomer at 200 µg orally could also suppress pentagastrin-(6 µg kg^{-1} i.m.) induced secretion (Karim *et al.*, 1973b). In addition, 16-diMePGE$_2$ either i.v. or orally could inhibit basal and pentagastrin-stimulated acid secretion (Karim *et al.*, 1973c). One awaits further confirmatory clinical data on the effects of these and other analogues on stimulated gastric juice. This series of compounds could open new possibilites in controlling gastric secretion in man.

9.2 MECHANISM OF ACTION OF PROSTAGLANDINS

The mechanism of the antisecretory action of the prostaglandins is not known. Prostaglandins have been evaluated for their effects on secretion and gastric mucosal blood flow (Jacobson, 1970; Wilson and Levine, 1972; Main and Whittle, 1972). Intravenous and intraarterial injections of PGE_1 and PGA_1 into the gastric vascular beds of dogs resulted in a marked decrease of peripheral vascular resistance and a decrease in gastric arterial perfusion pressure—that is, potent vasodilation of the gastric circulation (Nakano and Prancan, 1972). It is not clear that when secretion is increased or decreased, mucosal blood flow is altered in the same direction (see section 5.1) and that there is a direct relationship. Thus, Jacobson concludes that the primary antisecretory mechanism of PGE_1 in the dog is not necessarily by altering gastric mucosal blood flow. A similar conclusion was drawn for the action of several prostaglandins on rat antisecretory mucosal blood flow relations (Main and Whittle, 1972; 1973a; 1973b). Prostaglandins of the E and A series by the i.v. route in the rat can inhibit gastric acid secretion and either increase or decrease mucosal blood flow depending on the dose and the secretory state of the stomach. The secondary action of affecting mucosal blood flow is also shown where PGE_1 is an effective antisecretory agent on isolated gastric mucosa of frog where blood flow is not a factor (Way and Durbin, 1969).

Extensive evidence has accumulated that the prostaglandins act through a cyclic 3′,5′-adenosine monophosphate (cAMP) system. The relationship between cAMP and gastric secretion has been reviewed (Samir Amer, 1972). The stimulatory effects of various secretagogues on cAMP (Bersimbaev et al., 1971; Salganik et al., 1972) is presented in the scheme below. Gastrin and histamine stimulate cAMP which is considered to be the second messenger in the action of hormones. The hormones stimulate while several xanthine derivatives reduce the rate of metabolism of cAMP.

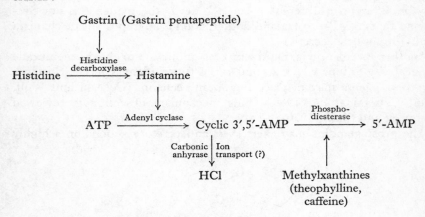

Scheme for the regulation of HCl secretion

The prostaglandins affect cAMP differently in different species. The accumulated evidence indicates that stimulation of gastric secretion in certain species (rabbit, dog) if regulated by cAMP, is possibly related to a decrease rather than an increase in the intracellular levels of the nucleotide. Thus both the prostaglandins and exogenous cAMP are capable of reducing the secretory volume and acid output in the dog (Levine, 1971). A more direct experiment has been reported (Bieck et al., 1973). The infusion of prostaglandin E_2 (1 μg kg^{-1} min^{-1}) into dogs with Heidenhain pouches significantly decreased histamine-induced secretions as well as the amount of cAMP secreted into the gastric juice. Other experimental studies (Mao *et al.*, 1972) have failed to demonstrate that cAMP is involved in secretory mechanisms in the stomach of the dog.

In contrast, cAMP increased acid production in frog gastric mucosa (Harris *et al.*, 1969; Way and Durbin, 1969). However, PGE_1 could antagonize gastrin- or histamine- but *not* cAMP-induced secretion in the frog preparation (Way and Durbin, 1969). Cyclic AMP çan also stimulate gastric secretion in the rat (Salganik *et al.*, 1972; Whittle, 1972). This secretion is partially antagonized by PGE_2 (Whittle, 1972). Histamine, pentagastrin and carbachol can increase cAMP levels in the gastric mucosa of theophylline-treated rats (Narumi and Maki, 1973; Bersimbaev *et al.*, 1971; Domschke *et al.*, 1973). A series of natural and cyclic nucleotides were evaluated for their secretory action on the rat (Jawaharlal and Berti, 1972). In this study, cAMP was inactive while dibutyryl-cAMP and HD-233 (C_6-piperidinopurin-ribosid-3',5'-AMP) stimulated secretion that could be antagonized by PGE_1. Thus the interaction of prostaglandins with adenyl cyclase and alteration of cyclic AMP may be different in different species. Indeed, the evidence is not convincing that cAMP-prostaglandin interaction is an important mechanism in altering gastric secretion.

Another speculation is that the prostaglandins act to change membrane permeability to ions which secondarily activate adenyl cyclase. Specifically these agents may displace membrane calcium (Coceani and Wolf, 1966; Coceani *et al.*, 1969). This mechanism of action is reviewed (Ramwell and Shaw, 1970).

The prostaglandins may exert their antisecretory actions on a highly

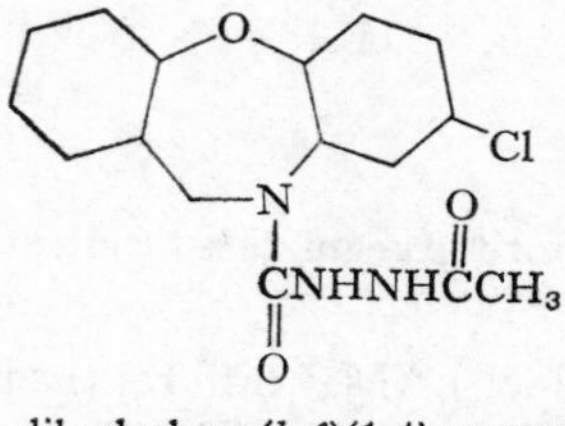

1-Acetyl-2-(8-chloro-10,11-dihydrobenz(*b*,*f*)(1,4)oxazepine-10-carbonyl)hydrazine

SC-19,220

(25)

specific receptor mechanism. As demonstrated for histamine and catecholamines, different blocking agents may be needed to alter the various biological effects of prostaglandins. Several compounds have been synthesized that block various prostaglandin actions. The chemical SC-

19220 (25) competitively antagonized the stimulatory action of several prostaglandins (PGE_1, PGE_2, and PGF_1) on isolated guinea-pig ileum (Sanner, 1969; 1972) and could prevent PGE_2-induced diarrhea in mice (Sanner, 1972). In contrast, SC-19220 was ineffective in blocking the antisecretory action of PGE_1 (Engel *et al.*, 1973). Thus a selective antagonist is available against certain prostaglandin actions. Can a prostaglandin analogue be developed that specifically inhibits gastric secretions and will ultimately be useful for treating patients with peptic ulcers?

10 Enterogastrones and other endogenous substances

The body contains several substances that can either increase or decrease gastric secretion. Recent isolation in pure form and synthesis of some of these hormones have resulted in unravelling the complexities of their actions. These biological substances are released by several mechanisms and possess multiple actions. The hormones, nerves and gastrointestinal secretions are involved in complex feedback systems. The complexity of these interactions matches the relationships described for the pituitary, thyroid, and adrenal glands. Some of these substances, or their derivatives, may ultimately find a place in the therapeutic regimen of controlling hypersecretion or treating peptic ulcers. This topic has been presented in symposia and reviews (Katz, 1973; Demling, 1972; Johnson and Grossman, 1971).

Several biological substances have been characterized to inhibit gastric secretion. These have been obtained from the urine, saliva, gastric juice and the small bowel and gastric mucosa. Thus the gut is an endocrine organ. Currently, several substances obtained from the small bowel have been best characterized for their inhibitory effects on secretion. These small bowel substances are referred to as enterogastrones and have been defined as any hormone released from the intestine which inhibits gastric secretions (Gregory, 1967; Johnson and Grossman, 1971). Enterogastrones which have been isolated and purified are secretin, cholecystokinin (CCK), glucagon, and gastric inhibitory polypeptide (GIP). These intestinal substances can be released by either nerve impulses or material entering the lumen, e.g. acid, fat, and hypertonic solutions. The actions of these substances were first characterized in the dog by perfusing the small bowel with acid or fat and monitoring the inhibition of secretion from a Heidenhain pouch. This period of study was followed by research with crude intestinal extracts. Finally, purification and synthesis of these substances has permitted the current flurry of research activity with this group of hormones.

Other substances have been extracted from various tissues and substances of the body. These have been partially purified and referred to by the suffix "-gastrone". These include sialogastrone from saliva, gastrone from gastric juice and urogastrone from urine. Extensive studies have been done on these various substances, though no useful, clinical candidate has been developed. The antisecretory properties of endogenous catecholomines (p. 234) and pepsin inhibitors (p. 258) have been discussed.

10.1 PURIFIED ENTEROGASTRONES

It has been postulated that the polypeptides, gastrin, cholecystokinin and secretin may affect gastric secretions by action on a common receptor (Grossman, 1970; Gadacz and Way, 1972). The receptor has two sites— one site with an affinity for gastrin and CCK which have chemically similar active fragments, the other site with an affinity for secretin. When two substances compete for the same receptor site, one of two possible effects may be seen. If the two agents have equal intrinsic activities (efficacies), an additive effect will be seen until the maximum response is reached. Secondly, if the agents have unequal intrinsic activities, competitive inhibition may be observed between them. By intrinsic activity one means that various agonists that apparently act on the same receptor site may produce maximal responses of different magnitudes. Similarly, two agents acting on different receptor sites will demonstrate either an additive effect if both are stimulatory or noncompetitive inhibition if one is inhibitory. If two noncompetitive agonists stimulate their respective receptor sites, their combined effect can be greater than that to either agent alone.

With the intestinal hormones, CCK is a competitive inhibitor of gastrin-stimulated acid secretion in certain species (Johnson and Grossman, 1970) and secretin is a noncompetitive inhibitor of gastrin- or CCK-stimulated acid secretion (Johnson and Grossman, 1969). A competitive interaction may also exist between glucagon and secretin since they are chemical homologues. This interaction has not been quantified. Thus, several of the purified enterogastrones and gastrin can be assessed in quantitative pharmacological terms.

10.2 SECRETIN

Several reviews describe the properties of secretin (Jorpes, 1968; Johnson and Grossman, 1971; Uvnäs, 1971; Hubel, 1972). The hormone has been isolated from the small intestine and synthesized. It consists of twenty-seven aminoacid residues. Fourteen of the twenty-seven aminoacids occupy the same position as in glucagon which has twenty-nine aminoacids. This structural similarity may suggest some pharmacological interactions. All twenty-seven aminoacids must be present in secretin to demonstrate biological activity (Ondetti *et al.*, 1968). Evidently, secretin activity is dependent on a helical, tertiary configuration (Bodansky *et al.*, 1969). This is in contrast to gastrin and CCK where portions of each molecule retain activity.

Secretin was first implicated in decreasng gastric secretion in 1957 (Greenlee *et al.*, 1957). Intravenous injections of impure secretin could decrease the response to feeding in dogs with a Heidenhain pouch. Secretin could also decrease the response to the endogenous release of gastrin. It could not block histamine-induced secretions. The ability of secretin to block gastrin-induced secretions has been confirmed (Gillespie and Grossman, 1964; Wormsley and Grossman, 1964; Gurll *et al.*, 1966). The antisecretory activity of secretin has been confirmed by the use of synthetic secretin (Vagne *et al.*, 1968; Johnson and Grossman, 1968; Bedi *et al.*, 1971) which indicates that in earlier studies the antisecretory action was not due to the presence of a contaminating substance. A dose–response study between gastrin and secretin using dogs with Heidenhain pouches revealed a noncompetitive inhibition (Johnson and Grossman, 1969). This study was interpreted as evidence that secretin acts at a receptor site different from the one affected by gastrin. Secretin will also reduce gastrin-induced secretions in the cat (Stening *et al.*, 1969b), the rat (Tumpson and Johnson, 1969; Johansson *et al.*, 1972; Chey *et al.*, 1973; Schmidt *et al.*, 1973) and man (Brooks and Grossman, 1970; Konturek, 1970; Wormsley, 1970; Chey *et al.*, 1970). The species sensitivity to secretion inhibition of gastrin-induced secretion is dog = rat > man ≫ cat.

Several studies on the dog have confirmed the work of Greenlee *et al.* (1957) that histamine-induced secretions are not blocked by secretin (Gillespie and Grossman, 1964; Wormsley and Grossman, 1964; Gurll *et al.*, 1966; Lucien *et al.*, 1970). Nor does secretin block histamine-induced secretion in the cat (Konturek *et al.*, 1969), rat (Johnson and Tumpson, 1970), or man (Johnson and Duthie, 1966; Chey *et al.*, 1970). In contrast, secretin can block histamine-induced secretions in the conscious rat (Chey *et al.*, 1973). This latter positive response may be due to the relative doses of the agonist and antagonist used. In addition, secretin did not block insulin- or 2-deoxy-D-glucose-induced secretion in the dog (Way, 1970). In addition to acting at the parietal cell, secretin may prevent the release of gastrin. Secretin caused a decrease in serum gastrin levels in five of six fasting patients with duodenal ulcers, and postprandial serum gastrin levels in nine of nine controls as well as six of six patients with duodenal ulcers. Secretin also decreased serum gastrin in four fasting dogs (Bunchman *et al.*, 1971; Thompson *et al.*, 1972). Thus secretin is selective in blocking gastrin- but not histamine- or cholinergic-induced secretions and may also prevent the release of gastrin.

In contrast to its effect on acid secretion, secretin causes pepsin secretion. This stimulation of pepsin output has been reported in the dog (Magee and Nakajima, 1968; Stening *et al.*, 1969a), cat (Gillespie and Grossman, 1964), rat (Johansson *et al.*, 1972), and man (Brooks *et al.*, 1969; Berstad and Petersen, 1970).

10.3 GLUCAGON

Glucagon is present in both the pancreas and the small bowel (Heding, 1971; Unger *et al.*, 1968). It has been shown to inhibit basal acid secretion in dog and man (Aylett, 1962; Robinson *et al.*, 1957; Becker *et al.*, 1973), secretion induced by meals in the dog (Lin and Benslay, 1962; Lin *et al.*, 1963; Becker *et al.*, 1973), insulin-induced secretion in the dog (Lin and Benslay, 1962; Lin *et al.*, 1963; Lin and Spray, 1968; Lin and Warrick, 1971; Von Heimburg and Hallenbeck, 1964), rat (Lin and Spray, 1971), and man (Dotevall *et al.*, 1969), and secretion induced in the dog by sham feeding and distension of the pylorus (Lin *et al.*, 1963). Glucagon in antagonizing the gastrin-induced secretion could reduce secretory volume and acid concentration. This was independent of its effect on mucosal blood flow (Lin and Warrick, 1971). Most studies indicate that glucagon does not block histamine-induced secretions in the dog (Melrose, 1960; Clarke *et al.*, 1960), or man (Dotevall and Westling, 1960; Dotevall *et al.*, 1969), or at best can only minimally reduce histamine-induced secretions (Dreiling and Janowitz, 1959; Lin *et al.*, 1970; Lin *et al.*, 1973). Glucagon can decrease the output of pepsin (Dreiling and Janowitz, 1959). Glucagon is also capable of reducing serum basal gastrin levels in dog and man or gastrin levels increased by food in healthy people, dogs and people with duodenal ulcers (Becker *et al.*, 1973). Thus, glucagon, like secretin, has similar effects in its ability to markedly reduce gastrin-induced secretions while having minimal or no effects on histamine-induced secretions. In contrast to secretin, most studies indicate that glucagon can inhibit insulin-induced secretions. Glucagon may also exert an indirect effect on secretions by blocking the release of gastrin from the gastrointestinal tract. The similarity in aminoacid sequence and structure between glucagon and secretin may indicate a common site of action. Could these two substances be antagonistic to each other at the receptor site? This study has not been performed. In any event, two enterogastrones are able to inhibit acid secretion and have a similar spectrum of activity against several agonists.

GASTRIC ANTISECRETORY AND ANTIULCER AGENTS 291

10.4 CHOLECYSTOKININ

A crude extract of intestinal mucosa was found to cause contraction of the gallbladder and was named cholecystokinin which is abbreviated CCK (Ivy and Oldburg, 1928). Fifteen years later, a similar extract was found to stimulate pancreatic enzyme release and was named pancreozymin (Harper and Raper, 1943). Careful isolation and identification revealed that both biological activities are elicited by one compound—which was designated as cholecystokinin-pancreozymin (Jorpes, 1968; Mutt and Jorpes, 1968). Since all of the gastrointestinal hormones are currently being implicated in multiple biological actions, it has been suggested that only the initially described name be used (Johnson and Grossman, 1971). Thus, this substance has reverted to its original name of cholecystokinin (CCK) rather than cholecystokinin-pancreozymin (CCK-PZ). The hormone is a single-chain polypeptide of thirty-three aminoacids (Mutt and Jorpes, 1968; Ondetti et al., 1970). Several shorter fragments of the molecule possess biological activity. The C-terminal octapeptide (OP-CCK) also identified as SQ-19,844, is several times more potent than the natural hormone on either a weight or a molar basis (approximately 10 and 2·5 times, respectively) in stimulating the gallbladder contraction, pancreatic enzyme secretions or acting as a gastric acid secretagogue (Rubin et al., 1969; Rubin and Engel, 1974). This implies that the partly purified hormone may still be contaminated with some unknown material. Indeed the careful study between OP-CCK and tissue extract of CCK does reveal quantitative difference between synthetic, purified material and the tissue extract (Rubin and Engel, 1974). Another dog study varifies the differences between the two CCK preparations (Gadacz and Way, 1972).

The effects of CCK on gastric secretions are both secretory and antisecretory. Chemically, the C-terminal pentapeptide sequence of CCK is identical to gastrin. Thus, when CCK is given alone in small amounts it is a weak stimulant of gastric acid secretion (Preshaw and Grossman, 1965; Murat and White, 1966; Nakamura et al., 1968; Rubin and Engel, 1974); however, it is a competitive inhibitor of gastrin. The hormone can antagonize gastrin-induced secretion in the dog (Gillespie and Grossman, 1964; Bedi et al., 1968; 1971; Stening et al., 1969b; Johnson and Grossman, 1970) and man (Wormsley, 1968; Brooks and Grossman, 1970; Chey et al., 1970). The administration of small secretory inhibitory doses of secretin with CCK resulted in at least an additive effect of the two hormones against pentagastrin-induced secretions in the dog (Bedi et al., 1971). The data is suggestive of potentiation of inhibition between the two hormones.

The action of CCK against histamine-induced secretions in the dog is complex. CCK can either inhibit or enhance histamine action which depends on the dose of the antagonist and whether CCK is infused or injected (Stening *et al.*, 1969b; Johnson and Grossman, 1969; Lucien *et al.*, 1970; Rubin and Engel, 1974). It also depends on the purity of the CCK (Lucien *et al.*, 1970). The cat responds differentially to CCK (Svensson and Emås, 1971). The hormone, CCK, given by a rapid i.v. injection, can increase secretory response to low or half maximal histamine-induced secretions as well as inhibit close to maximal responses of histamine.

In the rat, both natural CCK and the synthetic octapeptide (OP-CCK) exert a potent secretagogue action (Schmidt *et al.*, 1973; Rubin and Engel, 1974). The OP-CCK did not alter pentagastrin- or histamine-stimulated secretions (Chey *et al.*, 1973). The action of CCK with histamine depends on the dose of histamine. In the presence of a low dose of histamine the secretory effects of CCK would simply be additive with histamine. At maximal histamine response, the weak effects of CCK are no longer visible.

The action of CCK against gastrin- or pentagastrin-stimulated acid secretions is most pronounced in dogs, intermediate in man and insignificant in the cat or rat. When given alone, CCK increases secretion in the dog. When given with gastrin, it occupies receptors normally available to the gastrin molecules which appear to have a greater intrinsic activity in the dog. The species differences may be due to differences in intrinsic activities (efficacies) of CCK and gastrin in each species. Thus, in the dog the intrinsic activity for the secretory effect is higher for gastrin than for CCK. When CCK is available to the receptors, it competitively inhibits the secretory effect of gastrin. In the cat or rat, both gastrin and CCK are potent secretagogues and each has a similar intrinsic activity. Thus in these latter two species there is no competitive inhibition of the effect of gastrin by CCK.

10.5 GASTRIC INHIBITORY POLYPEPTIDE

Another enterogastrone, named gastric inhibitory polypeptide (GIP), was obtained from one of the fractions separated during the purifying procedure for CCK (Brown *et al.*, 1969; Brown and Pederson, 1970). This substance was devoid of gallbladder stimulating properties but could reduce endogenous gastrin-induced acid and pepsin output in the dog. Further work (Brown *et al.*, 1970; Brown and Dryburth, 1971) showed that this material was a polypeptide containing forty-three aminoacids with a molecular weight of 5105. There are similarities in the aminoacid sequence among GIP, gastrin and other enterogastrones. Porcine gastrin and GIP contain the same aminoacid sequence in the first 15 positions from the N-terminal of the molecule. Similarly, nine of the first 26 aminoacids of secretin and GIP occur in the same positions. This similarity in structure may reflect a possible weak agonist or competitive antagonist action of GIP for gastrin secretin receptors.

The polypeptide GIP does possess a broader spectrum of antisecretory activity than secretin. Unlike secretin, GIP at a dose as low as $4.0 \mu g$ $kg^{-1} h^{-1}$ could give a 40 per cent inhibition of histamine-induced acid secretion and 75 per cent inhibition of pepsin secretion in the dog (Pederson and Brown, 1972). The dose of histamine used could elicit a 60 per cent of maximum response. As with secretin, GIP can reduce pentagastrin- and insulin-induced acid and pepsin secretions. GIP was more effective against pentagastrin- than histamine-induced secretions. Others, using similar methods of extraction of small-bowel mucosa and purification have isolated a similar inhibitory substance (Lucien et al., 1969; Ichimura, 1971). This material, apparently not as pure as GIP, could also inhibit histamine-induced secretions in the dog (Lucien et al., 1970) or reduce pyloric ligated rat secretions (Ichimura, 1971). A substance extracted from the mucosa of the duodenal bulb could inhibit gastrin-stimulated secretions. This material was named Bulbogastrone (Uvnäs, 1971). No details on methods of extraction or chemical properties of this latter material have been revealed. Thus, other enterogastrones, like GIP and bulbogastrone, await further study on the gastrointestinal tract.

10.6 CRUDE GASTRIC ANTISECRETORY SUBSTANCES

Multiple groups have attempted to purify various extracts of biological material that demonstrate gastric antisecretory activity. Much of this work is bedeviled by contamination of the extracts by bacterial endotoxins (pyrogens) which cause fever and/or vomiting in the test animals (Cowley, 1973). Bacterial endotoxins can inhibit gastric secretions (Meyer et al., 1918). However, different antisecretory characteristics are frequently seen between some of these crude extracts and the bacterial material. The lack of purity of the antisecretory material negates any conclusion on the clinical usefulness or physiological role of these extracts.

Extensive work has been performed on the inhibitory activities of material in gastric juice or gastric mucosa. This topic has been reviewed (Code, 1967; Jerzy Glass and Code, 1968; Semb, 1969a). The material named gastrone, and occasionally referred to as gastric inhibitory substance (GIS), has been obtained from human and dog gastric juice and human and dog mucosa. It is more inhibitory when obtained from an acid gastric juice and still more potent from the juice of patients with pernicious anemia or gastric cancer. The presence of gastrone was first described by Brunschwig and co-workers between 1939–1942 (Brunschwig et al., 1942). This demonstrated that gastric juice from patients with different diseases, canine gastric juice and simple extracts of human gastric mucosa could inhibit food-induced secretions in dogs with Heidenhain pouches.

Code and his associates continued the attempt to characterize the properties of gastrone (Jerzy Glass and Code, 1968), as did others (Menguy and Smith, 1960; Katzka and Riss, 1962; Semb, 1966). The material was bioassayed either in the dog or pyloric ligated rat preparation. Research efforts have been developed to fractionate and purify gastrone. Currently, two crude materials have been identified as gastrone A—a large molecular weight (> 100 000) mucous substance with certain electrophoretic properties and gastrone B—a glycoprotein with a molecular weight between 10 000–40 000. The former can inhibit 50 per cent of the gastric secretions in the rat at doses of 0·2 to 0·5 mg, while gastrone B gives a 50 per cent inhibition at 7 to 48 μg. Gastrone B is also active in the Heidenhain pouch dog assay at approximately 100 μg. Potent inhibitory material, characterized as a glyco-protein, has also even been obtained from the stomach and intestinal mucosa of the whale (Kabeno et al., 1971). Could the gastrointestinal tract contain a clinically useful antisecretory glycoprotein?

In a careful recent study, assay of Gastrone B revealed that the antisecretory effects are associated with pyrexia in the dogs (Cowley, 1973). Bacteria could be cultured from the gastrone. Thus partial purification of gastrone has failed to remove the pyrogenic activity. Contamination may still be a major problem in identifying specific endogenous antisecretory agents. In another study with several of these inhibitory substances, the relationship between elevated temperature and secretory inhibition was not always correlated (Semb, 1969b). This author concluded that pyrexia was not a factor in the antisecretory action of the extracts. Yet, in the majority of the studies, this does appear to be a factor. Hood et al. (1953) calculated a significant correlation ($r = 0·56$) between increased body temperature and inhibition of secretion.

Antisecretory activity has been characterized for secretions from the dog's intestinal loop (Rudick et al., 1966; Semb, 1969b), and substances in saliva which have been named sialogastrone (Smith et al., 1958; Code, 1967; Menguy and Berlinski, 1967; Baume et al., 1968). As assayed in the rat, the highest inhibition of secretion was obtained from the saliva of people with gastric ulcers (71–73 per cent) and gastric carcinoma (66–80 per cent), less from the saliva of normals (59–73 per cent) and lowest from the saliva of people with duodenal ulcers (40–58 per cent) (Menguy et al., 1964). This material has been semipurified and identified as a polysaccharide or mucopolysaccharide which would be related to gastrone A (Baume *et al.*, 1967). Extracts of the submaxillary glands of several species also contain antisecretory substances (Kobayashi and Yamamoto, 1972; Kobayashi *et al.*, 1972). The salivary glands of the rat may even possess secretory materials (Levine, 1965b). Fasting dog thoracic duct lymph is also inhibitory to histamine- or gastrin-induced gastric secretions in dogs (Rudick *et al.*, 1966). Are all of these substances true endogenous secretory inhibitors or are they biological contaminants? Sterile body fluids like synovial fluid and ovarian cyst fluid were devoid of any antisecretory activity (Smith *et al.*, 1958). Thus, the physiological and/or pathological significance of these partially purified materials are still unidentified.

The literature contains many articles describing the antisecretory activity of various tissue extracts (Grossman, 1950). The early descriptions of crude preparations of secretin and CCK were of course done with tissue extracts. The injection of intestinal mucosa extracts (enterogastrone) were repeatedly shown to decrease secretion and protect against gastric lesions. A dog surgical preparation, named the Mann–Williamson dog, was frequently used to evaluate the antiulcer properties of tissue extracts. The preparation is one in which the jejunum is anastomosed to the stomach, which results in the development of jejunal ulcers, perforations and death in untreated animals. The lesions are assumed to be due to corrosive action of the unbuffered acid bathing the mid portion of the small bowel. Several reports indicate that mucosal extracts can protect against lesions in this type of dog preparation (Hands *et al.*, 1942; Greengard *et al.*, 1946). Indeed an "immunity" developed in some dogs and they were protected for one year after treatment had stopped. These animals lost their prolonged secretory response to histamine or alcohol which is characteristic of untreated Mann–Williamson dogs (Grossman *et al.*, 1944). It was speculated that the mucosal extract did not depress the stomach acid secretory ability but may have removed all abnormal stimulants to secretion. It was shown that the extracts had no specific action on acid output but did alter secretory rates which subsequently affected acidity (Linde *et al.*, 1952). These extracts had no oral activity in protecting against the production of lesions in the Mann–Williamson dog (Saltzstein *et al.*, 1947; 1949). The substance did not protect against gastric lesions in the pyloric ligated rat (Morris *et al.*, 1947; Benditt *et al.*, 1949). Several negative reports are also published on the parenteral ineffectiveness in dog and man of the mucosal extract (Saltzstein *et al.*, 1949; Ferayorni *et al.*, 1948).

In 1944, a new remedy for peptic ulcers was introduced in Switzerland under the name of Robuden® (Schmassman, 1944). This consisted of an aqueous extract of stomach and intestinal walls of animals. It was admini-

stered by mouth or injection. Various combinations were used for either
duodenal or gastric ulcers. This commercial preparation was quickly
accepted by the clinician as a solution for peptic ulcer disease. By 1958,
over 45 publications described the action of this preparation. About
forty of these studies described the effects of Robuden® on the clinical
course of peptic ulcers, success being claimed in 37 of these studies. The
references are tabulated (Jerzy Glass and Schwartz, 1959). Two negative
double-blind clinical studies are referenced as samples of this literature
(Evans, 1954; Stolte, 1950). Attempts to identify Robuden® indicate
that it contains several mucous substances, pepsin and alkali materials of
unknown nature (Jerzy Glass and Schwartz, 1959). The agent does not
alter acid secretions but can stimulate the production of mucus. The extract has failed to produce consistent, beneficial animal or clinical evidence of usefulness. Clearly, a more purified preparation is needed before
lasting clinical benefits can be claimed for such a crude extract.

Crude extracts of urine have also been studied. One of these preparations has been described as possessing antiulcer activity in the Mann–
Williamson dog preparation without decreasing gastric secretions. This
was called Anthelone. It consisted of extracts of urine obtained either from
pregnant women, non-pregnant women (Sandweiss and Friedman, 1942),
men (Gray et al., 1939), or dogs (Culmer et al., 1939b). The urinary extracts obtained from pregnant women was specifically called antuitrin-S
which was presumably gonadotropic hormone (Sandweiss et al., 1938;
Saltzstein et al., 1949). Urine collected from patients with duodenal
ulcers did not contain the antiulcer factor. The urinary extracts that decreased the acid secretion of the dog was named urogastrone and was
marketed under the name Kutrol®. Urogastrone is not an enterogastrone
since its output is not decreased by resection of the entire small bowel of
dogs (Gray et al., 1940). Both positive (Page and Heffner, 1948) and
negative clinical results have been reported (Kirsner et al., 1948; Dailey
and Benefiel, 1953; Bercovitz, 1954). Several attempts have been made to
purify these urinary extracts (Gray et al., 1942; Gregory, 1955;
Corbellini et al., 1966; Morimoto and Yamamoto, 1969; Lawrence et al.,
1971; Lucchetti, 1973). The history and properties of these urinary extracts have been published (Sandweiss, 1945; Sandweiss et al., 1954).
The former reference states: ". . . more purified and more concentrated
products are yet to be prepared. Larger series of patients are yet to be
treated and observed for much longer periods of time." This statement
essentially summarizes the fate of many substances introduced into
medicine for treating patients with peptic ulcers.

Chronologically, the indication that the gastrointestinal tract contains
substances that can influence gastric secretions was first demonstrated by

placing certain materials into the tract. Certain constituents of chyme, variations in the ionic composition of the material, or intestinal acidification of the small bowel decreased gastric secretions. Whether the endogenous substances released by these techniques are identified enterogastrones or possibly some unidentified substances has not been completely resolved. Even the physiological role of the identified substances has not been settled. The classically established role of the hormone secretin as a pancreas stimulator for bicarbonate release is open to question (Wormsley, 1973). Indeed, a neurological component to the hormonal effects on acid secretion may also be involved (Johnston and Duthie, 1969; Konturek and Johnson, 1971). Predictably, the list of chemically identified intestinal hormones will be expanded. Both the early (Grossman, 1950) and more recent progress (Sircus, 1958; Andersson, 1971; Johnson and Grossman, 1971) in the identification and characteristics of gastrointestinal hormones has been reviewed. The specificity of releasing agents, like specific fatty acids, certain aminoacids and acid has been reported. Several of the known endogenous substances like secretin and CCK may be differentially released to augment each other's principle actions (Meyer and Grossman, 1972).

The endocrine system of the body possesses multiple actions on the secretory process of the stomach. Hypophysectomy in rats reduced gastric secretions and reduced the incidence of susceptability to prednisolone-induced lesions (Robert et al., 1966). A hormone like ACTH may decrease and alter mucus production leading to impaired defense mechanisms (Desbaillets and Menguy, 1967). Calcitonin is antisecretory in man (Hesch et al., 1971). An interaction between calcium and several hormones can exert an effect on gastric secretion (Barreras, 1973). Hormones from pituitary gland, pancreas, sex glands and parathyroids all exert a profound effect on the stomach. The gastrointestinal tract response to a number of hormones (Crean, 1963) and the actions of the adrenocortical steroids on the stomach (Cook, 1967) have been critically reviewed. Some of these actions have been discussed within this paper. The reader is left to see the review articles for further details.

11 Miscellaneous agents

Many substances can inhibit gastric secretion. This section will describe agents that have not received extensive study, agents that affect secretions or reduce ulcer incidence secondarily to their major pharmacological actions and agents listed in patents that claim antisecretory or antiulcer activity among their biological activities.

A series of imidazoles have been characterized for their analgesic, antiinflammatory, antipyretic, and anticonvulsive activity (Alimirante *et al.*, 1965). Zolimidine (**26**), possesses the above spectrum of activity as well as a marked protective action in animals against induced gastric lesions (Camarri *et al.*, 1972). It can also increase the production of gastric

2-(*p*-Methylsulfonylphenyl)imidazo(1,2-*a*)pyridine
zolimidine

(**26**)

mucus in animals and man. Clinically, 1200 mg daily for eight days had no effect on mucus production (mucoprotein concentration—mean 94·5 mg per 100 ml gastric juice) in normals. (Mucoprotein concentration in gastric juice was calculated by determining the amount of tryosine.) However, in seven people with gastric ulcers, in which mucoprotein concentration was low (46·1 mg per 100 ml), the drug at 800 or 1200 mg daily for 30–40 days could elevate the mucoprotein to normal (85·3 mg ml^{-1} gastric juice). Similarly, thirteen patients with duodenal ulcers under similar therapy demonstrated a gastric mucoprotein elevation from 63·8 to 88·2 mg per 100 ml of secretion. Thus zolimidine did not affect the mucoprotein concentration in the gastric juice of healthy individuals but consistently "normalized" the mucus in ulcer patients. The value of this action of the drug will have to be assessed for its ability to relieve pain and prevent the recurrence of peptic ulcers.

Another substance which increases mucus production is ϵ-*p*-chlorobenzyl-oxycarbonyl-L-lysin-OMe-HCl, KL-11 (Ezer and Szporny, 1970; Ridley *et al.*, 1971). This drug was demonstrated to incorporate labelled SO_4 into the gastric mucosa of rats. It could also protect rats against gastric lesions induced by six hours of pyloric ligation or guinea-pigs against betazole-induced duodenal lesions.

Vitamin A is claimed to be important in maintaining the integrity of the mucus secreting cells in the gastrointestinal tract (DeLuca and Wolf, 1969; DeLuca *et al.*, 1969). Vitamin A, administered to rats prior to restraint, could not protect against the induced gastric lesions (Rasche and Butterfield, 1973). Clinically, there is a marked depression of serum Vitamin A in severely injured patients. Massive parenteral Vitamin A could reduce the bleeding and stress ulcer incidence but didn't alter the incidence of mortality in this small group of patients (Chernov *et al.*, 1971). Vitamin E can also protect rats against stress-induced gastric lesions (Kangas *et al.*, 1972). The mechanism of action and therapeutic value of these two vitamins in either stress-induced, or conventional ulcers should be assessed.

[1-(o-Chloro-α-phenylbenzyloxy)ethyl]-4-(o-methylbenzyl)piperazine
Chlorbenzoxamine
(27)

Chlorbenzoxamine, UCB 1474, or Libratar® (27) at doses of 0·1 to 1 mg kg⁻¹ subcutaneously, intraduodenally or orally could protect against gastric lesions in pyloric ligated rats (Levis *et al.*, 1957; Levis *et al.*, 1959). It could also protect the guinea-pig against histamine-induced lesions, and reduce gastric secretion in an acute dog preparation. The drug could protect against several other lesion-producing situations, for example, serotonin, cortisone, reserpine, or restraint (Levis and Beersaerts, 1960; Radouco-Thomas *et al.*, 1960; Hillyard and Grandy, 1963). The protective effect seems critically dependent on dose. Protection from the various challenges was seen with chlorbenzoxamine at 1 mg kg⁻¹. Higher doses were significantly less protective. The drug from 0·04 to 10 mg kg⁻¹ does not decrease secretory volume in the rat (Hillyard and Grandy, 1963). Hypophysectomy in the rat abolished the antiulcer effect in the pyloric ligated preparation. The drug could protect against histamine-induced lesions in the dog. This was seen at daily oral doses of 0·5 mg kg⁻¹ but not at 0·25 or 2·5 mg kg⁻¹.

In two clinical trials, chlorbenzoxamine, at 30 mg four times a day in 30 ulcer patients (type of ulcer not indicated) showed no marked improvement (Jain, 1962). In a proper double-blind study, on gastric and duodenal ulcer patients, 60 mg chlorbenzoxamine three times a day produced no roentgenological improvement of the lesion or reduction in subjective symptoms in comparison to a placebo (Varis *et al.*, 1972). The ability of chlorbenzoxamine to protect against experimental gastric and small bowel lesions seems evident. This action in animals may be a central mechanism. However, the limited clinical trials did not confirm the usefulness of this drug. Again, one sees the inability to use currently available animal models for clinical ulcer disease. Are these models inadequate or are the clinical trials improperly designed to prove a useful clinical candidate?

Other agents have demonstrated protection in experimental models. Protection in the 18-hour pyloric ligated rat was obtained with 4-amino-3-hydroxybutyric acid (Nagai *et al.*, 1971). In a study on a series of aminoacids for their effect against stress-induced lesions in the rat, glutamine gave the highest degree of protection. Other less effective aminoacids were tyrosine, ornithine and methionine. No protection was seen with lysine, proline, or threonine (Takagi and Okabe, 1968). Glutamine could also increase the hexosamine content of mucosa over that of controls in the stressed rat or cortisone-treated rat (Takagi and Yano, 1972). In a small double-blind study on peptic ulcer patients (presumably gastric ulcers), 1·6 g of glutamine daily could enhance the healing rate (Shive *et al.*, 1957). Again, confirmation by other clinical studies is lacking. Solcoseryl, a mixture of low-molecular substances from the deproteinized blood of young calves, protected against reserpine- or serotonin-and/or stress-induced lesions in the rat (Ito *et al.*, 1972).

Gastric antisecretory activity has been reported for the antimalarials, quinine, quinacrine, chlorguanide and related compounds (Babkin and Karp, 1947; Burn and Vane, 1948), maleimides (Fletcher *et al.*, 1959), 3-amino-4-chromanones (Huckle *et al.*, 1969), doxapram and AHR-619 (Alphin *et al.*, 1969). Even the mercury salt, mercury acetate, is antisecretory (Seijffers *et al.*, 1963). Other agents have been demonstrated to possess experimental antiulcer activity. These are 3,4,5-trimethoxy-benzoyl-N'-oxyalkylpiprazine derivatives (Toldy and Tóth, 1964), dioxatrine, 1-benzyl-4-(2,6-dioxo-3-phenyl-3-piperidyl)-piperidine hydrochloride (Niemegeers and Janssen, 1964), a series of p-aminobenza-midopyridines (Moffett *et al.*, 1971), benzamidopiperidine derivatives (Irikura and Kasuga, 1971) and a series of sulfonylurea derivatives (McColl *et al.*, 1963). The latter is surprising since an hypoglycemic agent, tolbutamide, a sulfonylurea, stimulates gastric secretions in man (Weiss and Sciales, 1961).

The biochemical mechanisms of hydrogen ion secretion have not been elucidated. The enzyme, carbonic anhydrase (see scheme in section 9) has been implicated in one of the mechanisms for transporting the hydrogen ion (Maren, 1967). Presently, the quantitative contribution of this system to acid secretion has not been clarified. The enzyme has an ubiquitous distribution in the body. Thus any agent developed to date that inhibits carbonic anhydrase has antisecretory as well as other biological actions, for example, diuresis. Are there isoenzymes of carbonic anhydrase that may be selectively inhibited in the gastric mucosa? No specific gastric carbonic anhydrase inhibitors have been developed. The prototype carbonic anhydrase inhibitor, acetazolamide, has been studied for its effect on gastric secretions. It can inhibit histamine-induced secretions in the dog (Janowitz *et al.*, 1952; Powell *et al.*, 1962), cat (Emås, 1962), as well as in man (Janowitz *et al.*, 1957; Hirschowitz *et al.*, 1959) and isolated frog mucosa (Hersey and High, 1971). In addition it can decrease the secretory response to gastrin-induced secretion in the cat (Emås, 1962), and protect against histamine-induced ulcers in the guinea-pig (Djahanguiri and Hemmati, 1968). Two possible mechanisms have been suggested for acetazolamide. The drug primarily inhibits chloride transport which short circuits the tissue. This effect decreases the electro-chemical gradient which results in a reduction of acid secretion (Hogben, 1965). The more acceptable hypothesis is that acetazolamide decreases the availability of hydrogen for transport in the gastric mucosa by inhibiting carbonic anhydrase (Maren, 1967) which is functionally linked to magne-sium-dependent adenosine triphosphatase (Narumi and Kanno, 1973).

Enzymatic therapy for peptic ulcer patients was suggested for a pre-paration called carbamine which contains effervescent citrate and urea. The urea and carbon dioxide were supposedly the substrate for gastric urease and carbonic anhydrase. It was speculated that these two enzymes promoted the healing of peptic ulcers. Clinical trials suggest usefulness (Kelly, 1960; Goodfriend *et al.*, 1960)!

The two secretagogues, histamine and methylxanthines, have an imi-dazole ring as a common structural feature. Several imidazole derivatives have been shown to be antisecretory on the isolated frog stomach (Alonso *et al.*, 1965), and the rat (Méhes *et al.*, 1966). Imidazole itself as well as N-methylimidazole, 2-methylimidazole, 4(5)-methylimidazole and benzimidazole reduced basal acid secretion. The 2-methylimidazole could also decrease histamine-induced acid secretion in the dog (Harris and Silen, 1964). The compound 1-(2-piperidinoethyl)benzimidazole, or H-635 can decrease acid secretion in the rat (Mehes *et al.*, 1966). These chemicals have not been demonstrated to specifically block a histamine mechanism on the gastric mucosa.

Substances like nitrite, ammonium, cyanate, thiocyanate, or methyl thiocyanate, can suppress gastric secretions (LeFevre *et al.*, 1964; Wong *et al.*, 1969). These agents have been used as pharmacological tools for exploring the mode of secretion of the hydrogen ion. For example, thio-cyanate may be antisecretory to the isolated frog mucosa by competing with chloride for an active anion transport system (Durbin, 1964). Thiocyanate will decrease secretion in the rat or dog, possibly by increas-ing the back diffusion of the hydrogen ion (Moody and Davis, 1970; Narumi and Kanno, 1972). On a biochemical basis, antisecretory action may be due to inhibition of carbonic anhydrase (Davenport, 1940) or more directly by inhibiting magnesium-dependent adenosine triphos-phatase (Narumi and Kanno, 1973). The other actions of these inorganic substances, for example, cyanate decreases thyroid function, preclude their use in lowering acid secretion in man.

Nicotine may be another substance that may alter secretory processes. It has been shown that on chronic administration up to 14 days to rats, nicotine, via a central mechanism, can increase secretions (Thompson and George, 1972). In contrast, single injections are antisecretory (Thompson and Brückner, 1970). An adverse effect of nicotine may be due to its ability to decrease pancreatic bicarbonate output in the dog (Konturek et al., 1971). Cigarette smoking has also been related to the decrease in bicarbonate secretion into the small bowel of man (Bynum et al., 1972). Cigarette smokers have a higher incidence of duodenal ulcers than non-smokers (Edwards et al., 1959; Monson, 1970). The disease morbidity is directly related to the quantity and duration of smoking (Edwards et al., 1959). This effect could lower the endogenous effect of small-bowel secretions and possibly potentiate the ulcerogenic effect of non-neutralized gastric effluent. Nicotine has been shown to reinforce the ulcer-forming action of prolonged infusions of gastrin and carbachol (Robert, 1972). The suggestion that pancreatic bicarbonate secretion is important in preventing duodenal ulcers could open a new approach to treating this disease. Is it practical to develop drugs that could increase the alkalinity of the upper small bowel?

A central nervous system link to gastric secretory function has been well documented (Brooks, 1967; Reigel et al., 1971). Over a century ago, Beaumont noted the effect of emotional conflict on the color and secretion of the stomach (Beaumont, 1833, republished, 1959). The detailed pathway and mechanism have not been described. It is not surprising that drugs with primary actions in the brain can influence gastric secretion. One of the nonspecific actions of the anesthetics is to markedly decrease acid secretions. This topic was recently reviewed (Bennett and Bass, 1972). In the dog, pentobarbital could decrease secretions that were spontaneous or induced by histamine, alcohol or sham feeding (Powell and Hirschowitz, 1967). Anesthetics can also act on the isolated frog stomach. Amytal, methoxyflurane, chloroform and halothane can inhibit secretory processes (Villegas, 1969; Mackrell and Schwartz, 1969; Schwartz and Mackrell, 1969). In the rat, pentobarbital, chloralose and urethane were antisecretory while ether stimulated secretions (Lee and Thompson, 1967). In contrast, a detailed study on the antisecretory action of ether anesthesia has been reported (Dai and Ogle, 1973). Several anesthetics, urethane, barbitone, halothane and ether were shown to alter secretory action to various secretagogues in the rat (Barrett et al., 1966). Pentobarbital and the defunct sedative thalidomide can protect rats against restraint-induced ulcers (Hanson and Brodie, 1960;

Martindale, *et al.*, 1960; Brodie *et al.*, 1963). However, the protective dose and lethal dose of pentobarbital in rats were almost identical (Chen and Bass, 1964). A similar relationship was obtained for meprobamate. In man, the chronic use of phenobarbital had no short- or long-term influence on the healing of gastric ulcers in people (Truelove, 1960). Thus, nonspecific depressants like the anesthetics can influence experimental results. This influence may be by a central or a local action.

Centrally acting drugs with more specific loci of action can also influence the secretion and mucosa of the stomach. Chlorpromazine and benactyzine decrease restraint-induced ulcers in the rat (Hanson and Brodie, 1960). Though serotonin and 5-hydroxytryptophan can decrease acid secretion in the rat, neither lysergic acid diethylamide (LSD) nor brom-lysergic acid diethylamide alter secretions (Shay *et al.*, 1958). The anticonvulsant drug 3-ethyl-2-methyl-2-phenylsuccinimide, CI-419, could protect against stress-induced gastric lesions in the rat (Chen and Bass, 1964). The use of the benzodiazepines may be a practical approach to reduce the CNS component in people with ulcers. Chlordiazepoxide (Librium®) can reduce stress-induced lesions in rats (Haot *et al.*, 1964). Diazepam can decrease basal and night secretions in patients with duodenal ulcers (Birnbaum *et al.*, 1971) as well as decrease acid secretion in several rat preparations (Birnbaum *et al.*, 1973).

Two neuroleptic drugs, metoclopramide and sulpiride, was introduced to medicine as antiemetics. Clinically, metoclopramide has been shown to prevent the recurrence of duodenal ulcers. In a one year double-blind study on patients with duodenal ulcers, metoclopramide at 10 mg four times a day and at bedtime effectively prevented relapse in 41 of 51 patients. In contrast, the placebo treated group had 25 of 39 people with a recurrence of symptoms. Metoclopramide was ineffective in treating the acute exacerbations of duodenal ulcers (Moshal, 1973). In another double-blind study, metoclopramide (10 mg three times a day) was compared to carbenoxolone sodium (100 mg three times a day) for treating gastric ulcers in 28 out-patients (Hoskins, 1973). In this five-week trial, metoclopramide was as good as carbenoxolone in healing gastric ulcers. Sulpiride at 100 mg i.v. could moderately reduce (18 per cent) acid output induced by a continuous infusion of pentagastrin ($2 \mu g \ kg^{-1} \ h^{-1}$) (Aune and Stadaas, 1972). It is intriguing that two agents that possess antiemetic actions are useful for ulcer therapy. Metoclopramide has been demonstrated to enhance the rate of stomach emptying. Does this remove the "ulcerogenic factors" from the stomach and sweep them through the small bowel? Could the drug cause a rapid emptying of acid content, or alternately, prevent the reflux of small bowel contents? Antacids, in addition to neutralizing stomach contents, enhance the emptying rate of the stomach. These studies point to the possibility that gastro-intestinal motility may be a factor in ulcerogenesis. Alternately, are the neurolepic drugs acting through a central mechanism? A specific search for a centrally acting drug could be fruitful. This would eliminate one of the controlling parameters of the complex biological interaction that modulates gastric secretion.

Patents are issued with claims for gastric antisecretory or gastric anti-ulcer activity among their biologic actions. The following structures are samples of chemical structures claimed for gastrointestinal therapeutics (28, 29). Most of these patents do not include the biological data

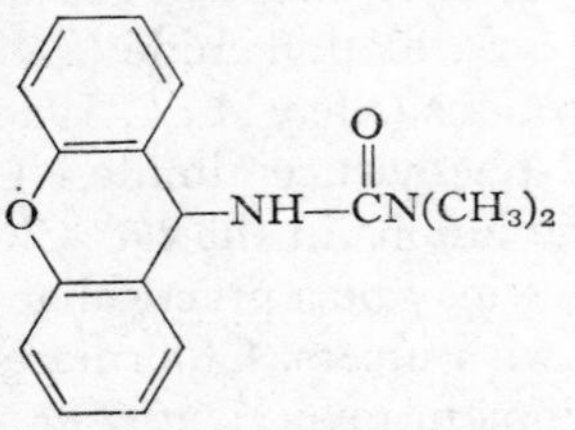

Netherlands 6,711,975 (1967)
(Boots Co. Ltd)

(28)

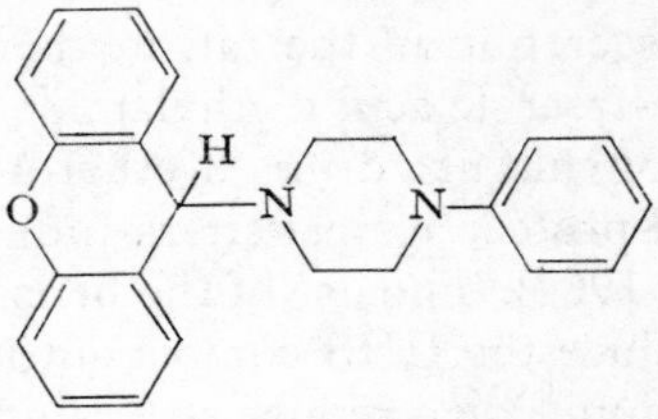

U.S. Pat. 3,356,681 (1967)
(G. D. Searle and Co.)

(29)

supporting their claim. Therefore, evaluation of the pharmacologic activity and therapeutic potential of agents claimed in patents must be postponed until sufficient data are published.

12 Summary

Peptic ulcers (esophageal, gastric, and duodenal ulcers), though possibly caused by the presence of acid and/or pepsin, may be induced by different biological situations. Experimentally, chemical, surgical, and manipul-ative stress procedures can alter secretion and mimic lesion production in the stomach. Duodenal experimental lesions are more difficult to produce and assess. Since the clinical disease is of unknown etiology, one cannot select a specific animal model for the clinical gastric or duodenal ulcer. The variability of the symptoms and history of the clinical disease make it difficult to assess a drug that will reduce the lesions and delay or prevent recurrences.

Due to the vagaries of the disease, many preparations and chemicals have been searched for and tried. Empirical animal screening for gastric antisecretory and antiulcer substances have resulted in demonstrating that many chemicals can affect the gastric parameters in animals, but few have been confirmed in man. Attempts to enhance the healing rate of gastric or duodenal lesions has produced at least two substances, gefarnate and carbenoxolone, that have been extensively used in man. These substances appear more effective on gastric than duodenal ulcers—the less common of the two lesions. Equally important, both substances were initially introduced clinically with minimal animal studies or toxicity evaluation. Is our knowledge of gastrointestinal function so meager that so many animal models are inadequate? The clinical evaluation of therapy in a disease which is characterized by unpredictable remissions and recurrences is difficult. The objectivity of double-blind therapeutic trials and objective measurements with fiberscopes is a welcome to gastroenterology research for evaluating therapeutic agents.

Endogenous substances can exacerbate or reduce gastric secretions and lesions. The understanding of the function of endogenous substances could lead to a rational approach to controlling ulcerogenic conditions. The search is on for substances that could block gastrin and/or histamine! In general, the medicinal chemist has not been very successful in developing peptide inhibitors, for example, antigastrin substances. The blockade of endogenous amines has been more successful. The recent characterization of H_2-receptors and the pharmacological characterization of burimamide and metiamide as H_2-receptor antagonists is indeed very promising for the development of a gastric antisecretory agent. As stated at a recent symposium, "H_2-receptor antagonists are the most likely candidates to succeed (as therapeutic agents) which have been developed since the discovery that the stomach secretes acid" (Code, 1973). Another promising approach is to develop a prostaglandin analogue with prolonged antisecretory action and minimal side effects. Will a better understanding of the role of the adrenergic nervous system and cAMP lead to an approach for controlling acid and pepsin secretion? Of the other endogenous substances, will one of the enterogastrones prove to be clinically useful? Any rational approach to developing drugs that affect endogenous substances will have to be specific for the secretory mechanisms and possess minimal side effects.

Both acid and pepsin appear to be involved in the ulcer disease. Inhibition of the action of pepsin seems possible. The ability of several peptides (e.g. pepstatin) to inhibit the proteolytic substances on a molar basis is a major breakthrough in controlling pepsin. These types of inhibitory substances should enable us to assess the role of pepsin in producing ulcers. If pepsin has a role, its control appears close at hand.

The role of stomach emptying and smooth muscle activity in ulcerogenesis is not understood. The value of neutralizing gastric effluent or removing it from the proximal small bowel has yet to be assessed. The retropulsion of bile into the stomach may be important in generating or maintaining a gastric lesion. Basic studies relating motility to ulcer production are lacking.

One is impressed with the multifacet pharmacological approach to a common disease entity. Success in pharmacologically controlling the acute exacerbation as well as the recurrence of the disease seems close at hand. Clinically, which of the agents presently available or to be developed will prove useful? Peptic ulcer still remains an enigmatic disease, but should lend itself to drug therapy.

REFERENCES

Aarsen, P. N. (1973). *Arzneim.-Forsch.* **23**, 1346.

Acheson, G. H. (1966). *Pharmacol. Rev.* **18**, 1.

Adami, E., Marazzi-Uberti, E. and Turba, C. (1962). *Med. Exp.* **7**, 171.

Adami, E., Marazzi-Uberti, E. and Turba, C. (1964). *Arch. Int. Pharmacodyn. Ther.* **147**, 113.

Adami, E., Fanti, G. and Presia, P. (1966). *In* "Proceedings of the 3rd World Congress of Gastroenterology, Tokyo", **2**, 134.

Ader, R. (1971). *In* "Advances in Psychosomatic Medicine" (Ed. H. Weiner), vol. **6**, p. 1. S. Karger, Basel.

Albinus, M. and Sewing, K. F. (1969). *J. Pharm. Pharmacol.* **21**, 656.

Albinus, M. and Sewing, K. F. (1973a). *Arch. Int. Pharmacodyn. Ther.* **279**, 417.

Albinus, M. and Sewing, K. F. (1973b). *Ag. Actions*, **3**, 172.

Alimirante, L., Polo, L., Mugnaini, A., Provinciali, E., Rugarli, P., Biancotti, A., Gamba, A. and Murmann, W. (1965). *J. Med. Chem.* **8**, 305.

Alonso, D., Rynes, R. and Harris, J. B. (1965). *Amer. J. Physiol.* **208**, 1183.

Alphin, R. S. and Ward, J. W. (1969). *Eur. J. Pharmacol.* **6**, 61.

Alphin, R. S., Franko, B. V. and Ward, J. W. (1969). *Arch. Int. Pharmacodyn. Ther.* **180**, 180.

Alphin, R. S., Vocac, J. A. and Droppleman, D. A. (1972). *Experientia*, **28**, 53.

Amer, M. S. (1969). *Clin. Res.* **17**, 524.

Amure, B. O. (1970). *Gut*, **11**, 171.

Amure, B. O. and Ginsberg, M. (1964). *Brit. J. Pharmacol. Chemother.* **22**, 520.

Amure, B. O. and Omole, A. A. (1970). *Gut*, **11**, 641.

Amy, J. J., Jackson, D. M., Adaikan Ganesan, R. and Karim, S. M. M. (1973). *Brit. Med. J.* **iii**, 208.

Anderson, W. (1961). *J. Pharm. Pharmacol.* **13**, 139.

Anderson, W. (1965). *Arch. Int. Pharmacodyn. Ther.* **157**, 181.

Anderson, W. (1969). *J. Pharm. Pharmacol.* **21**, 264.

Anderson, W. and Harthill, J. E. (1973). *Nature*, **243**, 417.

Anderson, W. and Soman, P. D. (1963). *Nature*, **199**, 389.

Anderson, W. and Soman, P. D. (1965a). *J. Pharm. Pharmacol.* **17**, 92.

Anderson, W. and Soman, P. D. (1965b). *J. Pharm. Pharmacol.* **17**, 121.

Anderson, W. and Soman, P. D. (1966a). *J. Pharm. Pharmacol.* **18**, 825.

Anderson, W. and Soman, P. D. (1966b). *J. Pharm. Pharmacol.* **18**, Suppl. 142S.

Anderson, W. and Watt, J. (1959). *J. Pharm. Pharmacol.* **11**, 1739.

Anderson, W., Marcus, R. and Watt, J. (1962). *J. Pharm. Pharmacol.* **14**, 119.
Anderson, W., Baillie, A. J. and Harthill, J. E. (1968). *J. Pharm. Pharmacol.* **20**, 715.
Andersson, S. (1971). *Gastroenterology*, **61**, 778.
Andersson, S., Bárány, F., Caboclo, J. L. F. and Mizuno, T. (1971). *Scand. J. Gastroenterol.* **6**, 683.
Anichkov, S. V. and Grechishkin, L. L. (1969). *Arch. Int. Pharmacodyn. Ther.* **180**, 281.
Antonsen, S. (1967). *Acta Pharmacol. Toxicol.* **25**, 405.
Antonsen, S. (1968). *Acta Pharmacol.* **26**, Suppl. 2, 1.
Aoyagi, T., Morishima, H., Nishizawa, R., Kunimoto, S., Takeuchi, T. and Umezawa, H. (1972). *J. Antibiot.* **25**, 689.
Ash, A. S. F. and Schild, H. O. (1966). *Brit. J. Pharmacol. Chemother.* **27**, 427.
Ashford, C. A. and Heller, H. (1949). *Brit. J. Pharmacol. Chemother.* **4**, 157.
Assem, E. S. K., Schild, H. O. and Wan, B. Y. C. (1973). *J. Physiol.* **234**, 75p.
Atik, M., Balart, L. A., Isla, F. and McHardy, G. (1965). *J. Amer. Med. Ass.* **191**, 114.
Aune, S. and Stadaas, J. O. (1972). *Scand. J. Gastroenterol.* **7**, 713.
Aures, D., Davidson, W. D. and Håkanson, R. (1969). *Eur. J. Pharmacol.* **8**, 100.
Avery Jones, F. and Sullivan, F. M. (1972). "Carbenoxolone in Gastroenterology". Butterworths, London.
Aylett, P. (1962). *Clin. Sci.* **22**, 179.
Babkin, B. P. (1950 2nd ed.). *In* "Secretory Mechanism of the Digestive Glands", p. 252. Paul B. Hoeber, Inc., New York.
Babkin, B. P. and Karp, D. (1947). *Can. Med. Ass. J.* **56**, 137.
Balmforth, G. V., Samuel, R. de K. G. and Kerridge, D. (1964). *Brit. Med. J.* i, 355.
Bank, S., Marks, I. N., Palmer, P. E. S., Groll, A. and van Eldik, E. (1967). *S. Afr. Med. J.* **41**, 297.
Bapna, J., Neff, N. H. and Costa, E. (1970). *Neuropharmacol.* **9**, 333.
Barnes, W. A., Redo, S. F., Ecker, R. R. and Wenig, J. (1967). *Amer. J. Surg.* **113**, 27.
Baron, J. H. and Sullivan, F. M. (1970). "Carbenoxolone Sodium". Butterworths, London.
Baron, J. H., Nabarro, J. D. N., Slater, J. D. H. and Tuffley, R. (1969). *Brit. Med. J.* ii, 793.
Barreras, R. F. (1973). *Gastroenterology*, **64**, 1168.
Barrett, A. M., Raventos, J. and Siddall, R. A. (1966). *Brit. J. Pharmacol. Chemother.* **28**, 51.
Barth, H., Niemeyer, I. and Lorenz, W. (1973). *Ag. Actions*, **3**, 138.
Bass, P. and Patterson, M. A. (1967). *J. Pharmacol. Exp. Ther.* **156**, 142.
Bass, P., Purdon, R. A. and Patterson, M. A. (1966a). *J. Pharmacol. Exp. Ther.* **153**, 292.
Bass, P., Purdon, R. A., Patterson, M. A. and Butler, D. E. (1966b). *J. Pharmacol. Exp. Ther.* **152**, 104.
Bass, P., Butler, D. E., Patterson, M. A. and Purdon, R. A. (1967). *Arch. Int. Pharmacodyn. Ther.* **169**, 131.
Basso, N., Umeda, N., Roth, J. L. A., Passaro, Jr., E. and Pfeiffer, C. J. (1971). *Gastroenterology*, **61**, 207.
Bateson, P. R. (1954). *Med. Illus.* **8**, 370.

Baume, P. and Powell, K. C. (1966). *Med. J. Aust.* **2**, 596.

Baume, P., Baxter, C. H. and Nicholls, A. (1967). *Amer. J. Dig. Dis.* **12**, 965.

Baume, P., Baxter, C. H. and Nicholls, A. (1968). *Aust. Ann. Med.* **17**, 42.

Beaumont, W. (1959). "Experiments and Observations on the Gastric Juice and the Physiology of Digestion". Dover Publications Inc., New York.

Becker, M. and Sewing, K. F. (1971). *J. Pharm. Pharmacol.* **23**, 434.

Becker, H. D., Reeder, D. D. and Thompson, J. C. (1973). *Gastroenterology*, **65**, 28.

Bedi, B. S., Gillespie, G. and Gillespie, I. E. (1967a). *Lancet*, **i**, 1240.

Bedi, B. S., Gillespie, G. and Gillespie, I. E. (1967b). *Lancet*, **ii**, 841.

Bedi, B. S., Govaerts, J. P. and Master, S. P. (1968). *Scand. J. Gastroenterol.* **2**, 68.

Bedi, B. S., Debas, H. T., Wasunna, A. E. O., Buxton, B. F. and Gillespie, I. E. (1971). *Gut*, **12**, 968.

Benditt, E., Kirsner, J. and Rowley, D. (1949). *Gastroenterology*, **13**, 330.

Benfey, B. G., Ledoux, G. and Melville, K. I. (1959a). *Brit. J. Pharmacol. Chemother.* **14**, 142.

Benfey, B. G., Ledoux, G. and Segal, M. (1959b). *Brit. J. Pharmacol. Chemother.* **14**, 380.

Bennett, A. and Fleshler, B. (1970). *Gastroenterology*, **59**, 790.

Bennett, A., Friedman, C. A. and Vane, J. R. (1967). *Nature*, **216**, 873.

Bennett, A., Murray, J. G. and Wyllie, J. H. (1968). *Brit. J. Pharmacol. Chemother.* **32**, 339.

Bennett, A., Stamford, I. F. and Unger, W. G. (1972). *J. Physiol.* **226**, 96P.

Bennett, A., Stamford, I. F. and Unger, W. G. (1973a). *J. Physiol.* **229**, 349.

Bennett, A., Stamford, I. F. and Unger, W. G. (1973b). *In* "Advances in the Biosciences", vol. 9, p. 265. Pergamon Press, Vieweg, Braunschweig.

Bennett, D. R. and Bass, P. (1972). *In* "Handbook of Experimental Pharmacology" (Ed. M. B. Chenoweth),vol. 30, p. 299. Springer-Verlag, New York.

Bercovitz, Z. T. (1954). *Gastroenterology*, **26**, 230.

Berg, B. N., Zucker, T. F. and Zucker, L. M. (1949). *Proc. Soc. Exp. Biol. Med.* **71**, 374.

Bergman, J., Persson, K. Ö. U. and Westling, H. (1962). *Acta Med. Scand.* **172**, 637.

Bergström, S., Carlson, L. A. and Weeks, J. R. (1968). *Pharmacol. Rev.* **20**, 1.

Bersimbaev, R. I., Argutinskaya, S. V. and Salganik, R. I. (1971). *Experientia*, **27**, 1389.

Berstad, A. (1972). *Scand. J. Gastroenterol.* **7**, 129.

Berstad, A. and Petersen, H. (1970). *Scand. J. Gastroenterol.* **5**, 647.

Bertaccini, G., Erspamer, V. and Impicciatore, M. (1973). *Brit. J. Pharmacol. Chemother.* **49**, 437.

Bertellini, G. A., Butti, A., Piantanida, G., Prino, A., Riva, A., Rossi, A. and Rossi, S. (1971). *Arzneim.-Forsch.* **21**, 244.

Berthet, G. (1961). *Gaz. Med. France*, **68**, 2789.

Bhana, D., Karim, S. M. M., Carter, D. C. and Ganesan, P. A. (1973). *Prostaglandins*, **3**, 307.

Bhargava, K. P., Gupta, M. B. and Tangri, K. K. (1973). *Eur. J. Pharmacol.* **22**, 191.

Bianchi, R. G. and Cook, D. L. (1964). *Gastroentrology*, **47**, 409.

Bianchi, R. G. and Saccabusi, E. (1969). *Minerva Med.* **60**, 1044.

Bieck, P. R., Oates, J. A. and Adkins, R. B. (1971). *Clin. Res.* **19**, 387.

Bieck, P. R., Oates, J. A., Robison, G. A. and Adkins, R. B. (1973). *Amer. J. Physiol.* **224**, 158.

Binder, B. and Sewing, K. F. (1973). *Naunyn-Schmiedeberg's Arch. Pharmakol. Exp. Pathol.* **278**, 425.

Birnbaum, D., Karmeli, F. and Tefera, M. (1971). *Gut*, **12**, 616.

Birnbaum, D., Karmeli, F. and Wauku, S. Y. (1973). *Rend. Gastroenterol.* **5**, 1.

Bitch, V. (1966). *Scand. J. Clin. Lab. Invest.* **18**, 357.

Black, J. W., Duncan, W. A. M., Durant, C. J., Ganellin, C. R. and Parsons, E. M. (1972). *Nature*, **236**, 385.

Black, J. W., Duncan, W. A. M., Emmett, J. C., Ganellin, C. R., Hesselbo, T., Parsons, M. E. and Wyllie, J. H. (1973). *Ag. Actions*, **3**, 133.

Blair, D. W. and Forrest, A. P. M. (1960). *Exp. Surg.* **47**, 428.

Blum, A. J., Hirschowitz, B. I., Helander, H. F. and Sachs, G. (1971). *Biochim. Biophys. Acta*, **241**, 261.

Bodanszky, A., Ondetti, M. A., Mutt, V. and Bodanszky, M. (1969). *J. Amer. Chem. Soc.* **91**, 944.

Boissier, J. R., Giudicelli, J. F., Larno, S. and Fichelle, J. (1970). *J. Pharmacol.* **1**, 109.

Bonfils, S., Hardouin, J. P. and Delbarre, F. (1954). *C. R. Soc. Biol.* **148**, 881.

Bonfils, S., Dubrasquet, M. and Lambling, A. (1959). *Med. Exp.* **1**, 239.

Bonfils, S., Dubrasquet, M. and Lambling, A. (1960). *Rev. Fr. Etud. Clin. Biol.* **5**, 71.

Bonfils, S., Kaess, H. and Lambling, A. (1961). *Gastroenterologia*, **96**, 91.

Bonfils, S., Dubrasquet, M. and Lambling, A. (1962a). *J. Appl. Physiol.* **17**, 299.

Bonfils, S., Dubrasquet, M. and Lambling, A. (1962b). *Gastroenterologia*, **98**, 217.

Bonfils, S., Dubrasquet, M., Gorostiaga-Pirotta, A. and Lambling, A. (1965). *Arch. Mal. App. Dig. Nutr.* **54**, 467.

Borella, L. E. and Herr, F. (1971). *Gastroenterology*, **61**, 345.

Borellini, D. and Milvio, C. (1969). *Minerva Med.* **60**, 1053.

Borsy, J., Andrasi, F. and Farkas, L. (1970). *In* "Abstracts of the 4th World Congress of Gastroenterology" (Eds P. Riis, P. Anthonisen and H. Baden), p. 304. Danish Gastroenterology Association, Copenhagen.

Bower, R. J. and Myerson, R. M. (1964). *Amer. J. Gastroenterol.* **42**, 515.

Brady, J. V. (1964). *Trans. N.Y. Acad. Sci.* **26**, 483.

Brady, J. V., Porter, R. W., Conrad, D. G. and Mason, J. W. (1958). *J. Exp. Anal. Behav.* **1**, 69.

Brodie, D. A. (1968). *Gastroenterology*, **55**, 125.

Brodie, D. A. (1970). *In* "Progress in Gastroenterology" (Ed. G. B. J. Glass), vol. 2, p. 92. Grune and Stratton, New York.

Brodie, D. A. and Hooke, K. F. (1971). *Digestion*, **4**, 193.

Brodie, D. A. and Valitski, L. S. (1963). *Proc. Soc. Exp. Biol. Med.* **113**, 998.

Brodie, D. A., Hanson, H. M., Sines, J. O. and Ader, R. (1963). *J. Neuropsychiat.* **4**, 388.

Brooks, F. P. (1967). *In* "Handbook of Physiology" Section 6, Alimentary Canal (Ed. C. F. Code), vol. 2, p. 805. Williams and Wilkins, Maryland.

Brooks, A. M. and Grossman, M. I. (1970). *Gastroenterology*, **59**, 114.

Brooks, A. M., Isenberg, J. and Grossman, M. I. (1969). *Gastroenterology*, **57**, 159.

Brown, J. C. and Dryburgh, J. R. (1971). *Can. J. Biochem.* **49**, 867.

Brown, J. C. and Pederson, R. A. (1970). *Scand. J. Gastroenterol.* **5**, 537.

Brown, D. D., Tomchick, R. and Axelrod, J. (1959a). *J. Biol. Chem.* **234**, 2948.

Brown, J. C., Mutt, V. and Pederson, R. A. (1970). *J. Physiol.* **209**, 57.

Brown, J. C., Pederson, R. A., Jorpes, E. and Mutt, V. (1969). *Can. J. Physiol. Pharmacol.* **47**, 113.

Brown, H. M., Christie, G. B., Colin-Jones, E., Finney, R. S. H., MacGreigor, W. C., Smith, J. M., Smith, W. O., Sullivan, F. M., Tárnoky, A. L., Turner, E. E., Walton, D. E. M. and Watkinson, G. (1959b). *Lancet,* **ii**, 492.

Burnschwig, A., Rasmusser, R. A., Camp, E. J. and Moe, R. (1942). *Surgery,* **12**, 887.

Bunchman II, H. H., Reeder, D. R. and Thompson, J. C. (1971). *Surg. Forum,* **22**, 303.

Burchell, H. D. and Varco, R. L. (1942). *J. Pharmacol. Exp. Ther.* **75**, 1.

Burn, J. H. and Vane, J. R. (1948). *Brit. J. Pharmacol. Chemother.* **3**, 346.

Butler, D. E., Purdon, R. A. and Bass, P. (1970). *Amer. J. Dig. Dis.* **15**, 157.

Butler, D. E., Bass, P., Nordin, I. C., Hauck, Jr., F. P. and L'Italien, Y. J. (1971). *J. Med. Chem.* **14**, 575.

Bynum, T. E., Solomon, T. E., Johnson, L. R. and Jacobson, E. D. (1972). *Gut,* **13**, 361.

Camarri, E., Zaccherotti, L. and D'Alonzo, D. (1972). *Arzneim.-Forsch.* **22**, 768.

Cameron, A. J. (1971). *Surg. Clin. N. Amer.* **51**, 893.

Caren, J. F., Aures, D. and Johnson, L. R. (1969). *Proc. Soc. Exp. Biol. Med.* **131**, 1194.

Carsten, M. E. and Pierce, J. G. (1957). *J. Biol. Chem.* **229**, 61.

Cass, R. and Spriggs, T. L. B. (1961). *Brit. J. Pharmacol. Chemother.* **17**, 442.

Cayer, D. and Ruffin, J. M. (1967). *Ann. N.Y. Acad. Sci.* **140**, 744.

Chasseaud, L. F., Fry, B. J., Saggers, V. H., Sward, I. P. and Hathway, D. E. (1972). *Biochem. Pharmacol.* **21**, 3121.

Chen. G. and Bass, P. (1964). *Arch. Int. Pharmacodyn. Ther.* **152**, 115.

Cheney, G. (1940). *Proc. Soc. Exp. Biol. Med.* **45**, 190.

Cheney, G. (1950). *Stanford Med. Bull.* **8**, 144.

Chernov, M. S., Hall, H. W. and Wood, M. (1971). *Amer. J. Surg.* **122**, 674.

Chey, W. Y., Hitanant, S., Hendricks, J. and Lorber, S. H. (1970). *Gastroenterology,* **58**, 820.

Chey, W. Y., Sivasomboon, B. and Hendricks, J. (1973). *Amer. J. Physiol.* **224**, 852.

Clark, D. H. (1953). *Brit. Med. J.* **i**, 1254.

Clark, D. H. (1957). *Scot. Med. J.* **2**, 392.

Clarke, S. D., Neill, D. W. and Wellbourn, R. B. (1960). *Gut,* **1**, 146.

Classen, M., Koch, H., Deyhle, P., Weidenhiller, S. and Demling, L. (1970). *Klin. Wochenschr.* **48**, 876.

Classen, M., Koch, H., Bickhardt, J., Topf, G. and Demling, L. (1971). *Digestion,* **4**, 333.

Cliff, J. M. and Milton-Thompson, G. J. (1970). *Gut,* **11**, 167.

Coceani, F. and Wolfe, L. S. (1966). *Can. J. Physiol. Pharmacol.* **44**, 933.

Coceani, F., Pace-Asciak, F., Volta, F. and Wolfe, L. S. (1967). *Amer. J. Physiol.* **213**, 1056.

Coceani, F., Pace-Asciak, C. and Wolfe, L. S. (1968). *In* "Prostaglandin Symposium of the Worcester Foundation for Experimental Biology" (Eds P. W. Ramwell and J. E. Shaw), p. 39. John Wiley, New York.

Coceani, F., Dreifuss, J. J., Puglisi, L. and Wolfe, L. S. (1969). *In* "Prostaglandins, Peptides and Amines" (Eds P. Mantegazza and E. W. Horton), p. 73. Academic Press, London and New York.

Cocking, J. B. (1972). *Gastroenterology*, **62**, 6.
Cocking, J. B. and MacCaig, J. N. (1969). *Gut*, **10**, 219.
Code, C. F. (1951). *Physiol. Rev.* **3**, 59.
Code, C. F. (1965). *Fed. Proc.* **24**, 1311.
Code, C. F. (1967). *In* "Gastric Secretion—Mechanisms and Control" (Eds T. K. Shnitka, J. A. L. Gilbert and R. C. Harrison), p. 377. Pergamon Press, Toronto.
Code, C. F. (1973). *In* "International Symposium of Histamine H_2-Receptor Antagonists" (Eds C. J. Wood and M. A. Simkins), p. 313. Smith, Kline and French Lab. Ltd., Welwyn Garden City.
Code, C. F., Maslinski, S. M., Mossini, F. and Navert, H. (1971). *J. Physiol.* **217**, 557.
Connell, A. M., Fletcher, J., Howel Jones, J. and Pygott, F. (1966). *Gut*, **7**, 717.
Connell, A. M., Sircus, W., Hill, R. A., Macleod, I. B. and Thomson, C. G. (1967). *Lancet*, **ii**, 720.
Connell, A. M., Hill, R. A. Macleod, I. B., Sircus, W. and Thomson, C. G. (1968). *Gut*, **9**, 641.
Cook, A. R. (1967). *Gastroenterology*, **52**, 272.
Cook, D. L. and Bianchi, R. G. (1967). *Life Sci.* **6**, 1381.
Cook, D. L. and Drill, V. A. (1967). *Ann. N.Y. Acad. Sci.* **140**, 724.
Cook, D. L., Eich, S. and Cammarata, P. S. (1963). *Arch. Int. Pharmacodyn. Ther.* **144**, 1.
Coppi, G., Bonardi, G. and Martinelli, E. (1969). *Arzneim.-Forsch.* **19**, 1519.
Corbellini, A., Lugaro, G., Lupi, I. and Crespi, E. (1966). *Ital. J. Biochem.* **15**, 151.
Cowley, D. F. (1973). *Gastroenterology*, **65**, 43.
Crane, J. T., Lindsay, S. and Dailey, M. E. (1947). *Amer. J. Dig. Dis.* **14**, 56.
Crean, G. P. (1963). *In* "Vitamins and Hormones" (Eds R. S. Harris, I. G. Wool and J. A. Loraine), vol. 21, p. 215. Academic Press, New York and London.
Croft, D. N. and Ingelfinger, F. J. (1969). *Clin. Sci.* **37**, 491.
Cross, S. and Rhodes, J. (1972). *Gastroenterology*, **62**, 737.
Culmer, C. U., Atkinson, A. J. and Ivy, A. C. (1939a). *Endocrinology*, **24**, 631.
Culmer, C. U., Atkinson, A. J. and Ivy, A. C. (1939b). *Amer. J. Physiol.* **126**, 472.
Curwain, B. P. and Holton, P. (1972). *Brit. J. Pharmacol. Chemother.* **46**, 225.
Curwain, B. P., Holton, P. and Spencer, J. (1972). *Brit. J. Pharmacol. Chemother.* **46**, 566p.
Curwain, B. P., Holton, P. and Spencer, J. (1973a). *J. Physiol.* **230**, 33p.
Curwain, B. P., Holton, P. and Spencer, J. (1973b). *Brit. J. Pharmacol. Chemother.* **48**, 341.
Dai, S. and Ogle, C. V. (1973). *Life Sci.* **13**, 327.
Dailey, M. E. and Benefiel, W. (1953). *Gastroenterology*, **24**, 535.
Dale, H. H. and Laidlaw, P. P. (1910). *J. Physiol.* **41**, 318.
Danhof, I. E. (1967). *Minerva Med.* **58**, 3670.
Danhof, I. E. (1969). *Rev. Med.* **49**, 107.
Danhof, I. E. and Geumei, A. (1972). *Brit. J. Pharmacol. Chemother.* **46**, 170.
Davenport, H. W. (1940). *Amer. J. Physiol.* **129**, 505.
Davenport, H. W. (1968). *Gastroenterology*, **54**, 175.
Davenport, H. W. and Chavré, V. J. (1950). *Gastroenterology*, **15**, 467.
Dean, A. C. B. (1968). *In* "A Symposium on Carbenoxolone Sodium" (Eds J. M. Robson and F. M. Sullivan), p. 33. Butterworths, London.
DeLuca, L. and Wolf, G. (1969). *Amer. J. Clin. Nutr.* **22**, 1059.

DeLuca, L., Little, E. P. and Wolf, G. (1969). *J. Biol. Chem.* **244**, 701.
de Marcos Perez, V. M. (1967). *Rev. Espan. Enferm. Ap. Dig.* **26**, 3.
Demling, L. (1972). *In* "Gastrointestinal Hormones". Georg Thiem, Verlag, Stuttgart.
Desbaillets, L. and Menguy, R. (1967). *Amer. J. Dig. Dis.* **12**, 582.
Deutsch, E. and Christian, H. J. (1959). *J. Amer. Med. Ass.* **169**, 2012.
Deutsch, E. and Thaler, H. (1951). *Virchows Arch. Pathol. Anat.* **320**, 1.
Djahanguiri, B. (1969a). *J. Pharm. Pharmacol.* **21**, 541.
Djahanguiri, B. (1969b). *Pharmacology*, **2**, 14.
Djahanguiri, B. and Hemmati, S. (1968). *Pharmacology*, **1**, 111.
Djahanguiri, B., Hemmati, S., Sadeghi, D. and Firouzabadi, A. (1967). *Med. Pharmacol. Exp.* **17**, 427.
Djahanguiri, B., Sadeghi, Dj., Pousti, A., Hemmati, S. and Firouzabadi, A. (1968b). *Eur. J. Pharmacol.* **2**, 315.
Djahanguiri, B., Sadeghi, Dj. and Hemmati, S. (1968a). *Arch. Int. Pharmacodyn. Ther.* **173**, 154.
Djahanguiri, B., Pousti, A. and Hemmati, M. (1969). *Pharmacology*, **2**, 243.
Djahanguiri, B., Taubin, H. L. and Landsberg, L. (1973). *J. Pharmacol. Exp. Ther.* **184**, 163.
Doll, R., Hill, I. D., Hutton, C. and Underwood, D. J. (1962). *Lancet*, **ii**, 793.
Doll, R., Hill, I. D. and Hutton, C. F. (1965). *Gut*, **6**, 19.
Doll, R., Langman, M. J. S. and Shawdon, H. H. (1968a). *Gut*, **9**, 42.
Doll, R., Langman, M. J. S. and Shawdon, H. A. (1968b). *Gut*, **9**, 46.
Dombro, R. and Ragins, H. (1967). *Nature*, **216**, 1225.
Domenjoz, R. and Theobald, W. (1959). *Arch. Int. Pharmacodyn. Ther.* **120**, 450.
Domschke, W., Domschke, S., Classen, M. and Demling, L. (1972). *Scand. J. Gastroenterol.* **7**, 647.
Domschke, W., Domschke, S., Classen, M. and Demling, L. (1973). *Nature*, **241**, 454.
Doscherholmen, A. (1949). *Acta Med. Scand.* **135**, 195.
Doteuchi, M. (1968). *Jap. J. Pharmacol.* **18**, 175.
Dotevall, G. and Westling, H. (1960). *Scand. J. Clin. Lab. Invest.* **12**, 489.
Dotevall, G., Kock, N. G. and Walan, A. (1969). *Scand. J. Gastroenterol.* **4**, 713.
Downer, H. D., Galloway, R. W., Horwich, L. and Parke, D. V. (1970). *J. Pharm. Pharmacol* **22**, 479.
Doyle, J. S., Egan, E. L. and Griffin, J. F. (1968). *J. Ir. Med. Ass.* **61**, 239.
Dozois, R. R. and Kelly, K. A. (1971). *Amer. J. Physiol.* **221**, 113.
Dreiling, D. A. and Janowitz, H. (1959). *Gastroenterology*, **36**, 580.
Durbin, R. P. (1964). *J. Gen. Physiol.* **47**, 735.
Dutta, N. K. and Tamhane, R. G. (1953). *Indian J. Med. Res.* **41**, 45.
Dyck, W. P., Werther, J. L., Rudick, J. and Janowitz, H. D. (1969). *Gastroenterology*, **56**, 488.
Eagleton, G. B. and Watt, J. (1965). *J. Pathol. Bacteriol.* **90**, 679.
Eagleton, G. B. and Watt, J. (1967). *J. Pathol. Bacteriol.* **93**, 694.
Eagleton, G. B., Watt, J. and Marcus, R. (1968). *J. Pharm. Pharmacol.* **20**, 970.
Eagleton, G. B., Watt, J. and Marcus, R. (1969). *J. Pharm. Pharmacol.* **21**, 123.
Eckenfels, A. and Vane, J. R. (1972). *Brit. J. Pharmacol.* **45**, 451.
Editorial (1962). *Nutr. Rev.* **20**, 30.
Editorial (1971). *Food Cosmet. Toxicol.* **9**, 561.
Edwards, F., McKeown, T. and Whitefield, A. G. (1959). *Lancet*, **i**, 196.

Ellenbogen, L., Kelly, R. G., Taylor, Jr., R. J. and Stubbs, Jr., C. S. (1973). *Biochem. Pharmacol.* **22**, 939.

Ellis, C. and Nicoloff, D. M. (1969). *Gastroenterology*, **56**, 1155.

Emås, S. (1962). *Gastroenterology*, **43**, 557.

Emås, S., Swan, K. G. and Jacobson, E. D. (1967). *In* "Handbook of Physiology" Section 6, Alimentary Canal (Ed. C. F. Code), vol. 2, p. 743. Williams and Wilkins, Maryland.

Emmelin, N. and Frost, J. (1947). *Acta Physiol. Scand.* **13**, 75.

Engel, J. J., Scruggs, W. and Wilson, D. E. (1973). *Prostaglandins*, **4**, 65.

Engqvist, A., Von Feilitzen, F., Pyk, E. and Reichard, H. (1973). *Gut*, **14**, 711.

Esposito, S. and Nicolini, E. (1961). *Gazz. Med. Ital.* **120**, 485.

Evans, P. R. C. (1954). *Brit. Med. J.* **1**, 612.

Evans, P. R. C., Nowell, S. and Thomas, I. A. P. (1965). *Postgrad. Med. J.* **41**, 48.

Evers, P. W. and Ridley, P. T. (1971). *In* "Annual Reports in Medicinal Chemistry" (Ed. C. K. Cain), p. 68. Academic Press, New York and London.

Eyre, P. and Wells, P. W. (1973). *Brit. J. Pharmacol. Chemother.* **49**, 364.

Ezer, E. and Szporny, L. (1970). *J. Pharm. Pharmacol.* **22**, 143.

Fantozzi, R., Mannaioni, P. F. and Moroni, F. (1973). *Brit. J. Pharmacol. Chemother.* **49**, 361.

Feldman, H. and Gilat, T. (1971). *Gut*, **12**, 449.

Ferayorni, R. R., Code, C. F. and Morlock, C. G. (1948). *Gastroenterology*, **11**, 730.

Ferguson, W. W., Edmonds, A. W., Staring, J. R. and Wangensteen, S. L. (1973). *Ann. Surg.* **177**, 648.

Ferrando, R. J. and Lozzio, B. B. (1957). *Med. Parma*, **17**, 235.

Figueroa, R. B. and Klotz, A. P. (1963). *Curr. Ther. Res.* **5**, 70.

Finlay, T. H., Dharmgrongartama, E. D. and Perlmann, G. E. (1973). *J. Biol. Chem.* **248**, 4827.

Finney, R. S. H. and Tárnoky, A. L. (1960). *J. Pharm. Pharmacol.* **12**, 49.

Flavell Matts, S. G. and Swan, C. H. J. (1965). *Postgrad. Med. J.* **41**, 109.

Fletcher, T. L., Dahl, A. W., Jesseph, J. E., Steinbock, H. L. and Harkins, H. N. (1957). *Proc. Soc. Exp. Biol. Med.* **95**, 559.

Fletcher, T. L., Buchman, H. L., Dahl, A. W., Jesseph, J. E. and Harkins, H. N. (1959). *J. Med. Pharm. Chem.* **1**, 275.

Fletcher, T. L., Pitts, C. L., Everett, M. T. and Griffith, C. A. (1969). *Proc. Soc. Exp. Biol. Med.* **132**, 205.

Fogelson, S. J. (1931). *J. Amer. Med. Ass.* **96**, 673.

Forrest, A. P. M. and Code, C. F. (1954). *J. Pharmacol. Exp. Ther.* **110**, 447.

Franco-Browder, S., Masson, G. M. C. and Corcoran, A. C. (1959). *J. Allergy*, **30**, 1.

Fraser, P. M., Doll, R., Langman, M. J. S., Misiewicz, J. J. and Shawdon, H. H. (1972). *Gut*, **13**, 459.

Friesen, S. R., Baronofsky, I. D. and Wangensteen, O. H. (1946). *Proc. Soc. Exp. Biol. Med.* **63**, 23.

Gadacz, T. R. and Way, L. W. (1972). *Amer. J. Surg.* **123**, 143.

Gaetani, M. and Debeus, R. (1972). *Digestion*, **7**, 302.

Galloway, R. (1968). *In* "A Symposium on Carbenoxolone Sodium" (Eds J. M. Robson and F. M. Sullivan), p. 203. Butterworths, London.

Ganellin, C. R. (1973a). *J. Pharm. Pharmacol.* **25**, 787.

Ganellin, C. R. (1973b). *J. Med. Chem.* **16**, 616.

Ganellin, C. R. (1973c). *J. Med. Chem.* **16**, 620.
Ganellin, C. R. and Pepper, E. S. (1973). *J. Med. Chem.* **16**, 610.
Garattini, S., Giachetti, A., Jori, A., Pieri, L. and Valzelli, L. (1962). *J. Pharm. Pharmacol.* **14**, 509.
Garcia, M. F. (1960). *Rev. Brasil. Gastroenterol.* **12**, 263.
Gassman, R. and Forster, G. (1963). *Ther. Umsch.* **20**, 306.
Gáti, T., Keszler, P., Zelles, T. and Pucsok, J. (1971). *Acta Physiol. Acad. Sci. Hung.* **40**, 393.
Geismar, P. and Mosbech, J. (1970). *In* "Carbenoxolone Sodium" (Eds J. H. Baron and F. M. Sullivan), p. 83. Butterworths, London.
Geismar, P., Mosbech, J. and Myren, J. (1973). *Scand. J. Gastroenterol.* **8**, 251.
Geumei, A., Issa, I., el-Gendi, M. and Abd-el-Samie, Y. (1969). *Surgery*, **66**, 663.
Geumei, A., Issa, I., el-Gendi, M. and Abd-el-Samie, Y. (1972a). *Amer. J. Dig. Dis.* **17**, 55.
Geumei, A., Issa, I. and Abd-el-Samie, Y. (1972b). *Pharmacology*, **7**, 29.
Ghosh, M. N. (1959). *J. Physiol.* **147**, 585.
Ghosh, M. N. and Schild, H. O. (1958). *Brit. J. Pharmacol.* **13**, 54.
Gilg, E. (1948). *Acta Pharmacol.* **4**, 81.
Gillespie, I. E. and Grossman, M. I. (1964). *Gut*, **5**, 342.
Gillespie, G., McCusker, V. I., Bedi, B. S., Debas, H. T. and Gillespie, I. E. (1968). *Gastroenterology*, **55**, 81.
Giordano, G. and Comi, L. (1967). *Minerva Med.* **58**, 3688.
Goady, P. and Phillips, E. A. (1973). *Brit. J. Pharmacol.* **49**, 368.
Gobbi, F. (1967). *Minerva Med.* **58**, 3685.
Goodale, R. L. Jr., Eyal, Z., Largiader, F. A. and Wangensteen, O. H. (1964). *J. Surg. Res.* **4**, 403.
Goodfriend, D. J., Vanderkleed, C. E. and Goodfriend, T. L. (1960). *Amer. J. Gastroenterol.* **33**, 80.
Goodier, T. E. W., Horwich, L. and Galloway, R. W. (1967). *Gut*, **8**, 544.
Goldstein, M., Lauber, E. and McKeregan, M. R. (1964). *Biochem. Pharmacol.* **13**, 1103.
Graham, A. H. (1964). *Gut*, **5**, 597.
Gray, J. S., Wieczorowski, E. and Ivy, A. C. (1939). *Science*, **89**, 489.
Gray, J. S., Culmer, C. U., Wieczorowski, E. and Adkinson, J. L. (1940). *Proc. Soc. Exp. Biol. Med.* **43**, 225.
Gray, J. S., Wieczorowski, E., Wells, J. A. and Harris, S. C. (1942). *Endocrinology*, **30**, 129.
Green, A. L. (1964). *Biochim. Biophys. Acta*, **81**, 391.
Greengard, H., Atkinson, A. J., Grossman, M. I. and Ivy, A. C. (1946). *Gastroenterology*, **7**, 625.
Greenlee, H. B., Longhi, E. H., Guerrero, J. D., Nelsen, T. S., el-Bedri, A. L. and Dragstedt, L. R. (1957). *Amer. J. Physiol.* **190**, 396.
Gregory, R. A. (1955). *J. Physiol.* **129**, 528.
Gregory, R. A. (1967). *In* "Gastric Secretion—Mechanisms and Control" (Eds T. K. Shnitka, J. A. L. Gilbert and R. C. Harrison), p. 467. Pergamon Press, Toronto.
Gregory, H. (1970). *Amer. J. Dig. Dis.* **15**, 141.
Gregory, R. A. and Ivy, A. C. (1941). *Quart. J. Physiol.* **31**, 111.
Grossman, M. I. (1950). *Physiol. Rev.* **30**, 33.
Grossman, M. I. (1970). *Lancet*, **i**, 1088.

Grossman, M. I., Greengard, H., Dutton, D. F. and Woolley, J. R. (1944). *Gastroenterology*, **2**, 437.

Grossman, M. I., Robertson, C. and Rosiere, C. E. (1952). *J. Pharmacol. Exp. Ther.* **104**, 277.

Gurll, N. J., Pelso, O. and Silen, W. (1966). *J. Surg. Res.* **6**, 373.

Håkanson, R. (1965). *Nature*, **208**, 793.

Håkanson, R. and Liedberg, G. (1971). *Expereintia*, **27**, 1045.

Håkanson, R. and Liedberg, G. (1972). *Eur. J. Pharmacol.* **18**, 31.

Håkanson, R., Liedberg, G. and Oscarson, J. (1973). *Brit. J. Pharmacol. Chemother.* **47**, 498.

Håkanson, R., Liedberg, G., Oscarson, J., Rehfeld, J. F. and Stadil, F. (1973). *Experientia*, **29**, 570.

Häkkinen, I. and Hartiala, K. (1966). *Acta Physiol. Scand.* **66**, 326.

Häkkinen, I., Hartiala, K. and Lang, H. (1966). *Acta Physiol. Scand.* **66**, 333.

Hallenbeck, G. A. (1943). *Amer. J. Physiol.* **139**, 329.

Halpern, B. and Martin, J. (1946). *C. R. Soc. Biol.* **140**, 830.

Hamor, G. H., Breslow, D. M. and Fisch, G. W. (1970). *J. Pharm. Sci.* **59**, 1752.

Hands, A. P., Greengard, H., Preston, F. W., Fauley, G. B. and Ivy, A. C. (1942). *Endocrinology*, **30**, 905.

Hanson, H. M. and Brodie, D. A. (1960). *J. Appl. Physiol.* **15**, 291.

Haot, J., Djahanguiri, B. and Richelle, M. (1964). *Arch. Int. Pharmacodyn. Ther.* **148**, 557.

Harjola, P. T. and Sivula, A. (1966). *Acta Chir. Scand.* **132**, 166.

Harper, H. A. and Raper, H. S. (1943). *J. Physiol.* **102**, 115.

Harris, J. B. and Silen, W. (1964). *Fed. Proc.* **23**, 214.

Harris, J. B., Nigon, D. and Alonso, D. (1969). *Gastroenterology*, **57**, 377.

Harrison, R. C., Lakey, W. H. and Hyde, H. A. (1956). *Ann. Surg.* **144**, 441.

Hase, T. and Scarborough, E. S. (1971). *J. Appl. Physiol.* **30**, 580.

Hausmann, W. and Tárnoky, A. L. (1966). *Brit. J. Pharmacol. Chemother.* **26**, 412.

Haverbach, B. J., Stevenson, T. D., Sjoerdsma, A. and Terry, L. L. (1955). *Amer. J. Med. Sci.* **230**, 601.

Hawkins, W. W. and Leonard, V. G. (1962). *J. Lab. Clin. Med.* **60**, 641.

Heding, L. G. (1971). *Diabetologia*, **7**, 10.

Henman, F. D. (1970). *Gut*, **11**, 344.

Hersey, S. J. and High, W. L. (1971). *Biochim. Biophys. Acta*, **233**, 604.

Hesch, R. D., Hüfner, M., Hasenhager, B. and Creutzfeldt, W. (1971). *Hormones Metab. Res.* **3**, 140.

Hess, H. J. (1969). *In* "Annual Reports in Medicinal Chemistry" (Ed. C. K. Cain), p. 56. Academic Press, New York and London.

Heymann, H., Ginsberg, T., Gulick, Z. R. and Mayer, R. L. (1959). *Proc. Soc. Exp. Biol. Med.* **100**, 279.

Hilliard, J. and West, P. M. (1957). *Endocrinology*, **60**, 797.

Hillyard, I. W. and Grandy, R. P. (1963). *J. Pharmacol. Exp. Ther.* **142**, 358.

Hirschowitz, B. I. (1967). *In* "Handbook of Physiology", Section 6, Alimentary Canal (Ed. C. F. Code), vol. 2, p. 889. Williams and Wilkins, Maryland.

Hirschowitz, B. I., London, J. A. and Wiggins, H. S. (1959). *J. Lab. Clin. Med.* **53**, 577.

Hoefke, W. and Kobinger, W. (1966). *Arzneim.-Forsch.* **16**, 1038.

Hoffmeister, W. and Hoffmeister, A. W. (1971). *Z. Gesamte. Exp. Med.* **156**, 195.

Hogben, C. A. M. (1965). *Fed. Proc.* **24**, 1353.

Hollander, E. (1960). *Amer. J. Gastroenterol.* **34**, 613.

Hood, Jr., R. T., Code, C. F. and Grindlay, J. H. (1953). *Amer. J. Physiol.* **173**, 270.

Horton, E. W., Main, I. H. M., Thomson, C. J. and Wright, P. M. (1968). *Gut*, **9**, 655.

Horwich, L. and Galloway, R. (1965). *Brit. Med. J.* **ii**, 1274.

Hoskins, E. O. L. (1973). *Postgrad. Med. J.* **49**, Suppl. 95.

Houck, J. C., Bhayana, J. and Lee, T. (1960). *Gastroenterology*, **39**, 196.

Howat, H. T. and Schofield, B. (1954). *J. Physiol.* **123**, 1.

Hubel, K. A. (1972). *Gastroenterology*, **62**, 318.

Huckle, D., Lockhart, I. M. and Wright, M. (1969). *J. Med. Chem.* **12**, 277.

Huidobro, F. (1954). *Arch. Int. Pharmacodyn. Ther.* **98**, 308.

Humphrey, M. J., Lindup, W. E., Parke, D. V. and Chakraborty, J. (1972). *Biochem. J.* **130**, 87P.

Hunt, J. N. (1948). *Biochem. J.* **42**, 104.

Hunt, T. (1972). *In* "Carbenoxolone in Gastroenterology" (Eds F. Avery Jones and F. M. Sullivan), p. 55. Butterworths, London.

Hunt, J. N. and Knox, M. T. (1968). *In* "Handbook of Physiology" Section 6, Alimentary Canal (Ed. C. F. Code), vol. 4, p. 1917. Williams and Wilkins, Maryland.

Hunt, J. N. and Ramsbottom, N. (1967). *Brit. Med. J.* **iv**, 386.

Husain, S. S., Ferguson, J. B. and Fruton, J. S. (1971). *Proc. Nat. Acad. Sci. U.S.A.* **68**, 2765.

Huszti, Z., Kasztreiner, E., Kürti, M., Fekete, M. and Borsy, J. (1973). *Biochem. Pharmacol.* **22**, 2253.

Ichiki, H. and Isoda, M. (1973). *Arzneim.-Forsch.* **23**, 461.

Ichimura, M. (1971). *Yakugaku Zasshi*, **91**, 245.

Impicciatore, M. and Grossman, M. I. (1973). *Amer. J. Dig. Dis.* **18**, 551.

Irikura, T. and Kasuga, K. (1971). *J. Med. Chem.* **14**, 357.

Isaza, J., Sugawara, K., Tiongco, R. and Eisenberg, M. M. (1970). *Surgery*, **67**, 462.

Isaza, J., Woodward, E. R. and Dragstedt, L. R. (1971). *Surgery*, **69**, 441.

Isenberg, J. I. and Grossman, M. I. (1969). *Gastroenterology*, **56**, 450.

Ishii, Y. (1968). *Arzneim.-Forsch.* **18**, 53.

Ishii, Y. (1969). *Jap. J. Pharmacol.* **19**, 125.

Ishii, Y. (1970). *Jap. J. Pharmacol.* **20**, 71.

Ito, R., Nishizaki, H., Uchiyama, T., Tokoro, Y. and Tosaka, K. (1972). *Arzneim.-Forsch.* **22**, 1510.

Iveson, P., Parke, D. V. and Williams, R. T. (1966). *Biochem. J.* **100**, 28P.

Ivey, K. J. and Gray, C. (1973a). *Gastroenterology*, **64**, 1101.

Ivey, K. J. and Gray, C. (1973b). *Aust. N.Z. J. Med.* **3**, 451.

Ivy, A. C. and Bachrach, W. H. (1966). *In* "Handbook of Experimental Pharmacology" (Eds O. Eicher and A. Farah), vol. 18, p. 810. Springer-Verlag, New York.

Ivy, A. C. and Liepins, K. W. (1958). *Amer. J. Physiol.* **195**, 521.

Ivy, A. C. and Oldberg, E. (1928). *Amer. J. Physiol.* **86**, 599.

Jacobson, E. D. (1961). *Fed. Proc.* **20**, 20.

Jacobson, E. D. (1964). *Amer. Heart. J.* **68**, 214.

Jacobson, E. D. (1970). *Proc. Soc. Exp. Biol. Med.* **133**, 516.

Jacobson, E. D., Konturek, S. J. and Johnson, L. R. (1971). *Gastroenterology*, **60**, 780.

Jaffe, B. M., Newton, W. T. and McGuigan, J. E. (1968). *Gastroenterology*, **54**, 1295.
Jain, A. C. (1962). *J. Ass. Physicians India*, **10**, 435.
Jankelson, I. R. and Jankelson, O. M. (1959). *Amer. J. Gastroenterol.* **32**, 636.
Janowitz, H. D., Colcher, H. and Hollander, F. (1952). *Amer. J. Physiol.* **171**, 325.
Janowitz, H. D., Dreilling, D. A., Rolbin, L. H. and Hollander, F. (1957). *Gastroenterology*, **33**, 378.
Jawaharlal, K. and Berti, F. (1972). *Pharmacol. Res. Commun.* **4**, 143.
Jerzy Glass, G. B. and Schwartz, S. A. (1959). *Amer. J. Dig. Dis.* **4**, 988.
Jerzy Glass, G. B. and Code, C. F. (1968). *In* "Progress in Gastroenterology" (Ed. G. B. Jerzy Glass), vol. 1, p. 221. Greene and Stratton, New York.
Johansson, I. L., Lundell, L. and Svensson, S. E. (1972). *Brit. J. Pharmacol. Chemother.* **46**, 94.
Johnson, L. R. and Grossman, M. I. (1968). *Amer. J. Physiol.* **215**, 885.
Johnson, L. R. and Grossman, M. I. (1969). *Amer. J. Physiol.* **217**, 1401.
Johnson, L. R. and Grossman, M. I. (1970). *Amer. J. Physiol.* **218**, 550.
Johnson, L. R. and Grossman, M. I. (1971). *Gastroenterology*, **60**, 120.
Johnson, L. R. and Tumpson, D. B. (1970). *Proc. Soc. Exp. Biol. Med.* **133**, 125.
Johnston, D. and Duthie, H. L. (1966). *Gut*, **7**, 58.
Johnston, D. and Duthie, H. L. (1969). *Scand. J. Gastroenterol.* **4**, 561.
Johnston, M. and Kahlson, G. (1967). *Brit. J. Pharmacol. Chemother.* **30**, 274.
Jorpes, J. E. (1968). *Gastroenterology*, **55**, 157.
Jow, E., Webster, D. R. and Skoryna, S. C. (1960). *Gastroenterology*, **38**, 732.
Kabeno, H., Honda, T., Koabayashi, Y. and Murata, T. (1971). *Chem. Pharm. Bull.* **19**, 1487.
Kahlson, G. and Rosengren, E. (1968). *Physiol. Rev.* **48**, 155.
Kahlson, G., Rosengren, E. and Thunberg, R. (1963). *J. Physiol.* **169**, 467.
Kahlson, G., Rosengren, E., Svahn, D. and Thunberg, R. (1964a). *J. Physiol.* **174**, 400.
Kahlson, G., Lilja, B. and Svensson, S. E. (1964b). *Lancet*, **ii**, 1269.
Kahlson, G., Rosengren, E. and Thunberg, R. (1967). *J. Physiol.* **190**, 455.
Kahlson, G., Rosengren, E. and Svensson, S. E. (1968). *Brit. J. Pharmacol. Chemother.* **33**, 493.
Kangas, J. A., Schmidt, K. M. and Solomon, G. F. (1972). *Amer. J. Clin. Nutr.* **25**, 864.
Karim, S. M. M., Carter, D. C., Bhana, D. and Ganesan, P. A. (1973a). *Brit. Med. J.* **i**, 143.
Karim, S. M. M., Carter, D. C., Bhana, D. and Ganesan, P. A. (1973b). "Advances in the Biosciences" (Ed. S. Bergström), vol. 9, p. 255. Pergamon Press, Vieweg, West Germany.
Karim, S. M. M., Carter, D. C., Bhana, D. and Ganesan, P. A. (1973c). *Prostaglandins*, **4**, 71.
Karppanen, H. O. and Westermann, E. (1973). *Naunyn-Schmiedebergs Arch. Pharmakol. Exp. Pathol.* **279**, 83.
Katz, J. (1973). *Med. Clin. N. Amer.* **57**, 893.
Katzka, I. and Riss, L. (1962). *Gastroenterology*, **43**, 71.
Kaufmann, H. J. and Spiro, H. M. (1968). *Gastroenterology*, **54**, 913.
Kawashima, K. (1972). *Jap. J. Pharmacol.* **22**, 155.
Kawashima, K. and Takagi, K. (1972). *Jap. J. Pharmacol.* **22**, 147.
Kawashima, K., Lee, E. B., Hirai, T., Takeuchi, K. and Takagi, K. (1972). *Chem. Pharm. Bull.* **20**, 755.

Kay A. W. and Forrest, A. P. M. (1956). *Exp. Surg.* **43**, 522.

Kelly, H. T. (1960). *Amer. J. Gastroenterol.* **34**, 589.

Kelly, P. and Robert, A. (1969). *Gastroenterology*, **56**, 24.

Kettering, R. F. (1971). *Surg. Clin. N. Amer.* **51**, 835.

Kier, L. B. (1968). *J. Med. Chem.* **11**, 411.

Kier, L. B. (1970). *In* "Fundamental Concepts in Drug-receptor Interactions" (Eds J. F. Danielli, J. F. Moran and D. J. Triggle), p. 28. Academic Press, New York and London.

Kier, L. B. (1971). *In* "Medicinal Chemistry" (Ed. A. DeStevens), vol. **10**, p. 174.

Kirsner, J. B. and Wolff, R. A. (1943). *Proc. Soc. Exp. Biol. Med.* **54**, 11.

Kirsner, J. B., Levin, E. and Palmer, W. L. (1948). *Gastroenterology*, **10**, 256.

Kim, K. S. and Shore, P. A. (1963). *J. Pharmacol. Exp. Ther.* **141**, 321.

Klotz, A. P. (1967). *Ann. N.Y. Acad. Sci.* **140**, 697.

Klotz, A. P. and Duvall, M. R. (1957). *J. Lab. Clin. Med.* **50**, 753.

Kobayaski, Y. and Maudsley, D. V. (1968). *Brit. J. Pharmacol. Chemother.* **32**, 428P.

Kobayashi, M. and Yamamoto, M. (1972). *Yakugaku Zasshi*, **92**, 226.

Kobayashi, M., Morimoto, T. and Yamamoto, M. (1972). *Yakugaku Zasshi*, **92**, 221.

Konturek, S. J. (1970). *Gut*, **11**, 158.

Konturek, S. J. and Johnson, L. R. (1971). *Gastroenterology*, **61**, 667.

Konturek, S. J. and Olesky, J. (1969). *Scand. J. Gastroenterol.* **4**, 13.

Konturek, S. J. and Radecki, T. (1963). *Biochem. Pharmacol.* **12**, Suppl., 134.

Konturek, S. J., Gabrys, B. and Dubiel, J. (1969). *Amer. J. Physiol.* **217**, 1110.

Konturek, S. J., Solomon, T. E., McCreight, W. G., Johnson, L. R. and Jacobson, E. (1971). *Gastroenterology*, **60**, 1098.

Kowalewski, K. (1967). *Arch. Int. Pharmacodyn. Ther.* **170**, 66.

Kowalewski, K., Lyon, R. K., Edwards, G. E. and Shnitka, T. K. (1958). *Can. J. Biochem. Physiol.* **36**, 977.

Kunimoto, S., Aoyagi, T., Morishima, H., Takeuchi, T. and Umezawa, H. (1972). *J. Antibiot.* **25**, 251.

Kunz, O. (1971). *Med. Klin.* **66**, 822.

Kuruvilla, J. T. (1971). *Gut*, **12**, 897.

Lai, K. S. (1964). *Gut*, **35**, 327.

Lambling, A., Bonfils, S., Kaess, H. and Simonpoli. Ch. (1961). *Gastroenterologia*, **95**, 85.

Lambling, A., Hardouin, J. P., Bonfils, S. and Laumonier, R. (1953). *Arch. Mal. App. Dig.* **42**, 417.

Langman, M. J. S. (1968a). *Postgrad. Med. J.* **44**, 603.

Langman, M. J. S. (1968b). *Gut*, **9**, 5.

Langman, M. J. S., Knapp, D. R. and Wakley, E. J. (1973). *Brit. Med. J.* **3**, 84.

Lawrence, A. J., Schild, H. O. and Smith, G. M. (1971). *Brit. J. Pharmacol. Chemother.* **41**, 8.

Lazar, J., Orth, H., Möhring, J. and Gross, F. (1972). *Naunyn-Schmiedeberg's Arch. Pharmacol.* **275**, 114.

Lee, Y. H. and Bianchi, R. G. (1972). Fifth International Congress on Pharmacology, 136.

Lee, Y. H. and Thomson, J. H. (1967). *Amer. J. Physiol.* **213**, 1331.

Lee, Y. H. and Thompson, J. H. (1968). *Eur. J. Pharmacol.* **3**, 366.

Lee, Y. H. and Thompson, J. H. (1969). *Amer. J. Dig. Dis.* **14**, 14.

Lee, Y. H., Mollison, K. W. and Cheng, W. D. (1971). *Arch. Int. Pharmacodyn. Ther.* **191**, 370.

Lee, Y. H., Phillips, E. and Sause, H. W. (1972). *Arch. Int. Pharmacodyn. Ther.* **195**, 402.

Lee, Y. H., Cheng, W. D., Bianchi, R. G., Mollison, K. and Hansen, J. (1973). *Prostaglandins*, **3**, 29.

LeFevre, M. E., Gohmann, E. J. Jr. and Rehm, W. S. (1964). *Amer. J. Physiol.* **207**, 613.

Lenz, J., Hartel, W. and Schuster, G. (1971). *Med. Klin.* **66**, 553.

Lerner, H. J. and Thompson, J. C. (1963). *Proc. Soc. Exp. Biol. Med.* **112**, 730.

Levey, S. and Sheinfeld, S. (1954). *Gastroenterology*, **27**, 625.

Levine, R. J. (1965a). *Fed. Proc.* **24**, 1331.

Levine, R. J. (1965b). *Life Sci.* **4**, 959.

Levine, R. J. (1968). *Fed. Proc.* **27**, 1310.

Levine, R. (1971). *Ann. N.Y. Acad. Sci.* **180**, 336.

Levine, R. J., Sato, T. L. and Sjoerdsma, A. (1965). *Biochem. Pharm.* **14**, 139.

Levis, S. and Beersaerts, J. (1960). *Arch. Int. Pharmacodyn. Ther.* **126**, 359.

Levis, S., Preat, S., Beersaerts, J., Dauby, J., Beelen, L. and Baugniet, V. (1957). *Arch. Int. Pharmacodyn. Ther.* **109**, 129.

Levis, S., Preat, S. and Beersaerts, J. (1959). *Arch. Int. Pharmacodyn. Ther.* **118**, 167.

Lilja, B. and Svensson, S. E. (1967). *J. Physiol.* **190**, 261.

Lim, R. K. S., Ivy, A. C. and McCarthy, J. E. (1925). *Quart. J. Exp. Physiol.* **15**, 13.

Lin, T. M. and Benslay, D. N. (1962). Proceedings of the International Physiological Congress, **2**, 283.

Lin, T. M. and Spray, G. F. (1968). *Gastroenterology*, **54**, 1254.

Lin, T. M. and Spray, G. F. (1971). *Arch. Int. Pharmacodyn. Ther.* **191**, 88.

Lin, T. M. and Warrick, M. W. (1971). *Gastroenterology*, **61**, 328.

Lin, T. M., Alphin, R. S., Henderson, F. G., Benslay, D. N. and Chen, K. K. (1962). *Ann. N.Y. Acad. Sci.* **99**, 30.

Lin, T. M., Benslay, D. N. and Tust, R. H. (1963). *Physiologist*, **6**, 225.

Lin, T. M., Evans, D. C., Spray, G. F. and Benslay, D. N. (1970). *Arch. Int. Pharmacodyn. Ther.* **188**, 332.

Lin, T. M., Evans, D. C. and Spray, G. F. (1973). *Arch. Int. Pharmacodyn. Ther.* **202**, 314.

Linde, S. (1950). *Acta Physiol. Scand.* **21**, Suppl. 74.

Linde, S., Obrink, K. J. and Uhlefendahl, H. (1952). *Acta Physiol. Scand.* **25**, 82.

Lindmar, R. and Muscholl, E. (1961). *Arch. Exp. Pathol. Pharmacol.* **242**, 214.

Lipkin, M. and Ludwig, W. (1968). *In* "A Symposium on Carbenoxolone Sodium" (Eds J. M. Robson and F. M. Sullivan), p. 41. Butterworths, London.

Lippmann, W. (1968a). *Experientia*, **15**, 1151.

Lippmann, W. (1968b). *Experientia*, **15**, 1153.

Lippmann, W. (1969a). *Biochem. Pharmacol.* **18**, 2517.

Lippmann, W. (1969b). *J. Pharm. Pharmacol.* **21**, 335.

Lippmann, W. (1970a). *J. Pharm. Pharmacol.* **22**, 387.

Lippmann, W. (1970b). *J. Pharm. Pharmacol.* **22**, 568.

Lippmann, W. (1970c). *Arch. Int. Pharmacodyn. Ther.* **188**, 28.

Lippmann, W. (1970d). *J. Pharm. Pharmacol.* **22**, 65.

Lippmann, W. (1971a). *Arch. Int. Pharmacodyn. Ther.* **193**, 340.

Lippmann, W. (1971b). *Ann. N.Y. Acad. Sci.* **180**, 332.
Lippmann, W. (1973). *Experientia*, **29**, 990.
Lippmann, W. and Seethaler, K. (1973). *Experientia*, **29**, 993.
Littman, A. (1972). *Gastroenterology*, **62**, 141.
Littman, A. and Chalmers, T. C. (1970). *Gastroenterology*, **58**, 913.
Loew, E. R. and Chickering, O. (1941). *Proc. Soc. Exp. Biol. Med.* **48**, 65.
Loew, E. R., Kaiser, M. E. and Moore, V. (1945). *J. Pharmacol. Exp. Ther.* **85**, 120.
Loew, E. R., MacMillan, R. and Kaiser, M. E. (1946). *J. Pharmacol. Exp. Ther.* **86**, 229.
Longhi, E. H., Greenlee, H. B., Bravo, J. L., Guerrero, J. D. and Dragstedt, L. R. (1957). *Amer. J. Physiol.* **191**, 64.
Lösel, H. (1964). *Med. Welt*, **13**, 709.
Lucchetti, G. (1973). *Farmaco, Ed. Prat.* **28**, 339.
Lucien, H. W., Itoh, Z., Sun, D. C. H., Meyer, J., Carlton, N. and Schally, A. V. (1969). *Arch. Biochem. Biophys.* **134**, 180.
Lucien, H. W., Itoh, Z. and Schally, A. V. (1970). *Gastroenterology*, **59**, 707.
Lynch, T. A., Highley, W. L. and Worton, A. G. (1964). *J. Pharm. Sci.* **53**, 1077.
MacCraig, J. N. (1970). *In* "Carbenoxolone Sodium" (Eds J. H. Baron and F. M. Sullivan), p. 91. Butterworths, London.
MacDougall, J. D. B., Carr, A. J. and Blair, D. W. (1964). *Brit. J. Surg.* **51**, 937.
Mackrell, T. N. and Schwartz, M. (1969). *Amer. J. Physiol.* **216**, 572.
Magee, D. F. and Nakajima, S. (1968). *Experientia*, **24**, 689.
Main, I. H. M. and Whittle, B. J. R. (1972). *Brit. J. Pharmacol. Chemother.* **44**, 331P.
Main, I. H. M. and Whittle, B. J. R. (1973a). *Brit. J. Pharmacol. Chemother.* **49**, 428.
Main, I. H. M. and Whittle, B. J. R. (1973b). *In* "Advances in the Biosciences", vol. **9**, p. 271. Pergamon Press, Vieweg, Braunschweig.
Malen, C. E., Danree, B. H. and Pascaud, X. B. L. (1971). *J. Med. Chem.* **14**, 244.
Malis, J. L. (1966). *Pharmacologist*, **8**, 186.
Mann, F. C. and Williamson, C. S. (1923). *Ann. Surg.* **77**, 409.
Mao, C. C., Shanbour, L. L., Hodgins, D. S. and Jacobson, E. D. (1972). *Gastroenterology*, **63**, 427.
Marazzi-Uberti, E. and Turba, C. (1961). *Med. Exp.* **4**, 284.
Marciniszyn, J. P. and Kassell, B. (1971). *J. Biol. Chem.* **246**, 6560.
Maren, T. J. (1967). *Physiol. Rev.* **47**, 732.
Margolis, S., Kang, S. and Green, J. P. (1971). *Int. J. Clin. Pharmacol.* **5**, 270.
Markowitz, J., Archibald, J. and Downie, H. G. (1959, 4th ed.). *In* "Experimental Surgery", p. 191. Williams and Wilkins, Baltimore.
Marks, N., Grynbaum, A. and Lajtha, A. (1973). *Science*, **181**, 949.
Martin, F., Vuez, J. L., Berard, A., Andre, C. and Lambert, R. (1968). *Digestion*, **1**, 165.
Martindale, K., Somers, G. F. and Wilson, C. W. M. (1960). *J. Pharm. Pharmacol.* **12**, Suppl. 153T.
Marullo, U. and Cuzzocrea, D. (1964). *Arch. Atti. Soc. Med. Chir. Messina*, **8**, 3.
Maudsley, D. V., Kobayashi, Y., Williamson, E. and Bovaird, L. (1973). *Nature New Biology*, **245**, 148.
McCarthy, J. D., Evans, S. O. and Dragstedt, L. R. (1954). *Gastroenterology*, **27**, 275.

McColl, J. D., Lee, C. F. and Hajdu, A. (1963). *Arch. Int. Pharmacodyn. Ther.* **141**, 179.

McCoy, E. J. and Bass, P. (1963). *Amer. J. Physiol.* **205**, 439.

McDonald, I. (1956). *Gastroenterology*, **30**, 602.

McGavack, T. H., Elias, H. and Boyd, L. J. (1946). *Gasteroenterology*, **6**, 439.

McGuigan, J. E. (1968a). *Gastroenterology*, **55**, 315.

McGuigan, J. E. (1968b). *Fed. Proc.* **27**, 1337.

McGuigan, J. E. (1968c). *Gastroenterology*, **54**, 1005.

Méhes, J., Decsi, L., Várszegi, M. K., Hideg, H. and Hankovszky, O. H. (1966). *J. Pharm. Pharmacol.* **18**, 551.

Melchiorri, P. and Sopranzi, N. (1971). *Ag. Actions*, **2**, 58.

Melrose, A. G. (1960). *Gut*, **1**, 142.

Menguy, R. and Berlinski, M. (1967). *Amer. J. Dig. Dis.* **12**, 1.

Menguy, R. and Smith, W. O. (1960). *Proc. Soc. Exp. Biol. Med.* **105**, 238.

Menguy, R. and Thompson, A. E. (1967). *Ann. N.Y. Acad. Sci.* **140**, 797.

Menguy, R., Masters, Y. F. and Gryboski, W. (1964). *Gastroenterology*, **46**, 32.

Menon, M. K., Clark, W. G. and Aures, D. (1971). *Life Sci.* **10**, 1097.

Meyer, J., Cohen, S. J. and Carlson, A. J. (1918). *Arch. Int. Med.* **21**, 354.

Meyer, J. H. and Grossman, M. I. (1972). *In* "Gastrointestinal Hormones" (Ed. L. Demling), p. 43. Georg Thieme Verlag, Stuttgart.

Meyer, R. F., Cummings, B. L., Bass, P. and Collier, H. O. J. (1965). *J. Med. Chem.* **8**, 515.

Middleton, W. R. J., Cooke, A. R., Stephen, D. and Skyring, A. P. (1965). *Lancet*, **i**, 1030.

Millar, R. A., Keener, E. B. and Benfey, B. G. (1959). *Brit. J. Pharmacol. Chemother.* **14**, 9.

Miller, R. P., Poper, C. J., Wilson, C. W. and DeVito, E. (1972). *Biochem. Pharmacol.* **21**, 2941.

Misher, A., Pendleton, R. G. and Staples, R. (1969). *Gastroenterology*, **57**, 294.

Moersch, R. U. and Rivers, A. B. (1946). *Gastroenterology*, **7**, 91.

Moffett, R. B., Robert, A. and Skaletzky, L. L. (1971). *J. Med. Chem.* **14**, 963.

Mole, K. H. and Shepherd, D. M. (1972). *Arch. Int. Pharmacodyn. Ther.* **195**, 109.

Mole, K. H. and Shepherd, D. M. (1973). *J. Pharm. Pharmacol.* **25**, 609.

Monson, R. R. (1970). *Gastroenterology*, **58**, 337.

Montgomery, R. D. (1967). *Gut*, **8**, 148.

Montgomery, R. D., Lawrence, I. H., Manton, D. J., Mendl, K. and Rowe, P. (1968). *Gut*, **9**, 704.

Montgomery, R. D., Mehta, S. C. and Lawrence, I. H. (1969). *Practitioner*, **202**, 398.

Moody, R. G. and Davis, W. L. (1970). *Gastroenterology*, **59**, 350.

Moreno, O. M. and Brodie, D. A. (1962). *J. Pharmacol. Exp. Ther.* **135**, 259.

Mori, G., Boidi, G. P. and Fresia, P. (1964). *Acad. Med. Lombard*, **19**, 438.

Mori, G., Cova, G. and Ingrami, A. (1969). *In* "Proceedings of 8th International Congress of Gastroenterology" (Eds O. Gregor and O. Riedl), p. 67. Schattauer Verlag, Stuttgart.

Morimoto, T. and Yamamoto, M. (1969). *Yakugaku Zasshi*, **89**, 215.

Morishima, H., Takita, T., Aoyagi, T., Takeuchi, T. and Umezawa, H. (1970). *J. Antibiot.* **23**, 263.

Morley, J. S. (1968). *Fed. Proc.* **27**, 1314.

Morris, C. R., Grossman, M. I. and Ivy, A. C. (1947). *Amer. J. Physiol.* **148**, 382.

Moshal, M. G. (1973). *Postgrad. Med. J.* **49**, Suppl., 100.
Moss, M. L. and Mellon, M. G. (1942). *Ind. Eng. Chem.* **14**, 862.
Multicentre Trial, A. (1971). *Brit. Med. J.* **3**, 501.
Murari, G. (1964). *Med. Exp.* **11**, 361.
Murat, J. W. and White, T. T. (1966). *Proc. Soc. Exp. Biol. Med.* **123**, 593.
Mutt, V. and Jorpes, J. E. (1968). *Eur. J. Biochem.* **6**, 156.
Nagai, K., Sano, A., Yamaguchi, K. and Kodaira, Y. (1971). *Arzneim-Forsch.* **21**, 96.
Nakamura, M., Nakajima, S. and Magee, D. F. (1968). *Gut*, **9**, 405.
Nakano, J. and Prancan, A. V. (1972). *Proc. Soc. Exp. Biol. Med.* **139**, 1151.
Namekata, M. (1962a). *Chem. Pharm. Bull.* **10**, 171.
Namekata, M. (1962b). *Chem. Pharm. Bull.* **10**, 177.
Namekata, M. (1962c). *Chem. Pharm. Bull.* **10**, 182.
Namekata, M., Matsuo, A., Momose, A. and Takagi, M. (1967). *Yakugaku Zasshi*, **87**, 376.
Narumi, S. and Kanno, M. (1972). *Jap. J. Pharmacol.* **22**, 663.
Narumi, S. and Kanno, M. (1973). *Biochim. Biophys. Acta*, **311**, 80.
Narumi, S. and Maki, Y. (1973). *Biochim. Biophys. Acta*, **311**, 90.
National Liaison Committee (1967). *Gastroenterology*, **53**, 821.
Newcomb, P. B., Stone, W. D. and Richardson, D. C. (1970). *In* "4th World Congress Gastroenterology", p. 313. Danish Gastroenterol. Association, Copenhagen.
Nezamis, J. E., Robert, A. and Stowe, D. F. (1971). *J. Physiol.* **218**, 369.
Niada, R. and Prino, G. (1973). *Brit. J. Pharmacol. Chemother.* **48**, 550.
Niemegeers, C. J. E. and Janssen, P. A. (1964). *J. Pharm. Pharmacol.* **16**, 26.
Nikodijevic, B. and Vanov, S. (1960). *Experientia*, **16**, 464.
Oesterling, T. O., Morozowich, W. and Roseman, T. J. (1972). *J. Pharm. Sci.* **61**, 1861.
Ojha, K. N. and Wood, D. R. (1950). *Brit. J. Pharmacol. Chemother.* **5**, 389.
Okabe, S., Saziki, R. and Takagi, K. (1970). *Jap. J. Pharmacol.* **20**, 10.
Okabe, S., Roth, J. L. A. and Pfeiffer, C. J. (1971a). *Experientia*, **27**, 146.
Okabe, S., Roth, J. L. A. and Pfeiffer, C. J. (1971b). *Amer. J. Dig. Dis.* **16**, 277.
Ondetti, M., Sheehan, J. T. and Bodanszky, M. (1968). *In* "Pharmacology of Hormonal Polypeptides and Hormones" (Eds N. Back, L. Martini and R. Paoletti), p. 18. Plenum Press, New York.
Ondetti, M., Rubin, B., Engel, S. L., Pluscec, J. and Sheehan, J. T. (1970). *Amer. J. Dig. Dis.* **15**, 149.
Ottenjahn, R. and Rosch, W. (1970). *Med. Klin.* **65**, 74.
Pace-Asciak, C. (1972). *Biochim. Biophys. Acta* **280**, 161.
Pace-Asciak, C. and Wolfe, L. S. (1970). *Biochim. Biophys. Acta*, **218**, 539.
Pace-Asciak, C., Morawska, K. and Wolfe, L. S. (1970). *Biochim. Biophys. Acta*, **218**, 288.
Page, R. C. and Heffner, R. R. (1948). *Gastroenterology*, **11**, 842.
Parbhoo, S. P. and Johnston, I. D. A. (1966). *Gut*, **7**, 612.
Parke, D. V. (1967). *In* "Carbenoxolone Sodium" (Eds J. M. Robson and F. M. Sullivan), p. 15. Butterworths, London.
Parke, D. V. (1972). *In* "Carbenoxolone in Gastroenterology" (Eds F. Avery Jones and F. M. Sullivan), p. 19. Butterworths, London.
Parke, D. V., Humphrey, M. J., Chakraborty, J. and Lindup, W. E. (1972a). *In* "5th International Congress on Pharmacology", p. 176.
Parke, D. V., Hunt, T. C. and Iveson, P. (1972b). *Clin. Sci.* **43**, 393.
Parke, D. V., Pollock, S. and Williams, R. T. (1963). *J. Pharm. Pharmacol.* **15**, 500.

Pascaud, X. B. and Blouin, M. M. (1972). *In* "5th International Congress on Pharmacology", p. 177.
Pascaud, X. B. and Laubie, M. (1971). *Arzneim. Forsch.* **21**, 1547.
Pascaud, X. B., Poignant, J. C. and Malen, C. (1971). *C. R. Acad. Sci. Paris*, **273**, 1441.
Pastor Franco, A. (1966). *Rev. Clin. Espan.* **100**, 50.
Pederson, R. A. and Brown, J. C. (1972). *Gastroenterology*, **62**, 393.
Pendleton, R. G., Bartakovitz, P., Miller, D. A., Mann, W. A. and Ridley P. T. (1970). *J. Pharmacol. Exp. Ther.* **174**, 421.
Perkins, W. E. and Vars, L. (1973). *Brit. J. Pharmacol.* **47**, 847.
Persson, K. Ö. U. and Bunke, B. (1962). *Acta Pharmacol. Toxicol.* **19**, 219.
Peterson, P. V., Lassen, N., Hansen, V., Huld, T., Hjortkjaer, J., Holmblad, J., Moller-Nielsen, I., Nymark, M., Pedersen, V., Jorgensen, A. and Hours, W. (1966). *Acta Pharmacol. Toxicol.* **24**, 121.
Pe Thein, M. B. and Schofield, B. (1962). *Gastroenterology*, **43**, 436.
Pfeiffer, C. J. (1971). *In* "Peptic Ulcer". J. P. Lippincott Co., Philadelphia.
Pfeiffer, C. J. and Peters, C. M. (1969). *Gastroenterology*, **57**, 518.
Piper, D. W. (1960). *Gastroenterology*, **38**, 616.
Piper, D. W. and Fenton, B. (1961a). *Amer. J. Dig. Dis.* **6**, 134.
Piper, D. W. and Fenton, B. (1961b). *Gastroenterology*, **40**, 638.
Piper, D. W. and Heap, T. R. (1972). *Drugs*, **3**, 366.
Placer, Z., Roubal, Z. and Vokac, V. (1958). *Rev. Czech. Med.* **4**, 111.
Pletscher, A., Gey, K. F. and Burkard, W. P. (1966). *In* "Handbook of Experimental Pharmacology" (Eds O. Eichler and A. Farah), vol. 19, p. 593. Springer-Verlag, New York.
Porter, G. A. (1970). *In* "Carbenoxolone Sodium" (Eds J. H. Baron and F. M. Sullivan), p. 33. Butterworths, London.
Porter, R. W., Brady, J. V., Conrad, D., Mason, J. W., Galambos, R. and Rioch, D. M. (1958). *Psychosom. Med.* **20**, 379.
Powell, D. W. and Hirschowitz, B. I. (1967). *Amer. J. Physiol.* **212**, 1001.
Powell, D. W., Robbins, R. C., Boyett, J. D. and Hirschowitz, B. I. (1962). *Amer. J. Physiol.* **202**, 293.
Pradhan, S. N. and Wingate, H. W. (1962). *Arch. Int. Pharmacodyn. Ther.* **140**, 399.
Pradhan, S. N. and Wingate, H. W. (1966). *Arch. Int. Pharmacodyn. Ther.* **162**, 303.
Preshaw, R. M. and Grossman, M. I. (1965). *Gastroenterology*, **48**, 36.
Prino, G., Paglialunga, S., Nardi, G. and Lietti, A. (1971). *Eur. J. Pharmacol.* **15**, 119.
Prino, G., Paglialunga, S., Lietti, A. and Niada, R. (1972a). *Eur. J. Pharmacol.* **17**, 279.
Prino, G., Lietti, A. and Allegra, G. (1972b). *Amer. J. Dig. Dis.* **17**, 863.
Radouco-Thomas, C., Lataste-Dorolle, C., Rogg-Effron, C., Voluter, G., Meyer, M., Chaumontet, J. M. and Larue, D. (1960). *Arzneim.-Forsch.* **10**, 588.
Ragins, H. E., Benditt, E. T., Greenlee, H. B. and Dragstedt, L. R. (1958). *Gastroenterology*, **35**, 1.
Ramwell, P. W. and Shaw, J. E. (1970). *In* "Recent Progress in Hormone Research" (Ed. E. B. Astwood), vol. 26, p. 139. Academic Press, New York and London.
Rand, M. J. and Wilson, J. (1968). *Eur. J. Pharmacol.* **3**, 27.
Rasche, R. and Butterfield, W. C. (1973). *Arch. Surg.* **106**, 320.
Ravin, L. J., Baldinus, J. G. and Mazur, M. L. (1962). *J. Pharm. Sci.* **51**, 857.
Redford, M. and Schofield, B. (1965). *J. Physiol.* **180**, 304.

Redford, M., Savage, L. E. and Schofield, B. (1972). *J. Physiol.* **162**, 61P.
Reigel, D. H., Larson, S. J., Sances, Jr., A., Hoffman, N. E. and Switala, K. J. (1971). *Surgery*, **70**, 161.
Reitter, H. (1952). *Antihistaminica Z. klin. Med.* **149**, 553.
Rheault, M. J., Semb, L. S., Harkins, H. N. and Nyhus, L. M. (1965a). *Ann. Surg.* **161**, 587.
Rheault, M. J., Semb, L. S., Harkins, H. N. and Nyhus, L. M. (1965b). *Amer. J. Dig. Dis.* **10**, 128.
Rhodes, J. (1972). *Gastroenterology*, **63**, 171.
Rhodes, J., Barnardo, D. E., Phillips, S. F., Rovelstad, R. A. and Hofmann, A. F. (1969). *Gastroenterology*, **57**, 241.
Rider, J. A., Moller, H. C. and DeFelice, E. A. (1965). *Toxicol. Appl. Pharmacol.* **7**, 438.
Ridley, P. T., Klaiber, M. S. and Miller, D. A. (1971). *Pharmacologist*, **13**, 291.
Robert, A. (1968). *In* "Prostaglandin Symposium of the Worcester Foundation for Experimental Biology" (Eds P. W. Ramwell and J. E. Shaw), p. 47. John Wiley, New York.
Robert, A. (1972). *Proc. Soc. Exp. Biol. Med.* **139**, 319.
Robert, A. and Magerlein, B. J. (1973). "Advances in the Biosciences", vol. 9, p. 247. Pergamon Press, Vieweg, Braunschweig.
Robert, A., Phillips, J. P. and Nezamis, J. E. (1966). *Amer. J. Dig. Dis.* **11**, 546.
Robert, A., Nezamis, J. E. and Phillips, J. P. (1967). *Amer. J. Dig. Dis.* **12**, 1073.
Robert, A., Phillips, J. P. and Nezamis, J. E. (1968a). *Gastroenterology*, **54**, 1263.
Robert, A., Nezamis, J. E. and Phillips, J. P. (1968b). *Gastroenterology*, **55**, 481.
Robert, A., Stout, T. J. and Dale, J. E. (1970). *Gastroenterology*, **59**, 95.
Robert, A., Stowe, D. F. and Nezamis, J. E. (1971). *Nature*, **233**, 497.
Robinson, R. M., Harris, K., Hlad, C. J. and Eiseman, B. (1957). *Proc. Soc. Exp. Biol. Med.* **96**, 518.
Robson, J. M. and Sullivan, F. M. (1968). *In* "Symposium on Carbenoxolone Sodium". Butterworths, London.
Rosch, W. and Ottenjahn, R. (1971). *Med. Klin.* **66**, 383.
Rosengren, E. and Svensson, S. E. (1969). *Brit. J. Pharmacol. Chemother.* **37**, 659.
Rosoff, C. B. and Goldman, H. (1968). *Gastroenterology*, **56**, 212.
Rovati, A. L. (1969). *Minerva Med.* **60**, 1011.
Rovati, A. L., Casula, P. L. and Da Re, G. (1967a). *Minerva Med.* **58**, 3651.
Rovati, A. L., Casula, P. L. and Da Re, G. (1967b). *Minerva Med.* **58**, 3656.
Rovati, A. L., Casula, P. L. and Da Re, G. (1969). *Rev. Med.* **49**, 81.
Rubin, B. and Engel, S. L. (1974). *In* "Nobel Symposium 16; Frontier in Gastrointestinal Hormone Research" (Ed. S. Andersson). Alinquist and Wiksell, Uppsala.
Rubin, B., Engel, S. L., Drungis, A. M., Dzelzkalns, M., Grigas, E. O., Waugh, M. H. and Yiaca, E. (1969). *J. Pharm. Sci.* **58**, 955.
Rudick, J., Gajewski, A. F., Pitts, C. L., Semb, L. S., Fletcher, T. L., Harkins, H. N. and Nyhus, L. M. (1966). *Amer. Surg.* **32**, 513.
Rudick, J., Semb, L. S. and Nyhus, L. M. (1967). *J. Surg. Res.* **7**, 383.
Rudick, J., Finkelstein, J., Kark, A. E. and Dreiling, D. A. (1968). *Proc. Soc. Exp. Biol. Med.* **127**, 781.
Rudick, J., Finkelstein, J., Dreiling, D. A. and Kark, A. E. (1969). *Surgery*, **65**, 470.
Russell, R. I. and Dickie, J. E. N. (1968). *J. Ther. Clin. Res.* **2**, 2.

Salganik, R. I., Argutinskaya, S. V. and Bersimbaev, R. I. (1972). *Experientia*, 28, 1190.

Saltzstein, H. C., Sandweiss, D. J., Hammer, J., Hill, E. J. and Vandenberg, H. J. (1947). *Arch. Surg.* 55, 126.

Saltzstein, H. C., Sandweiss, D. J., Hill, E. J. and Hammer, J. (1949). *Gastroenterology*, 12, 122.

Samir Amer, M. (1972). *Amer. J. Dig. Dis.* 17, 945.

Sandweiss, D. J. (1945). *Gastroenterology*, 5, 405.

Sandweiss, D. J. and Friedman, M. H. F. (1942). *Amer. J. Dig. Dis.* 9, 166.

Sandweiss, D. J., Saltzstein, H. C. and Farbman, A. A. (1938). *Amer. J. Dig. Dis.* 5, 24.

Sandweiss, D. J., Saltzstein, H. C. and Farbman, A. A. (1939). *Amer. J. Dig. Dis.* 6, 6.

Sandweiss, D. J., Scheinberg, R. and Saltzstein, H. C. (1954). *Gastroenterology*, 27, 411.

Sanner, J. H. (1969). *Arch. Int. Pharmacodyn. Ther.* 180, 46.

Sanner, J. H. (1972). *Intra-Science Chem. Rept.* 6, 1.

Sachatello, C. R. and Tritsch, G. L. (1971). *Endocrinology*, 88, 1303.

Sachatello, C. R., Sedwick, J., Moriarty, C. L., Grahl-Nielsen, O. and Tritsch, G. L. (1971). *Endocrinology*, 88, 1300.

Schayer, R. W. (1956). *Amer. J. Physiol.* 187, 63.

Schayer, R. W. (1959). *Physiol. Rev.* 39, 116.

Schayer, R. W. (1961). *Chemotherapia*, 3, 128.

Schayer, R. W. (1966). *In* "Handbook of Experimental Pharmacology" (Eds O. Eicher and A. Farah), vol. 18, p. 688. Springer-Verlag, New York.

Schayer, R. W. (1973). *Ag. Actions*, 3, 191.

Schmassmann, H. (1944). *Schweiz. Med. Wochenschr.* 74, 576.

Schmidt, H. A., Goebell, H. and Johannson, F. (1973). *Acta Hepato-Gastroenterol.* 20, 51.

Schofield, B. (1957). *Gastroenterology*, 33, 714.

Schofield, B., Redford, M., Grabham, A. H. and Nuaimi, K. (1967). *In* "Gastric Secretion, Mechanisms and Control" (Eds T. K. Shnitka, J. A. L. Gilbert and R. C. Harrison), p. 91. Pergamon Press, New York.

Schumann, H. J. and Kroneberg, G. (1970). *In* "New Aspects of Storage and Release Mechanisms of Catecholamines". Springer-Verlag, New York.

Schwartz, J. C. (1971). *In* "Peptic Ulcer" (Ed. C. J. Pfeiffer), p. 190. J. P. Lippincott Co., Philadelphia.

Schwartz, J. C., Rönnberg, A. L., Cohen, Y. and Valette, G. (1969). *Pharmacol. Res. Commun.* 1, 89.

Schwartz, M. and Mackrell, T. N. (1969). *Proc. Soc. Exp. Biol. Med.* 130, 1048.

Scobie, B. A. (1966). *N.Z. Med. J.* 65, 308.

Seifter, J., Glassman, J. M. and Hudyma, G. M. (1962). *Proc. Soc. Exp. Biol. Med.* 109, 664.

Seijffers, M., Birnbaum, D. and Groen, J. J. (1963). *Gastroenterologia*, 99, 105.

Semb, L. S. (1966). *Scand. J. Gastroenterol.* 1, 253.

Semb, L. S. (1969a). *J. Oslo City Hosp.* 19, 73.

Semb, L. S. (1969b). *Acta Physiol. Scand.* 77, 385.

Seronde, J. Jr. (1963). *Yale J. Biol. Med.* 36, 141.

Sethbhakdi, S., Pfeiffer, C. J. and Roth, J. L. A. (1970a). *Amer. J. Dig. Dis.* 15, 261.

Sethbhakdi, S., Roth, J. L. A. and Pfeiffer, C. J. (1970b). *Amer. J. Dig. Dis.* 15, 1055.

Sewing, K. F., Gorinsky, P. D. and Lembeck, F. (1968). *Naunyn-Schmiedebergs Arch Pharmakol. Exp. Pathol.* **261**, 89.

Shaw, J. E. and Ramwell, P. W. (1968). *In* "Prostaglandin Symposium of the Worcester Foundation for Experimental Biology" (Eds P. W. Ramwell and J. E. Shaw), p. 55. John Wiley, New York.

Shay, H., Komarov, S. A., Fels, S. S., Merance, D., Gruenstein, M. and Siplet, H. (1945). *Gastroenterology*, **5**, 43.

Shay, H., Komarov, S. A., Siplet, H. and Gruenstein, M. (1947a). *Amer. J. Dig. Dis.* **14**, 99.

Shay, H., Komarov, S. A. and Siplet, H. (1947b). *Science*, **105**, 128.

Shay, H., Sun, D. C. H. and Gruenstein, M. (1958). *In* "Proceedings of the World Congress of Gasteroenterology", p. 108. Williams and Wilkins Co., Baltimore.

Sherman, G. P., Woods, R. J. and Buckley, J. P. (1968). *Eur. J. Pharmacol.* **2**, 326.

Shive, W., Snider, R. N., DuBilier, B., Rude, J. C., Clark, G. E. and Ravel, J. O. (1957). *Tex. State J. Med.* **53**, 840.

Shoch, D. and Fogelson, S. J. (1942). *Proc. Soc. Exp. Biol. Med.* **50**, 304.

Sircus, W. (1958). *Quart. J. Exp. Physiol.* **43**, 114.

Sircus, W. (1972). *Gut*, **13**, 816.

Skidmore, I. F. and Whitehouse, M. W. (1966). *Biochem. Pharmacol.* **15**, 1965.

Skoryna, S. C., Webster, D. R. and Kohn, D. S. (1958). *Gastroenterology*, **34**, 1.

Smith, W. O., Hoke, R., Landy, F., Caputto, R. and Wolf, S. (1958). *Gastroenterology*, **34**, 181.

Somogyi, I., Kukor, I. and Huoranszky, F. (1965). *Gastroenterologia*, **103**, 76.

Spiro, H. M., Schwartz, R. D. and Pilot, M. L. (1959). *Amer. J. Dig. Dis.* **4**, 289.

Stadelmann, V. O., Miederer, S. E. and Werner, C. (1972). *Fortschr. Med.* **90**, 123.

Stening, G. F. and Grossman, M. I. (1968). *Proc. Soc. Exp. Biol. Med.* **128**, 430.

Stening, G. F., Johnson, L. R. and Grossman, M. I. (1969a). *Gastroenterology*, **56**, 468.

Stening, G. F., Johnson, L. R. and Grossman, M. I. (1969b). *Gastroenterology*, **57**, 44.

Stolte, J. B. (1950). *Lancet*, **ii**, 858.

Sullivan, F. M. (1972). *In* "Carbenoxolone in Gastroenterology" (Eds F. Avery Jones and F. M. Sullivan), p. 3. Butterworths, London.

Sun, D. C. H. (1967a). *Ann. N.Y. Acad. Sci.* **140**, 685.

Sun, D. C. H. (1967b). *Ann. N.Y. Acad. Sci.* **140**, 747.

Sun, D. C. H. and Ryan, M. L. (1970). *Gastroenterology*, **58**, 756.

Sun, D. C. H. and Shay, H. (1959a). *Gastroenterology*, **36**, 245.

Sun, D. C. H. and Shay, H. (1959b). *J. Pharmacol. Exp. Ther.* **126**, 155.

Svensson, S. O. and Emås, S. (1971). *Scand. J. Gastroenterol.* **6**, 371.

Takagi, K. and Harada, M. (1969). *Yakugaku Zassi*, **89**, 879.

Takagi, K. and Ishii, Y. (1967). *Arzneim.-Forsch.* **17**, 1544.

Takagi, K. and Okabe, S. (1968). *Jap. J. Pharmacol.* **18**, 9.

Takagi, K. and Yano, S. (1972). *Chem. Pharm. Bull.* **20**, 1170.

Takagi, K., Okabe, S., Yano, S., Kawashima, K. and Saziki, R. (1969). *Jap. J. Pharmacol.* **19**, 327.

Takagi, K., Okabe, S. and Saziki, R. (1970). *Jap. J. Pharmacol.* **19**, 418.

Taylor, K. M. (1973). *Biochem. Pharmacol.* **22**, 2775.

Tewari, S. N. and Kirk Wilson, A. (1973). *Practitioner*, **210**, 820.

Tewari, S. N. and Trembalowicz, F. C. (1968). *Gut*, **9**, 48.

Texter, E. C., Chow, C-c., Laureta, H. C., Towne, J. C., Meyer, M. A. and Cosey, E. J. (1967). *Ann. N.Y. Acad. Sci.* **140**, 734.

Thayer, Jr., W. R. and Martin, H. F. (1967). *Amer. J. Dig. Dis.* **12**, 1050.

Thayer, Jr., W. R., Toffler, A. H., Chapo, G. and Spiro, H. M. (1965). *Yale J. Biol. Med.* **38**, 257.

Thompson, J. C. and Peskin, G. W. (1961). *Surg. Gynecol. Obstet.* **112**, 205.

Thompson, J. C., Davidson, W. D., Miller, J. H. and Davies, R. E. (1964). *Surgery*, **56**, 861.

Thompson, J. C., Lerner, H. J., Tramontana, J. A. and Miller, J. H. (1966a). *Surg. Gynecol. Obstet.* **122**, 264.

Thompson, J. C., Lerner, H. J. and Musicant, M. E. (1966b). *Surg. Gynecol. Obstet.* **122**, 751.

Thompson, J. C., Reeder, D. D., Bunchman, H. H., Becker, H. D. and Brandt, E. N. (1972). *Ann. Surg.* **176**, 384.

Thompson, J. H. and Brückner, W. (1970). *Eur. J. Pharmacol.* **9**, 261.

Thompson, J. H. and George, R. (1972). *Amer. J. Dig. Dis.* **17**, 513.

Tiede, R. N., Pfeiffer, C. J. and Gass, G. H. (1963). *Nature*, **199**, 1296.

Tiongco, R., Isaza, J., Sugawara, K. and Eisenberg, M. M. (1968). *Surg. Forum*, **19**, 280.

Toldy, L. and Tóth, I. (1964). *Naturwissenschaften*, **51**, 387.

Torgersen, O. (1961). *Acta Path. Microbiol. Scand.* **152**, Suppl. 148, 171.

Tournut, J. and Boisson, J. (1973). *Ann. Gastroenterol.* **9**, 99.

Troidl, H., Lorenz, W., Barth, H., Rohde, H., Feifel, G., Schmal, A., Goecke, K., Reimann-Huhnd, A. and Seidel, W. (1973). *Ag. Actions*, **3**, 157.

Truelove, S. C. (1960). *Brit. Med. J.* **ii**, 559.

Tumpson, D. B. and Johnson, L. R. (1969). *Proc. Soc. Exp. Biol. Med.* **131**, 186.

Türker, R. K. (1973). *Pharmacology*, **9**, 306.

Turner, M. D. (1968). *Gut*, **9**, 134.

Turner, M. D., Miller, L. L. and Segal, H. L. (1967). *Gastroenterology*, **53**, 967.

Turpie, A. G. G. and Thomson, T. J. (1965). *Gut*, **5**, 591.

Turpie, A. G. G., Runcie, J. and Thomson, T. J. (1969). *Gut*, **10**, 299.

Umeda, N., Roth, J. L. A. and Pfeiffer, C. J. (1971). *Toxicol. Appl. Pharmacol.* **18**, 102.

Umezawa, H., Aoyagi, T., Morishima, H., Matsuzaki, M., Hamada, M. and Takeuchi, T. (1970). *J. Antibiot.* **23**, 259.

Unger, R. H., Ohneda, A., Valverde, I., Eisenstrant, A. M. and Exton, J. (1968). *J. Clin. Invest.* **47**, 48.

Uvnäs, B. (1942). *Acta Physiol. Scand.* **4**, Suppl. 13.

Uvnäs, B. (1971). *Scand. J. Gastroenterol.* **6**, 113.

Vagne, M., Stening, G. F., Brooks, F. P. and Grossman, M. I. (1968). *Gastroenterology*, **55**, 260.

Vallejo, E. A., Diaz, G., Arranz, B. M. and Lozano, L. (1969a). *Minerva Med.* **60**, 1057.

Vallejo, E. A., Diaz, G., Arranz, B. M. and Lozano, L. (1969b). *Minerva Med.* **60**, 1063.

Van Meter, J. C. and Oleson, J. J. (1949). *Proc. Soc. Exp. Biol. Med.* **71**, 163.

Van Zwieten, P. A. (1973). *J. Pharm. Pharmacol.* **25**, 89.

Vane, J. R. (1971). *Nature New Biology*, **231**, 232.

Varis, K., Nyberg, O., Gorbatow, O., Pörsti, P., Aukee, S., Perttala, Y., Spoof, M. and Siurala, M. (1972). *Scand. J. Gastroenterol.* **7**, 547.

Varró, V. and Náfrádi, J. (1970). *Scand. J. Gastroenterol.* **5**, 273.

Villegas, L. (1969). *Biochim. Biophys. Acta*, **173**, 348.

Vocac, J. A. and Alphin, R. S. (1968). *Eur. J. Pharmacol.* **4**, 99.
Vocac, J. A. and Alphin, R. S. (1969). *Arch. Int. Pharmacodyn. Ther.* **177**, 150.
Von Heimburg, R. L. and Hallenbeck, G. A. (1964). *Gastroenterology*, **47**, 531.
Von Schiemann, W. H. L. (1972). *Z. Allg. Med.* **48**, 71.
Waller, S. L. (1973). *Gut*, **14**, 402.
Waton, N. G. (1971). *Amer. J. Dig. Dis.* **16**, 921.
Watt, J. and Anderson, W. (1961). *Gastroenterology*, **40**, 180.
Watt, J. and Eagleton, G. B. (1964). *J. Pharm. Pharmacol.* **16**, 83T.
Watt, J., Eagleton, G. B. and Marcus, R. (1966). *Nature*, **211**, 989.
Way, L. W. (1970). *Clin. Res.* **18**, 175.
Way, L. and Durbin, R. P. (1969). *Nature*, **221**, 874.
Weeks, J. R. (1972). *In* "Annual Review of Pharmacology" (Ed. H. W. Elliot), vol. 12, p. 317. Annual Reviews Inc., Palo Alto.
Weisbrodt, N. W., Wiley, J. N., Overholt, B. F. and Bass, P. (1969). *Gut*, **10**, 543.
Weiss, A. and Sciales, W. J. (1961). *Ann. Int. Med.* **55**, 407.
Weissbach, H., Lovenberg, W. and Udenfriend, S. (1961). *Biochim. Biophys. Acta*, **50**, 177.
Whittle, B. J. R. (1972). *Brit. J. Pharmacol. Chemother.* **46**, 546P.
Wilson, D. E. (1972). *Prostaglandins*, **1**, 281.
Wilson, D. E. (1973). *Ann. Int. Med.* **79**, 269.
Wilson, D. E. and Levine, R. A. (1972). *Amer. J. Dig. Dis.* **17**, 527.
Wilson, D. E., Phillips, C. and Levine, R. A. (1970). *Gastroenterology*, **58**, 1007.
Wilson, D. E., Phillips, C. and Levine, R. A. (1971). *Gastroenterology*, **61**, 201.
Wilson, J. A. C. (1972). *Brit. J. Clin. Pract.* **26**, 563.
Winkelstein, A. (1940). *J. Mt Sinai Hosp. New York*, **7**, 29.
Wolf, J. (1973). *Amer. J. Gastroenterol.* **60**, 23.
Wong, R. T., Kasbekar, D. K. and Forte, J. G. (1969). *Proc. Soc. Exp. Biol. Med.* **131**, 534.
Wong, R. C., Nakagawa, Y. and Perlmann, G. E. (1972). *J. Biol. Chem.* **247**, 1625.
Wood, D. R. (1948). *Brit. J. Pharmacol. Chemother.* **3**, 231.
Woodward, E. R. and Dragstedt, L. R. (1960). *Physiol. Rev.* **40**, 490.
Woodward, E. R., Lyon, E. S., Landor, J. and Dragstedt, L. R. (1954). *Gastroenterology*, **27**, 766.
Wormsley, K. G. (1968). *Scand. J. Gastroenterol.* **3**, 632.
Wormsley, K. G. (1970). *Scand. J. Gastroenterol.* **5**, 207.
Wormsley, K. G. (1973). *Gut*, **14**, 743.
Wormsley, K. G. and Grossman, M. I. (1964). *Gastroenterology*, **47**, 72.
Wyllie, J. H., Hesselbo, T. and Black, J. W. (1972). *Lancet*, **ii**, 1117.
Wyllie, J. H., Ealding, W. D. P., Hesselbo, T. and Black, J. W. (1973). *Gut*, **14**, 424.
Yamaguchi, I., Katsuki, S., Ohashi, T. and Kumada, S. (1973). *Jap. J. Pharmacol.* **23**, 523.
Zaidi, S. H. and Singh, G. B. (1958). *Indian J. Med. Res.* **46**, 411.
Zeljony, G. P. and Savich, V. V. (1911). (Quoted in 1950, 2nd ed.) *In* "Secretory Mechanism of the Digestive Glands". B. B. Bapkin, p. 470. Paul B. Hoeber, Inc., New York.
Zimmon, D. S. and Mazzola, V. (1973). *Gut*, **14**, 847.
Zimmon, D. S., Miller, G., Cox, G. and Tesler, M. A. (1969). *Gastroenterology*, **56**, 19.

Subject Index

329

Cumulative Index of Authors

Cumulative Index of Titles

DATE DUE
